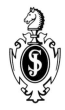

Isabel Stabile · Gedis Grudzinskas
Tim Chard (Eds.)

Spontaneous Abortion

Diagnosis and Treatment

With 32 Figures

Springer-Verlag
London Berlin Heidelberg New York
Paris Tokyo Hong Kong
Barcelona Budapest

Isabel Stabile, PhD, MRCOG
Center for Biomedical Research and Toxicology, Florida State University,
Tallahassee, Florida 32303, USA, and
Academic Unit of Obstetrics and Gynaecology, The Royal London Hospital,
Whitechapel, London E1 1BB, UK

J. G. Grudzinskas, MD, FRCOG, FRACOG
Academic Unit of Obstetrics and Gynaecology, The Royal London Hospital,
Whitechapel, London E1 1BB, UK

T. Chard, MD, FRCOG
Academic Unit of Reproductive Physiology, St Bartholomew's Hospital
Medical College, London EC1A 7BE, UK

Cover illustrations: Ch. 5, Fig. 5. TAS showing crumpled embryo surrounded by
reduced amniotic fluid volume. Ch. 5, Fig. 8. Histogram of ultrasonically diagnosed
complications of early pregnancy. (Adaptation.)

ISBN 3–540–19712–5 Springer-Verlag Berlin Heidelberg New York
ISBN 0–387–19712–5 Springer-Verlag New York Berlin Heidelberg

British Library Cataloguing in Publication Data
Spontaneous Abortion: Diagnosis and
Treatment
  I. Stabile, Isabel
  618.3
ISBN 3–540–19712–5

Library of Congress Cataloging-in-Publication Data
Spontaneous abortion: diagnosis and treatment/edited by Isabel
  Stabile, Gedis Grudzinskas, Tim Chard.
    p. cm.
  Includes index.
  ISBN 3–540–19712–5. – ISBN 0–387–19712–5
  1. Miscarriage. I. Stabile, Isabel, 1957–　. II. Grudzinskas.
J. G. (Jurgis Gediminas) III. Chard, T.
  [DNLM: 1. Abortion. WQ 225 S7636]
RG648.S683　1992
618.3′92—dc20
DNLM/DLC   92–2166
for Library of Congress   CIP

Typeset by Wilmaset Ltd, Wirral
Printed by Page Bros, Norwich. Bound by the Bath Press, Bath
28/3830–543210 Printed on acid-free paper

Preface

Spontaneous abortion is one of the commonest reasons for admission to gynaecology wards. This book brings together the experience of several distinguished workers in the field of early pregnancy failure.

The first chapters provide an overview of the classification of early pregnancy failure as well as the epidemiology, aetiology and pathology of spontaneous abortion. Later chapters focus on the diagnostic tools available to clinicians in the management of this condition with particular emphasis on abdominal and transvaginal ultrasound and biochemical tests. The relative predictive value of such tests is discussed in detail. The third part of the book describes specific categories of miscarriage such as recurrent and septic abortion and ectopic pregnancy. They also describe the knowledge developed as a result of the expansion of assisted conception techniques and the contribution of invasive procedures (chorion villus sampling and amniocentesis) to the problem of spontaneous miscarriage. The last part of the book focuses on treatment including surgical, immunological and endocrine techniques.

The aim of the book is to provide better understanding of questions such as:

What is the predictive value of symptoms and signs in the diagnosis of spontaneous miscarriage?

Can ultrasound be used confidently to diagnose spontaneous abortion?

Does ultrasound render biochemical tests obsolete in the management of spontaneous miscarriage?

What are the useful specific treatments available to women who are at risk of miscarrying?

What are the useful specific treatments available to women who have had recurrent spontaneous miscarriages?

What are the current strategies of treatment for women who are miscarrying?

Although it was intended to minimise repetition, which frequently mars multi-author volumes of this kind, we have chosen to permit a degree of overlap of views. Firstly, so that individual chapters may be read independently and secondly, although some of the views on specific treatment strategies may differ between various chapters, because of the authoritative stature of the writer, the debate may be of interest to the reader.

   Given the magnitude of the problem of spontaneous miscarriage, it is hoped that this book will stimulate further clinical research in this field.

London   Isabel Stabile
September 1991   Gedis Grudzinskas
                                                    Tim Chard

Contents

Contributors

Eva Alberman, MD, MRCP, FFCM, DPH
Wolfson Institute of Preventive Medicine, St. Bartholomew's
Hospital Medical College, London, EC1A 7BE, UK

Felicity Ashworth, MRCOG
Stoke Mandeville Hospital, Mandeville Road, Aylesbury, Bucks,
HP21 8AL, UK

Adam Balen, MRCOG
Cobbold Laboratories, The Middlesex Hospital, London, W1N 8AA,
UK

W. D. Billington, MA, BSc, PhD
Department of Pathology and Microbiology, The Medical School,
University of Bristol, University Walk, Bristol, BS8 1TD, UK

Stuart Campbell, FRCOG
Academic Department of Obstetrics and Gynaecology, King's
College Hospital, Denmark Hill, London, SE5 8RX, UK

Tim Chard, MD, FRCOG
Academic Unit of Reproductive Physiology, St. Bartholomew's
Hospital Medical College, London, EC1A 7BE, UK

Harold Fox, MD, FRCPath
Department of Pathology, University of Manchester, Stopford
Building, Oxford Road, Manchester, M13 9PT, UK

M. D. Griffith-Jones
Department of Obstetrics and Gynaecology, St. James's University
Hospital, Leeds, LS9 7TF, UK

J. G. Grudzinskas, MD, FRCOG, FRACOG
Academic Unit of Obstetrics and Gynaecology, The Royal London
Hospital, Whitechapel, London, E1 1BB, UK

Richard Lilford PhD, MRCOG
Department of Obstetrics and Gynaecology, St. James's University
Hospital, Leeds, LS9 7TF, UK

Adrian Lower, MRCOG
Academic Unit of Obstetrics and Gynaecology, The Royal London
Hospital, Whitechapel, London, E1 1BB, UK

Sir Malcolm Macnaughton, MD, FRCP, FRCOG
Department of Obstetrics and Gynaecology, University of Glasgow,
Glasgow, G31 2ER, UK

Lesley Regan, MD, MRCOG
Academic Department of Obstetrics and Gynaecology, St. Mary's
Hospital, London, W2 1PG, UK

Joe Leigh Simpson, MD
Department of Obstetrics and Gynaecology, University of Tennessee,
Memphis, Tennessee, 38163 USA

Isabel Stabile, PhD, MRCOG
Center for Biomedical Research and Toxicology, Florida State
University, Tallahassee, Florida, 32303 USA

John Yovich, MD, FRCOG, FRACOG, MAIBiol
Pivet Medical Centre, 166–168 Cambridge Street, Leederville, Perth
6007, Western Australia, Australia

1. Definitions and Clinical Presentation

Isabel Stabile, J. G. Grudzinskas and T. Chard

This chapter addresses the definitions of the major categories of spontaneous abortion and early pregnancy failure. A brief description of the pertinent clinical features of each condition is given as an introduction to the chapters that follow.

Spontaneous Abortion

In the United Kingdom spontaneous abortion is defined as the expulsion of a fetus without signs of viability before 28 weeks of pregnancy. The World Health Organization (WHO) definition also includes a weight criterion (less or equal to 500 g) and a gestational age cut-off limit of less than 22 weeks (FIGO News 1976). The 28-week definition demands revision in the light of substantial improvements in neonatal intensive care and the survival of many infants born before 28 weeks. The terms abortion and miscarriage are often used synonymously although miscarriage may be often used to describe spontaneous demise of first trimester pregnancies. Consistency in definition and terminology is essential for both clinicians and investigators.

Threatened Abortion

Most textbooks still define threatened abortion as painless vaginal bleeding prior to 28 weeks of pregnancy. However for practical purposes it is now applied only to bleeding before 24 weeks of pregnancy. This definition is consistent with the WHO nomenclature and with most epidemiological and pathological studies of threatened abortion. The condition is commoner in the first than in the second trimester. Perhaps a quarter of all pregnancies are complicated by threatened abortion, although many patients may be unaware of their pregnancy at the time they present with bleeding. It is one of the most common indications (together with suspected ectopic pregnancy) for emergency referral to obstetric ultrasound departments.

Can symptoms and/or clinical signs be used to predict outcome in threatened abortion? The consensus opinion is that the non-specific nature of abdominal pain, vaginal bleeding and pelvic tenderness hinder their prognostic use. However nausea and vomiting in otherwise normal early pregnancy are associated with a decreased risk of abortion. Weigel and Weigel (1989) studied a cohort of 903 West Coast American women. They demonstrated that vomiting is associated with a decreased abortion risk, while women who have nausea without vomiting have an abortion risk equal to that in the general population. Spontaneous abortion after vaginal bleeding was eightfold less common in women with vomiting in early pregnancy. Thus women who continue to experience morning sickness (but not nausea) during episodes of threatened abortion have a decreased risk of subsequent abortion.

Inevitable Abortion

Spontaneous abortion is a process rather than a single event. Once bleeding commences, several possible scenarios follow. The bleeding may resolve spontaneously in a few days, never to recur. It may continue, or stop and start over several days or weeks; this is known as threatened abortion. It is only when abdominal cramps supervene that the process moves in the direction of inevitability. At first the cervix remains closed; the process can still stop and the pregnancy continue. We do not know how often this occurs. However, if the cervix opens and cramps are severe (due to uterine contractions and cervical dilatation), then the abortion is inevitable. Symptoms alone are an unreliable predictor of outcome. Digital examination of the cervix is essential to determine what stage the abortion process has reached.

Inevitable abortion is complete or incomplete depending on whether or not all fetal and placental tissues have been expelled from the uterus. The typical features of incomplete abortion are heavy (sometimes intermittent) bleeding and cramps. If these symptoms improve spontaneously then complete abortion is likely. The number of spontaneous complete abortions is unknown because they are often not reported by the patient or her general practitioner. An ultrasound study of over 600 women with threatened abortion identified only four women with a complete abortion (Stabile et al. 1987). However, these figures probably underestimate the true extent of complete abortion (Chard 1991). The finding of a dilated cervix in the presence of continued pain and bleeding is usually diagnostic of an incomplete inevitable abortion. Occasionally, the cervix may close, a finding which should not of itself lead to the diagnosis of complete abortion. If available, ultrasound should always be used to ascertain that the uterus is in fact empty.

Missed Abortion

In missed abortion failure of pregnancy is identified before expulsion of the fetal and placental tissues. The diagnosis is usually made by failure to identify fetal heart action. Hard copy documentation of M Mode echocardiography should be included in the ultrasound records.

Fetal heart activity can be demonstrated from 6 weeks onwards using abdominal ultrasound. However using transvaginal ultrasound (TVS), Pennell et al. (1991) have demonstrated that one-third of normal embryos with a crown – rump length of less than 5 mm had no demonstrable cardiac activity. Thus the diagnosis of missed abortion (or early embryonic demise, the preferred term in the USA), should not be made in embryos smaller than this. In cases of doubt the ultrasound examination should be repeated a week later.

Anembryonic Pregnancy

The most common detectable cause of early pregnancy failure is anembryonic pregnancy (Stabile et al. 1987). The older term for this condition was blighted ovum; this should probably be abandoned. Current evidence suggests that apparently empty gestational sacs contained an embryo at some stage which subsequently was resorbed (Stabile 1991). This hypothesis is supported by the study of Meegdes et al. (1988). The incidence of avascular villi, fibrosis and cytotrophoblastic degeneration was the same in "anembryonic pregnancy" and missed abortion. These conditions may well represent two extremes of the same pathological process. The time elapsing between arrest of embryonic development and clinical presentation will determine the sonographic features.

Spontaneous Abortion of a Live Fetus

The true rate of pregnancy wastage is uncertain (Chard 1991). It will vary with maternal age (Wilson et al. 1986) and clinical circumstances. For example subclinical abortion rates i.e., before pregnancy is diagnosed clinically, biochemically or sonographically are probably in the order of 40%–60%; once a clinical diagnosis of pregnancy is made, the rate falls to around 15%–20%. Of greater practical value is the abortion rate after a live fetus is seen on scan. The consensus view appears to be that if fetal life is confirmed ultrasonically in the first trimester, 95%–98% of these women will progess to a normal outcome of pregnancy (Christiaens and Stoutenbeek 1984; Stabile et al. 1989). Moreover, the later viability is confirmed, the lower is the observed abortion rate. The figure is the same in women with clinically normal pregnancies. Thus bleeding in itself does not confer an additional risk of abortion, provided the fetus is actually alive.

In the first trimester 4%–5% of apparently normal pregnancies are destined to abort largely due to chromosomal abnormalities. This has important implications with regard to the safety of chorionic villus sampling which is generally performed only after fetal viability has been confirmed ultrasonically. The rate of loss related to the procedure ranges from 2%–4% in different studies.

Trophoblastic Tumours

Trophoblastic tumours include complete and partial hydatidiform moles, chorio-carcinoma and placental site tumour. The latter two conditions are true neoplasms whereas moles have been described as pathological conceptuses, resulting from errors at fertilisation (Szulman 1988). Hydatidiform moles are the most common type of trophoblastic disease.

The partial mole is typically a triploid conceptus while the complete mole has a diploid, totally paternally derived, genome. In complete mole there is generalised trophoblast hyperplasia and villous oedema producing the classical "bunch of grapes appearance" in the absence of an embryo. In partial mole there is focal trophoblast hyperplasia, trophoblastic inclusions and villous oedema in the presence of an embryo. The most important clinical distinction is the propensity for complete moles to become invasive, choriocarcinoma supervening in 2%–5% of cases. Although partial moles are much commoner in clinical practice, they are often undiagnosed pre-operatively. They typically present as inevitable abortion, the uterus being normal for gestational age. Prior to 8 or 9 weeks gestation, the fetus is usually still alive and the diagnosis is often missed even on ultrasound. The final diagnosis is usually made by the pathologist. Choriocarcinoma has not been described in association with a partial mole but follow-up with human chorionic gonadotrophin (hCG) should be performed to identify occasional cases of residual trophoblastic disease.

Septic Abortion

Septic abortion is said to occur when infection complicates abortion. Rarely this may follow incomplete spontaneous abortion. The diagnosis is based on features of pelvic infection (fever, suprapubic and pelvic pain, abdominal rigidity and uterine tenderness on bimanual palpation). The history of preceding interference may be witheld although evidence of lower genital tract injury should be sought. Bleeding and uterine contractions may be minimal and the cervix may remain closed. Early diagnosis and treatment of this complication are essential to prevent the tragedy of gross pelvic infection and consequent secondary infertility.

Recurrent Abortion

Recurrent abortion is defined as three or more consecutive spontaneous abortions. In mid trimester, incompetence of the internal cervical os may be the cause. These abortions are relatively painless and the membranes may bulge through the partly open cervix. Other causes include severe maternal systemic disease, fetal chromosomal and structural anomalies and uterine malformations. These factors are known to operate in the aetiology of sporadic spontaneous abortion, so what (if any) is the difference between sporadic and recurrent abortion? There is probably no difference from the morphological point of view. In a recent study the histopathological appearance of conception products from 44 women with recurrent abortion (prior to 16 weeks) were compared with those obtained from 105 women with sporadic abortion. Abnormal villi, suggestive of fetal chromosomal abnormalities, were found in approximately 60% of both groups (Houwert-de Jong et al. 1990). These figures are similar to those of Boué et al. (1975) in their analysis of 1500 karyotyped spontaneous abortions.

The demonstration that removal of the corpus luteum before the end of the seventh week of pregnancy leads to abortion which can be prevented by progesterone (Csapo et al. 1973), has led to the clinical use of progesterone treatment in cases of recurrent abortion. However, it is now generally believed that the reduction in hormone production is the effect rather than the cause of abortion.

Induced Abortion

Women usually refer to induced abortion (or termination of pregnancy) as abortion, preferring to refer to all other forms of early pregnancy failures as miscarriage. Approximately 25% of all pregnancies worldwide are deliberately terminated (Laferla 1986), the majority in the first trimester.

In the UK the legal grounds for termination are a risk to the physical or mental health of the pregnant woman or her existing children, providing the pregnancy does not exceed 24 weeks. This limit does not apply if there is a risk of grave permanent injury or death to the mother or a substantial risk of serious handicap in the child.

Ectopic Pregnancy

Trophoblast implants on extrauterine tissues more commonly than is generally recognised, though the true incidence is difficult to ascertain as the incidence is reported using denominators that are not comparable between populations. The often-quoted rate of 0.5%–1% of births is rising, with a fourfold increase in the USA from 1970 to 1985 (Center for Disease Control 1988). To some extent this reflects better diagnosis (Hemminki and Heironen 1987). Other factors are the increase in tubal damage due to sexually transmitted disease and the use of assisted reproductive techniques. Ectopic pregnancy still accounts for about 10% of maternal deaths, and remains the major cause of maternal mortality in the first trimester of pregnancy. Nevertheless better diagnosis and conservative treatment is reflected in the sevenfold lowering of the mortality rate, at least in the United States (Center for Disease Control 1988). The real challenge lies in preventing tubal damage by lowering the incidence of pelvic inflammatory disease.

Ectopic pregnancy can be very difficult to distinguish from pelvic inflammatory disease, ruptured corpus luteum, dysfunctional uterine bleeding and the various stages of spontaneous abortion. Thus accuracy of purely clinical diagnosis is only 50%. A review of the physical findings in 3500 cases of ectopic pregnancy (Stabile and Grudzinskas 1990) has demonstrated that abdominal pain is the most consistent symptom (90% of patients), while irregular vaginal bleeding and amenorrhoea were noted in 50%–80% of patients. The diagnosis rests on maintaining a high index of suspicion accompanied by the use of a few special tests.

Summary

Since symptoms and signs are unreliable indicators of the outcome of an abortion process, every woman who experiences pain or bleeding in early pregnancy should be offered an ultrasound scan. This both simplifies management and in most cases allows reassurance of the patient.

References

Boué J, Boué A, Lazar P (1975) Retrospective and prospective epidemiological studies of 1500 karyotyped spontaneous human abortions. Teratology 12:11–27
Center for Disease Control (1988) Ectopic pregnancy in the USA: 1970–1985. In: CDC Surveillance Summaries. Morb Mort Week Rev 37:9–18
Chard T (1991) Frequency of implantation and early pregnancy loss in natural cycles. In: Seppala M (ed) Implantation. Ballière's Clinical Obstetrics and Gynaecology, Vol 5, No 1. Ballière-Tindall, London, pp 179–189
Christiaens GCML, Stoutenbeek P (1984) Spontaneous abortion in proven intact pregnancies. Lancet ii:571–572
Csapo AI, Pulkkinen MO, Wiest WG (1973) Effects of luteectomy and progesterone replacement therapy in early pregnant patients. Am J Obstet Gynecol 115:759–765
FIGO News (1976) List of gynaecologic and obstetric terms and definitions. Int J Gynaecol Obstet 14:570–576
Hemminki E, Heironen PK (1987) Time trends of ectopic pregnancies. Br J Obstet Gynaecol 94:322–327
Houwert-de Jong MH, Bruinse HW, Eskes TKAB, Mantingh A, Terminjtelen A, Kooyman CD (1990) Early recurrent miscarriage histology of conception products. Br J Obstet Gynaecol 97:533–535
Laferla JJ (1986) Termination of pregnancy. W. B. Saunders, London
Meegdes BHLM, Ingenhoes R, Peeters LLH, Exalto N (1988) Early pregnancy wastage: relationship between chorionic vascularisation and embryonic development. Fertil Steril 49:216–219
Pennell RG, Needleman L, Pajak T, Baltarowich O, Vilaro M, Goldberg BB, Kurtz AB (1991)

Prospective comparison of vaginal and abdominal sonography in normal early pregnancy. J Ultrasound Med 10:63–67

Stabile I (1991) Anembryonic pregnancy. In: Chapman MG et al. (eds) The embryo: normal and abnormal development and growth. Springer-Verlag, London, pp 35–43

Stabile I, Grudzinskas JG (1990) Ectopic pregnancy: a review of incidence, etiology and diagnostic aspects. Obstet Gynecol Survey 45(6):335–347

Stabile I, Campbell S, Grudzinskas JG (1987) Ultrasound assessment in complications of first trimester pregnancy. Lancet ii:1237–1242

Stabile I, Campbell S, Grudzinskas JG (1989) Ultrasound and circulating placental protein measurements in complications of early pregnancy. Br J Obstet Gynaecol 96:1182–1191

Szulman AE (1988) Trophoblastic disease: clinical pathology of hydatidiform moles. In: Obstetric and Gynecology Clinics of North America 15:443–456

Weigel MM, Weigel RM (1989) Nausea and vomiting of early pregnancy and pregnancy outcome. An epidemiological study. Br J Obstet Gynaecol 96:1304–1311

Wilson RD, Kendrick V, Wittman BK, McGillivray B (1986) Spontaneous abortion and pregnancy outcome after normal first trimester ultrasound examination. Obstet Gynecol 67:352–355

2. Spontaneous Abortions: Epidemiology

Eva Alberman

Introduction

Between 10% and 20% of recognised pregnancies are spontaneously aborted, mostly some time after fetal death has occurred. The actual level of loss described varies with the definitions and methods of ascertainment used, and with the characteristics of the population under study. Embryonic losses in the earliest, clinically unrecognised, stages of pregnancy are considerably more common, but until recently their frequency could only be guessed at. Better estimates are now becoming possible using information from studies of in-vitro fertilisation (IVF) and from the use of very sensitive early pregnancy tests.

Clinically recognised spontaneous abortions are known to be heterogeneous, about one-half being chromosomally anomalous, the remainder including those due to known maternal causes, intrauterine infections and other environmental hazards and immunological feto-maternal incompatibilities. In a large proportion the cause remains unknown.

Problems of Definition and Ascertainment

Problems of definition arise firstly very early in pregnancy, where detection is possible only by chemical testing (Chard 1991), and towards the end of pregnancy where the distinction between a late spontaneous abortion, a still-birth or a neonatal death may depend on local judgement (Fenton et al. 1990) as well as current legislation. The situation in the UK at present is that any pregnancy ending in fetal death before 27 completed weeks, taken to be from the first day of the last menstrual period (LMP), is regarded as non-viable. For a live-born baby there is no lower gestational age or weight limit. Conversely a fetus expelled after 27 completed weeks, even when it has clearly been dead for some time, is technically a still-birth and therefore registrable as such. Different countries have different definitions of viability, thus making it difficult to compare spontaneous abortion rates between countries.

There are also problems in regard to definitions of gestational age of aborted fetuses. In general this is considered to be the age at the time of expulsion, and not at the probable time of fetal death. However some researchers have estimated fetal age from the stage of development reached, which may be misleading if fetal growth has been unduly slow, and some count it from the probable time of ovulation, thus making it on average two weeks shorter than if LMP is used. More recently the use of ultrasound measures which may differ both from calculated days, and from clinical estimates of fetal maturity, have introduced a new variability into the definitions used. The risk of fetal loss falls sharply from early pregnancy to later pregnancy, and in comparing gestational-age specific risks between different places and different times it is important that the same measures of fetal ageing are used. Moreover in early pregnancy the majority of losses are due to chromosomal anomalies, groups of which have characteristic distributions of gestational age at expulsion, and such patterns may be missed unless comparability is maintained.

Because of the marked fall in rate with every week of pregnancy (Fig. 2.1), estimates of the incidence of spontaneous loss vary considerably, depending on the methods of ascertainment used. Without screening for chemical indicators of early pregnancy, researchers are dependent on the ability of a mother to recognise, and report, early symptoms of pregnancy. This also depends on whether the mother is planning to conceive and is therefore alert to physiological change, or whether the conception is unexpected. In the elderly mother early signs of pregnancy may be confused with those of the menopause.

The fullest ascertainment, and therefore best estimates of incidence of fetal loss, is in self-selected groups intending to conceive who are repeatedly screened for signs of pregnancy until pregnancy is established, and are then followed until the pregnancy terminates. Even under ideal circumstances such a prospective

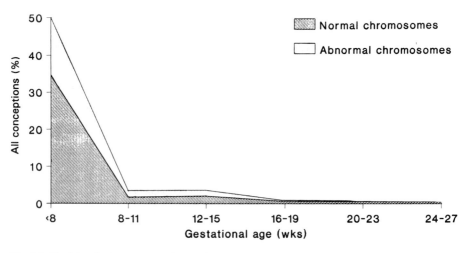

Fig. 2.1. Fetal loss by karyotype and gestational age. Derived from Kline et al. (1989b).

longitudinal study will still miss the earliest pre-implantation losses, where frequency can only be impugned from in-vitro studies. Moreover since these groups are so highly selected any extrapolation from the findings to the general population should be treated with caution.

The question of how the rate of fetal loss is calculated is also problematical. The use of longitudinal studies enable "life-tables" to be constructed, namely the length of survival of members of a cohort of pregnancies followed from the time these had been clinically recognised, or chemically detected. This makes possible the calculation, for each week of pregnancy, of the probability of loss of pregnancies thought to be alive at the beginning of that week. The earliest such studies were carried out in Hawaii (Yerushalmy et al. 1956). The calculated incidence rate will also depend on whether induced abortions, which may include an unduly high proportion of pregnancies at particular risk of fetal loss, are included in the denominator, or whether the latter only includes spontaneous abortions plus births. This is discussed fully by Narod and Khazen (1989).

Apart from missing unrecognised losses, studies which depend on the recall of the mother will be influenced by the time elapsing since the event, by the stage of gestation at which it occurred (late abortions being recalled better than early), and by the background of the mother, those with a medical background appearing to recall more such events than those without such training (Lindbohm and Hemminki 1988). Studies which depend on the abortion coming to the attention of a health care professional, or to hospital, will be even more selective, including cases later in pregnancy and probably more complicated. They will in general have considerably lower rates than those estimated from longitudinal or retrospective studies.

Current Estimates of Early Reproductive Loss

A critical review of the literature on the probabilities of early reproductive loss using prospectively collected cohort data is given in Kline et al. (1989a), and Chard (1991) adds more recent data derived from IVF findings. A reasonably coherent picture is emerging, which is summarised in Table 2.1 taken from Kline et al. (1989a). The estimates of loss rates between conception and implantation of 50% still rest largely on the observations by Hertig and Rock (1973) on pre-implantation ova retrieved at hysterectomy, but more recent data from IVF studies support the evidence for losses of this order of magnitude (Chard 1991).

The estimate of approximately 30% loss rates between implantation and the fetal stage of pregnancy lies somewhere between the risk of loss of those detectable only on human chorionic gonadotrophin (hCG) screening and those which are clinically recognisable. Kline and her colleagues draw upon the prospective study carried out by Wilcox et al. (1988) to estimate that of 100 post-implantation losses 70 are based only on biochemical diagnosis, and 30 are clinically recognised, and of those 30, 24 are lost at the pre-fetal stage and 6 reach the fetal stage (some 7 weeks) from the LMP. The estimates in Table 2.1 suggest that, overall, 50% of conceptions are lost and that once the pregnancy is clinically recognisable about 12% are subsequently lost.

Data assembled by Kline et al. (1989a) show that most retrospective enquiries

Table 2.1. Estimates of the probabilities of loss at successive stages of pregnancy

Stage	From fertilisation			From implantation		
	Number reaching stage	Number lost before next stage (%)	Cumulative loss %	Number reaching stage	Number lost before next stage (%)	Cumulative loss %
Conception	1000	272 (27)	–			
Implantation	728	160 (22)	27	1000	220 (22)	–
Clinically recognised pregnancy	568	54 (10)	43	780	74 (10)	22
Fetal stage	514	14 (3)	49	706	19 (3)	29
Live birth	500	–	50	687	–	31

From Kline et al. (1989a).

about previous pregnancy outcome report fetal death rates per 1000 pregnancies of between 11% and 16%, while two large studies of rates derived from hospital admissions for spontaneous abortions report rates between 6.8% and 7.2% (Narod and Khazen 1989) and between 7.8% and 10.2% (Lindbohm and Hemminki 1988) respectively.

The Role of Chromosomal Anomalies

Spontaneous abortions are a heterogeneous group and a large proportion, perhaps 40% (Kline et al. 1989b), are chromosomally abnormal.

It is not easy to estimate the precise contribution of chromosome abnormalities since these are probably maximal at the earliest, and least well documented, stages of pregnancy. Recent approaches include chromosomal studies of the germ cells, using oocytes available through IVF techniques, and the estimation of theoretical probabilities of the frequencies of different anomalies if these are involved in fertilisation. In-vitro studies also enable estimates to be made of anomalies at the earliest cleavage stages of the fertilised ovum. Any extrapolation from such results must be cautious, bearing in mind the unphysiological circumstances, the high degree of selectivity governing the choice of both the women (and to a lesser degree the men) contributing germ cells, and in the case of the oocytes the further selection for experimental culture. Full reviews of the results of such studies are given by Kline et al. (1989b) and by Jacobs (1990).

The interpretation of the findings is complex, and depends on a number of unproven assumptions. Very broadly, it seems likely that monosomies and trisomies other than those of the X and Y chromosomes arise from errors at gametogenesis, most being maternal errors; anomalies of the sex chromosomes arise in different ways, the common 45 X (Turner's syndrome) usually being of paternal origin.

The conclusion reached by Kline et al. (1989b) is that the proportion of chromosomally anomalous conceptions lost before the pregnancy is clinically recognisable is probably no higher than in the earliest embryos examined after expulsion. This may be of the order of 30%–40%; this rate rises to 50% or more in losses at 8–11 weeks and then falls. It must be remembered that this proportion depends on the balance of frequency and loss rate of fetuses of normal and abnormal chromosomal constitution at the same maturity, and little is known about the cause of early fetal loss in those of normal chromosomal constitution. Fig. 2.1 is a diagrammatic representation of the loss rate of chromosomally normal and abnormal conceptions at different stages of gestational age, based on the author's reading of the review data of Kline et al. (1989b).

From the studies of chromosomal constitution of clinically recognised spontaneous abortions, still-births and live births, a consensus has emerged regarding the frequency of the different anomalies and their likely survival (Kline et al. 1989b; Jacobs 1990). This is shown in Table 2.2, reporting different types of anomaly in 7 major studies, including 7000–8000 abortions. Trisomies form the majority of anomalies, with polyploidy and 45 X following in frequency. One of the most interesting questions, as yet unsolved, is why trisomies of certain chromosomes, such as 16, are unusually frequent in spontaneous abortions. This table also shows the remarkable difference in viability in the different karyotypes: trisomy 21 is remarkable for its relatively low lethality, accounting for its clinical importance in live births.

Table 2.2. Estimated frequencies and survival to birth: recognised pregnancies of different karyotype

Karyotype	% Distribution	% Survival (rounded)
Normal	52	92
Abnormal	48	7
45 X	8.6	7
Trisomy	26.8	6
16	7.5	0
13	1.1	3
18	1.1	5
21	2.3	22
22	2.7	0
Polyploidy	9.9	<1
Structural	2.0	variable
Other	0.7	–

Derived from Jacobs (1990).

Another unresolved question is the difference between gestational age at loss. Trisomies tend to abort at a modal age of 11–12 weeks, monosomies at 11–13 weeks, and triploidy losses are spread evenly between 7–18 weeks.

The Role of Malformations Other Than Those Caused by Chromosomal Anomaly

There is little doubt that the risk of spontaneous abortion is increased where there is a fetal malformation, more in some types than others. Since there has been no systematic search for malformations in fetal losses, and since in some cases the malformation is secondary to a chromosomal anomaly, it is very difficult to assess the size of the increased risk. Some attempt to quantify this was made for neural tube malformations, and it was suggested that perhaps 3% of chromosomally normal spontaneously aborted fetuses had such a malformation. At that time the risk in the same part of England in live births was of the order of 1.5 per thousand.

Sex Ratio

Most, but not all, studies have reported an excess of males in spontaneous abortions of normal chromosomal constitution at all stages of gestation. It is, of course, difficult to define a ratio in abortions of chromosomal anomalies, which include anomalies of the sex chromosomes. Kline et al. (1989b) review the literature on this question and conclude that there is a male excess at birth, which is "steadily depleted by the preferential attrition of males in the course of gestation and through the first week of life". This must, however, remain hypothetical since we do not know the sex ratio for most conceptions.

Multiple Pregnancies

It is probable that multiple conceptions are at increased risk of fetal loss, either very early resorption, post-implantation loss, or loss in the second trimester. The information on the level of these risks is unsatisfactory, but systematic early ultrasound findings should contribute to our knowledge.

Maternal Age and Parity

It has long been thought from the evidence of cross-sectional analyses that the risk of spontaneous abortion rises with parity, as well as with maternal age. However in recent years studies of fetal loss within families have revealed that the patterns are more complicated than at first thought (Alberman 1987). Within sibships of mothers of the same gravidity (i.e., having been pregnant the same number of times), the risk of fetal loss certainly does not rise with increasing birth order, and indeed shows a tendency to fall, particularly in the last pregnancy of each group (Fig. 2.2). This suggests that parents are more likely to stop reproduction after a live birth than after a spontaneous abortion. The apparent rise with parity found in cross-sectional studies is an artefact because women who are trying to compensate for repeated fetal losses are more likely to be found in the higher gravidity groups. There has been considerable discussion about the interpretation of such findings, and whether there is a true fall in risk with increasing birth order; this also may be an artefact produced when women who have finally achieved a successful pregnancy then stop trying to conceive.

This also leaves unanswered the question of the associated effect of maternal age on risk. However Fig. 2.3 presents for first pregnancies only (in women physicians) the percentage of spontaneous abortions by maternal age in relation to the corresponding live births plus spontaneous abortions. It appears that the risk remains largely unchanged until the age of 39 when it begins to rise.

This rise is found not only in abortions of abnormal chromosomal constitution,

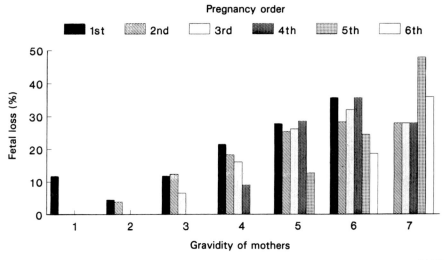

Fig. 2.2. Fetal loss by gravidity of mother and pregnancy order. Derived from Alberman (1987).

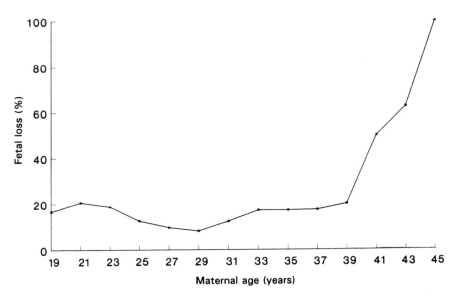

Fig. 2.3. The percentages of fetal loss in first pregnancies and maternal age. Derived from Alberman (1987).

particularly in trisomies, whose risk is known to increase with maternal age, but also in abortions of normal chromosomal constitution (Stein et al. 1980). In their data, from New York hospital patients, the rise of chromosomally normal abortions began at about 36 years, and the rise of trisomic abortions at about 34 years.

Outcome of Other Pregnancies in Sibships with Spontaneous Abortions

Studies of whole sibships (which include fetal losses) have been performed using the outcome of pregnancies reported by women doctors (Alberman et al. 1980). The findings suggest that the risk of fetal loss is not random: as clinical experience would predict, some mothers are more likely than others to have fetal losses, even if these do not meet the usual definition of recurrent aborters, namely those who have had three consecutive losses. Moreover it was found in the women doctors' study that the mean birth-weight of live births immediately preceding, as well as those following an early fetal loss was lower than in a sequence of live births. To what parental characteristics such a general heterogeneity of risk is attributable is not known, but it is probable that even within the high-risk mothers there are a variety of predisposing factors including maternal ill health and immunological incompatibilities.

Maternal Health

There is no doubt that the risk of fetal loss is influenced in many different ways by the health of the mother, or, on occasion, of the father. These may affect the risk of germ-cell anomalies, or possibly errors at early division of the zygote; maternal illness, genital malformations or exposure to environmental hazards may affect implantation or placentation, and maternal infections may pass through the placenta. In maternal scleroderma the risk of spontaneous abortion seems to be increased even before the onset of clinical disease (Silman and Black 1988) and in poorly controlled diabetes the rate of fetal loss can be correlated with biochemical indicators of levels of diabetic control. Fever of 100°F was a risk factor for the spontaneous abortion of chromosomally normal fetuses in the New York case-control study (Kline et al. 1989c). None of these factors is responsible for more than a small proportion of the overall incidence and in most cases the relationship is complicated and varies with the chromosomal constitution. It is probable that environmental factors are more likely to affect losses of normal chromosomal constitution, since those of abnormal constitution are likely to be lost under any circumstances.

Moreover the health of the parents as well as their risk of exposure to environmental hazards, and their abuse of tobacco and alcohol are all correlated with their educational level and the socio-economic conditions under which they live. Any studies of health and environmental effects need to take into account such potential confounding factors.

Maternal Smoking

There have been many studies of the effect of maternal smoking and alcohol consumption on the risk of spontaneous abortion of any conception, regardless of chromosome constitution, or on the risk of conceptions of specific chromosome defects, particularly trisomies. Not all these studies have taken into account the potential confounding factors listed above.

It is, therefore, not surprising that the published reports on these questions produce inconsistent and somewhat confusing results. Kline et al. (1989c) concluded that there is probably a real increase in the risk of spontaneous abortions of normal chromosome constitution with maternal smoking in pregnancy, but that the magnitude of the risk varies with socio-economic advantage. In their study of patients who were economically disadvantaged and were not treated privately this amounted to an odds ratio of 1.3 (95% confidence limits (CI) 1.1–1.6) for 1–13 cigarettes a day, and 1.6 (95% CI 1.2–2.0) with 14 or more cigarettes a day, after adjustment for maternal age, ethnic group, education and simultaneously for alcohol consumption. As one would expect, for the chromosomally abnormal group the risk was not significant, the odds ratio for 1–13 cigarettes a day being unity, and for 14 or more 1.2 (95% CI 0.9–1.7). For private patients no significant increase in risk was observed, the interpretation being that any such effect was "buffered" in those in better health.

Alcohol Consumption

Here even more than with smoking the reported results are confusing and again the New York studies report positive associations confined to "public" patients even after allowance for confounding factors. Kline et al. (1989c) remain cautious about concluding that there is any simple causal association. They point to the unexpected finding that the relationship with chromosomally abnormal losses was as strong as that with the normal losses as being evidence that the picture is not straightforward.

Oral Contraceptives, Spermicides and Intrauterine Devices

Both oral contraceptives and spermicides have been associated with an increased risk of fetal loss, and in particular with an increased risk of trisomic conceptuses, largely lost as spontaneous abortions. In the case of preconceptual use of oral contraceptives it now seems from a number of studies that this may be followed by a slightly reduced risk of spontaneous abortion (Royal College of General Practitioners' Oral Contraception Study 1976; Harlap et al. 1980), particularly those of normal chromosomal constitution. Where the incidence of chromosomally anomalous spontaneous abortions remains the same, this would lead to an increased ratio of abnormal to normal abortions (Alberman et al. 1976).

In the case of spermicides there is no evidence that their use increases the incidence of overall fetal loss, but there is a suspicion that they may increase the risk of fetal trisomy. In a detailed review Kline et al. (1989c) conclude that, with the exception of the results from a single study, there is no evidence for an increase in risk of trisomies compatible with life.

However, one of the few well-established risk factors for spontaneous abortions is the use of intrauterine devices for contraception, which may raise the risk two- to threefold for pregnancies conceived while the device is in situ (Vessey et al. 1979).

Previous induced abortion has also long been suspected as a risk factor for subsequent pregnancies, depending on the surgical techniques used (WHO Task Force 1979). It seems that improved methods of termination are no longer associated with a raised risk.

Other Environmental Hazards

Numerous other environmental hazards have been suspected as increasing the risk of reproductive loss. These hazards include exposure to anaesthetic gases, anticancer drugs, chemical hazards, irradiation and physical stress. Such exposures can be occupational or experienced by those living around their sources. The very extensive literature on occupational hazards has been reviewed recently by Taskinen (1990); that on environmental exposures is covered well by Kline et al. (1989c).

Occupational Hazards

Positive findings in respect of occupational risk and spontaneous abortion remain rare and inconsistent, particularly after allowing for difficulties in ascertainment and confounding factors. Workers from Finland (Taskinen 1990) and Canada (McDonald et al. 1988) found increased risks in women who worked in some occupations during pregnancy, but they were not always the same occupations. However, there was agreement that work involving heavy lifting and other physical stress increased the risk of spontaneous abortion and that those working with solvents were also at risk. Doctors and paramedical workers exposed to anaesthetic gases also may be at risk, although the statistical significance of the results varies in different studies. It may be that some of these long suspected hazards are disappearing with improvements in working conditions.

Environmental Risks

In Scandinavia there have been reports of increased risks of abortions in residents living near a copper smelter and in communities living near petrochemical works (Axelsson and Molin 1988). In neither case is the association large, and the methodological difficulties are sufficiently daunting to suggest that such results should be treated with caution.

There has been particular anxiety about the effects of environmental (or medical) radiation on reproduction. As with other hazards, the risk of spontaneous miscarriage is treated more as a marker for possible damage than as an adverse outcome *per se*. Indeed some may believe that if fetal damage results from environmental hazards, it is better that the fetuses are lost naturally than born impaired. The published data up to 1989 are reviewed by Kline et al. (1989c) and it is concluded that there is no evidence of an increase in spontaneous abortions. There is inconsistent evidence for an increase in trisomic conceptions with increased dose, particularly in older mothers. Recent reports, including one from Norway (Ulstein et al. 1990) relate increases in rates of hospital-treated spontaneous abortion with the Chernobyl disaster, although in Norway it was considered that the external radiation levels had been too small to account for the rise. The authors suggest that if it were true it might be secondary to contamination of drinking water or foodstuffs.

Conclusion

Spontaneous abortion is a common event, and losses before clinically recognised pregnancy are even more common. Abortion is an important mechanism for eliminating defective conceptions, and the study of spontaneous abortions is one of the most effective methods of gaining information about the prevalence and causes of fetal anomalies. Probably about one half of the losses are of potentially unimpaired fetuses, and further study of their causes would lead to better understanding of ways of preventing such loss. However it is clear that any study of purely environmental effects must make allowance for the complex interaction between relationships: socio-economic conditions with the frequency of exposure to parental smoking, maternal alcohol consumption, environmental pollution and occupational hazards. After such allowances have been made and when there are improved ways of detecting very early losses, a study of the trends in prevalence would be an important way of monitoring the effects of known or suspected reproductive hazards.

References

Alberman E (1987) Maternal age and spontaneous abortion. In: Bennett MJ et al. (eds) Spontaneous and recurrent abortion. Blackwell Scientific Publications, Oxford London Edinburgh Boston Palo Alto San Francisco, pp 77–89

Alberman E, Creasy M, Elliott M, Spicer C (1976) Maternal factors associated with chromosomal anomalies in spontaneous abortion. Br J Obstet Gynaecol 83:621–627

Alberman E, Roman E, Pharaoh POD, Chamberlain G (1980) Birthweight before and after a spontaneous abortion. Br J Obstet Gynaecol 87:275–280

Axelsson G, Molin I (1988) Outcome of pregnancy among women living near petrochemical industries in Sweden. Int J Epidemiol, 17:363–369

Chard T (1991) Frequency of implantation and early pregnancy loss in natural cycles. In: Seppala M (ed) Baillière's Clinical Obstetrics and Gynaecology, 5:179–189

Fenton AC, Field DJ, Mason E, Clarke M (1990) Attitudes to viability of preterm infants and their effect on figures for perinatal mortality. Br Med J 300:434–436

Harlap S, Shiono P, Ramcharan S (1980) Spontaneous fetal losses in women using different contraceptives around the time of conception. Int J Epidermiol 9:49–56

Hertig AT, Rock J (1973) Searching for early fertilized human ova. Gynecol Obstet Invest 4:121–139

Jacobs PA (1990) The role of chromosome abnormalities in reproductive failure. Reprod Nutr Dev Suppl 1:63s–74s

Kline J, Stein Z, Susser M (1989a) Conception to birth. Oxford University Press, New York, pp 43–68
Kline J, Stein Z, Susser M (1989b) Conception to birth. Oxford University Press, New York, pp 102–117
Kline J, Stein Z, Susser M (1989c) Conception to birth. Oxford University Press, New York, pp 81–101
Lindbohm ML, Hemminki K (1988) National data base on medically diagnosed spontaneous abortions in Finland. Int J Epidemiol 17:568–573
McDonald AD, McDonald JC, Armstrong B et al. (1988) Fetal death and work in pregnancy. Br J Ind Med 45:148–157
Narod SA, Khazen R (1989) Spontaneous abortions in Ontario, 1979 to 1984. Can J Public Health 80:209–213
Royal College of General Practitioners' Oral Contraception Study (1976) The outcome of pregnancy in former oral contraceptive users. Br J Obstet Gynaecol 83:621–627
Silman AJ, Black C (1988) Increased incidence of spontaneous abortion and infertility in women with scleroderma before disease onset: a controlled study. Ann Rheum Dis 47:441–444
Stein Z, Kline J, Susser E, Shrout P, Warburton D, Susser M (1980) Maternal age and spontaneous abortions. In: Porter IH et al. (eds) Human embryonic and fetal death. Academic Press, London Toronto New York Sydney San Francisco, pp 107–127
Taskinen HK (1990) Effects of parental occupational exposures on spontaneous abortion and congenital malformation. Scand J Work Environ Health 16:297–314
Ulstein M, Jensen TS, Irgens LM, Lie RT, Sivertsen E (1990) Outcome of pregnancy in one Norwegian county 3 years prior to and 3 years subsequent to the Chernobyl accident. Acta Obstet Gynecol Scand 69:277–280
Vessey MP, Meisler L, Flavel R, Yeates D (1979) Outcome of pregnancy in women using different methods of contraception. Br J Obstet Gynaecol 86:548–556
WHO Task Force (1979) Gestation, birthweight and spontaneous abortion in pregnancy after induced abortion. Lancet, 1:142–145
Wilcox AJ, Weinberg CR, O'Connor JF et al. (1988) Incidence of early loss of pregnancy. N Engl J Med 319:189–194
Yerushalmy J, Bierman JM, Kemp DH, Connors A, French FE (1956) Longitudinal studies of pregnancy on the island of Kauai, Territory of Hawaii. 1. Analysis of previous reproductive history. Am J Obstet Gynecol 71:80–96

3.   Aetiology of Pregnancy Failure

J. L. Simpson

Introduction

Genetic factors are the commonest cause of early embryonic loss. Here we systematically consider the genetic aetiology of pregnancy loss, updating previous publications (Carson and Simpson 1990; Simpson 1991a,b; Simpson and Carson 1992; Simpson and Golbus 1992).

Numerical Chromosomal Abnormalities (Aneuploidy and Polyploidy)

Preclinical Losses

Chromosomal abnormalities were observed in approximately 20% of in vitro fertilised embryos that are ostensibly normal (Angell et al. 1983; Rudak et al. 1985; Zenzes et al. 1985; Michelman et al. 1986; Plachot et al. 1987). The study of Plachot et al. (1987) is illustrative. Of 68 human embryos recovered at the 2 to 8 cell stages, 3 showed only a single pronucleus, presumably being haploid; 1 of the 3 was also monosomic for a C group chromosome. Of 15 embryos showing 3 or more pronuclei, 7 were grossly triploid, 3 triploid-diploid mosaics, 2 polyploid and only 3 grossly diploid. However, none of the 3 grossly diploid embryos could be verified by full chromosomal analysis to be normal. The 50 remaining embryos each showed 2 pronuclei and would be considered normal; thirty-seven (37) of these 50 could not be karyotyped. However, of the 13 that could be karyotyped, only 5 were cytogenetically normal. That chromosomal abnormalities are frequent in morphologically normal embryos suggested that the frequency would be higher yet in the early morphological abnormalities documented by Hertig and Rock. That is, the most likely explanation for morphological abnormalities is

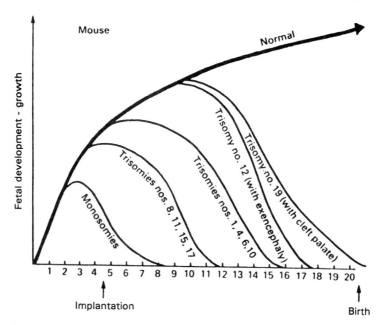

Fig. 3.1. Timing for loss of murine autosomal monosomy and murine autosomal trisomy (Gropp 1973).

genetic factors. Over many years Hertig and Rock (Hertig et al. 1956, 1959; Hertig and Rock 1973) recovered 8 pre-implantation embryos (less than 6 days from conception). Four of these embryos were morphologically abnormal. These embryos presumably would not have implanted or would not have survived long thereafter. Similarly, 9 of 26 implanted embryos (6–14 embryonic days) were morphologically abnormal, and also unlikely to develop further.

Consistent with this conclusion are animal studies of Gropp (1973, 1975). Mice heterozygous for various Robertsonian translocations were mated to produce various monosomies and trisomies. By selective mating and sacrifice of pregnant females, both survivability and phenotypic characteristics of the various aberrant complements could be determined. In the mouse, as in man, autosomal monosomy proved non-viable. Monosomies usually aborted within 4–5 days of conception (i.e., around implantation) (Fig. 3.1). Trisomies were lost later, with only a few (Nos 12 and 19) surviving until live birth.

First Trimester

Cytogenetic abnormalities are by far the most frequent explanation for the 12%–15% of clinically recognised pregnancy losses. The frequency of chromosomal abnormalities is approximately 50%. Among spontaneously expelled first trimester losses (Table 3.1), the frequency may even be higher.

One experimental difficulty is the impossibility of determining the status of abortuses that fail to grow in culture. Could failures be disproportionately represented by chromosomal abnormalities? Indeed, Guerneri et al. (1987)

Table 3.1. Chromosomal complements in spontaneous abortions: recognised clinically in the first trimester

Complement	Frequency	(%)
Normal		
46,XX or 46,XY		54.1
Triploidy		7.7
69,XXX	2.7	
69,XYX	0.2	
69,XXY	4.0	
Other	0.8	
Tetraploidy		2.6
92,XXXX	1.5	
92,XXYY	0.55	
Not Stated	0.55	
Monosomy X		8.6
Structural abnormalities		1.5
Sex chromosomal polysomy		0.2
47,XXX	0.05	
47,XXY	0.15	
Autosomal monosomy (G)		0.1
Autosomal trisomy		
Chromosome		22.3
No. 1	0	
No. 2	1.11	
No. 3	0.25	
No. 4	0.64	
No. 5	0.04	
No. 6	0.14	
No. 7	0.89	
No. 8	0.79	
No. 9	0.72	
No. 10	0.36	
No. 11	0.04	
No. 12	0.18	
No. 13	1.07	
No. 14	0.82	
No. 15	1.68	
No. 16	7.27	
No. 17	0.18	
No. 18	1.15	
No. 19	0.01	
No. 20	0.61	
No. 21	2.11	
No. 22	2.26	
Double trisomy		0.7
Mosaic trisomy		1.3
Other abnormalities or not specified		0.9
		100.0

Pooled data from several series, referenced elsewhere (Simpson and Bombard (1987)).

found a 77% frequency of chromosomal abnormalities in women studied immediately after ultrasound diagnosis of fetal demise and Ohno et al. (1991) found 76.9%. However, Eiben et al. (1987) found 48.6%. Tissue for analysis was obtained by chorionic villus sampling, rather than relying later in gestation upon recovery of spontaneously expelled products. A very high proportion of specimens proved informative. However, the gestational age in the sample of Guerneri et al. (1987) may also have been earlier than in other studies (Boué et al. 1975).

Second and Third Trimester

It would be of interest to know the prevalence of chromosomal abnormalities in losses occurring in pregnancies known to have been viable at 8 weeks' gestation. The high frequency of unrecognised missed abortion in the first trimester invalidates earlier reports that attempted to correlate precisely the frequency of chromosomal abnormalities with gestational interval. However, the frequency of chromosomal errors in losses recognised between 16 and 28 weeks is surely less than that observed in losses *recognised* earlier (Ruzicska and Cziezel 1971; Warburton et al. 1980). In the second trimester, one also observes chromosomal abnormalities more similar to those observed in live-born infants: trisomies 13, 18 and 21; monosomy X; sex chromosomal polysomies. Moreover, anatomical findings in such abortuses are reminiscent of those present in aneuploid live borns.

Pathological Findings in First Trimester Abortuses

Fetal Conditions

Autosomal Trisomy

Autosomal trisomies comprise the largest (53%) single class of chromosomal complements in cytogenetically abnormal spontaneous abortions. Frequencies of specific trisomies are listed in Table 3.1. Trisomy for every chromosome except No. 1 has been reported, and trisomy for that chromosome has been observed in an 8-cell embryo (Watt et al. 1987). The most common trisomy is No. 16. Some but not all trisomies show a maternal age effect, a relationship that is especially impressive for double trisomies.

Only a few trisomies show specific anatomical features. "Blighted ova" is claimed in trisomies 2, 3, 4 and 5, whereas Group C (6–12) trisomies usually show some fetal tissue (Boué et al. 1976). Cyclopia and other facial anomalies are observed in trisomy D (13–15, predominantly 13). Abnormal chorionic vessels, with or without arrest at the embryonic disc state, are often evident in trisomy 16.

Double autosomal trisomy occurs, but is lethal early in development.

Structural Chromosomal Rearrangement

Structural chromosomal rearrangements account for 1.5% of all abortuses (Table 3.1). Such abnormalities may either arise de novo (during gametogenesis), or be inherited from a parent carrying a "balanced" translocation or an inversion.

Phenotypic consequences depend upon the specific duplicated or deficient chromosomal segment. Although not a common cause of sporadic losses, inherited rearrangements are an important cause of repeated fetal wastage. We shall therefore return to this topic below.

Sex Chromosomal Polysomy (X or Y)

The complements 47,XXY and 47,XYY each occur in about 1 per 800 live-born males; 47,XXX occurs in 1 per 800 females. Howver, X or Y polysomies are observed in only 0.6% of abortuses' specimens (1.3% of chromosomally abnormal abortuses).

Chromosomal Translocations

Structural chromosomal abnormalities are a well-accepted explanation for repetitive abortions but a less common explanation for losses in general.

The most common structural rearrangement encountered is a translocation (Fig. 3.2). Individuals with balanced translocations are phenotypically normal, but abortuses or abnormal live borns may show duplications or deficiencies as a result of normal meiotic segregation.

If cytogenetic studies are routinely performed on all couples experiencing recurrent fetal losses, the frequency of translocations is about 2% of couples (Simpson et al. 1989). About 60% of these translocations are reciprocal, and 40% are Robertsonian. Investigations restricted to couples experiencing not only abortions but also still-born infants or anomalous live-born infants will yield relatively more translocations (Table 3.2). Females are about twice as likely as males to show a balanced translocation (Simpson et al. 1981). Questions that remain unanswered include (1) Are prevalence rates influenced by numbers of previous losses? (2) Does occurrence of both first- and second-trimester losses affect prevalence rates?

If a balanced translocation is detected, antenatal cytogenetic studies should obviously be offered in subsequent pregnancies. The frequency of unbalanced fetuses at 16 weeks (amniocentesis) is far lower if the balanced translocation is acertained through repetitive abortions (perhaps 3%) than if ascertained through an anomalous live born (approximately 12%) (Daniels et al. 1989).

In Robertsonian translocation, empiric risks are considerably less than theoretical risks (33% as shown in Fig. 3.3). The likelihood is 2% or less if the father carries a 14q21q translocation, and about 10% if the mother carries such a translocation (Boué and Gallano 1973; Daniels et al. 1989). For example, in t(13q;13q), the most common Robertsonian translocation found in normal individuals, the risks for a live born with trisomy 13 is 1% or less (Daniels et al. 1989).

Empirical data for specific reciprocal translocations are rarely available, but generalisations can be made on the basis of pooled data derived from many different translocations. Again, theoretical risks for abnormal offspring with unbalanced translocations are greater than empirical risks. The empirical risk is 12% for offspring of female heterozygotes and 12% for offspring of male heterozygotes (Daniels et al. 1989).

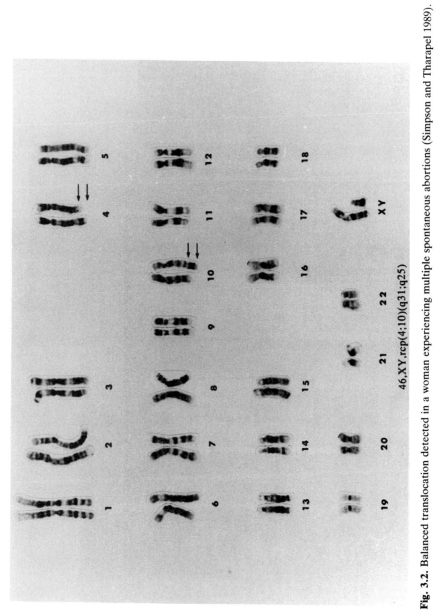

Fig. 3.2. Balanced translocation detected in a woman experiencing multiple spontaneous abortions (Simpson and Tharapel 1989).

46,XY,rcp(4;10)(q31;q25)

Table 3.2. Balanced translocations in couples experiencing repeated abortions

Repeated spontaneous abortions with or without normal live-born		Repeated spontaneous abortions with still-born or abnormal live-born		Repeated spontaneous abortions with no further subcategorisation	
Female	Male	Female	Male	Female	Male
89/3712	57/3651	20/432	7/409	100/3074	65/3009
2.4%	1.6%	4.6%	1.7%	3.3%	2.1%

Relationship between ascertainment and likelihood of detecting balanced translocations. Pooled data from Simpson et al. (1989).

Chromosomal Inversions

Another parental chromosomal rearrangement causing fetal loss is an inversion. In this intrachromosomal rearrangement the order of genes is reversed. This rearrangement usually occurs when two chromosomal breaks are followed by reinsertion in reverse order of the chromosomal segment produced by breaks. Inversions in which breakpoints exist on opposite sides of the centromere are *pericentric*; those in which breakpoints are on the same side of the centromere are *paracentric*.

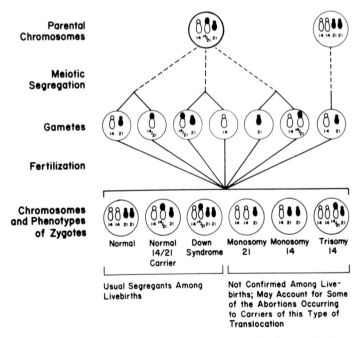

Fig. 3.3. Diagram of possible gametes and progeny of a phenotypically normal individual heterozygous for a Robertsonian translocation between chromosomes 14 and 21 (a form of D/G translocations). Three of the six possible gametes are incompatible with life. The likelihood that an individual with such a translocation would have a child with Down's syndrome is theoretically 33%. However, the empirical risk is considerably less (Gerbie and Simpson 1976).

28   Aetiology of Pregnancy Failure

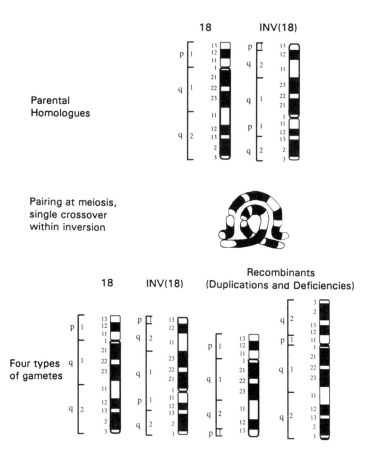

Fig. 3.4. Diagram illustrating the breakpoints leading to an inversion in chromosomes 18. The inversion loop resulting from pairing during meiosis is shown. As a result, crossing over at meiosis 1 would be expected to produce the four types of gametes shown. Two of the four would be genetically balanced, although one would show the same inversion present in the parent. In addition, two types of gametes would be genetically unbalanced, showing complementary duplications and deficiencies. It is the chromosomal region outside the inverted segment that appears as a duplication or deletion (Martin et al. 1983).

Heterozygotes for either pericentric or paracentric inversions may be normal if genes are not lost, gained, or altered as a result of the breaks leading to the inversion. However, individuals with inversions suffer abnormal reproductive consequences as a result of normal meiotic phenomena, namely crossing-over during meiosis I. In order for genes within inversions to pair, a loop must form during meiosis I. Crossing-over may or may not occur within an inversion loop, but it is likely to do so if the loop encompasses a large portion of the chromosome. If crossing-over occurs, certain gametes are unbalanced.

Inversions account for far less than 1% of couples experiencing repeated spontaneous abortion. Inversion is an infrequent cause of fetal loss, even among repeated aborters. However, inversions are highly deleterious and warrant prenatal studies (Martin et al. 1983; Sutherland et al. 1976). A single crossover within a *paracentric* inversion results in both dicentric and acentric products. Both acentric and dicentric gametes contribute to fetal wastage. Both outcomes are usually lethal; thus, paracentric inversions are rarely associated with anomalous live births.

Pericentric inversions are likely to cause not only abortions but anomalous live borns. After crossing-over, two of the four gametes represent the parental sequences (one normal, one inverted) (Fig. 3.4). The other two gametes represent recombinants, genes distal to one breakpoint deficient and genes distal to the other breakpoint duplicated. The prevalence of pericentric inversions among couples experiencing repetitive abortions is considerably lower than the prevalence of balanced translocations.

Genes Causing Aneuploidy

Numerical chromosomal abnormalities (aneuploidy) may also be responsible not only for sporadic losses but also for recurrent losses. Such reasoning is based on observations that the complements of successive abortuses in a given family are more likely to be either consistently normal or consistently abnormal (Table 3.3). That is, abortuses in a given family show non-random distribution with respect to chromosomal complements. If the complement of the first abortus is abnormal, the likelihood is 80% that the complement of the second abortuses will also be abnormal (Hassold 1980). The recurrent abnormality is usually trisomy, but it may also be monosomy or polyploidy. These data suggest that certain couples are predisposed towards chromosomally abnormal conceptions, most of which naturally result in spontaneous abortion. Presumably the mechanism involves mutant genes. In humans consanguinity has been said to increase the risk of aneuploidy (Alfi et al. 1981), but this claim is arguable. However, in rodents, frequency of aneuploidy varies by strain (Fabricant and Schneider 1978; Golbus 1981; Estop et al. 1986). Genes affecting meiosis are also well documented in plants and animals, and a variety of mechanisms by which genes could cause non-disjunction can be plausibly postulated. Although Warburton et al. (1987) believe that corrections for maternal age render the phenomenon of recurrent aneuploidy statistically non-significant, this author does not agree.

Table 3.3. The relationship between karyotypes of successive abortuses. Tabulated from Warburton et al. (1987)

Complement of first abortion	Complement of second abortion					
	Normal	Trisomy	Monosomy X	Triploidy	Tetraploidy	De novo rearrangement
Normal	142	18	5	7	3	2
Trisomy	31	30	1	4	3	1
Monosomy X	7	5	3	3	0	0
Triploidy	7	4	1	4	0	0
Tetraploidy	3	1	0	2	0	0
De novo rearrangement	1	3	0	0	0	0

The issue is clinically relevant because if a couple were predisposed to recurrent aneuploidy, they might logically be at increased risk for aneuploid live borns. The autosome trisomic in a subsequent pregnancy might not be character-ised by lethality (e.g., trisomy 16), but rather might be more compatible with life (e.g., trisomy 21). Available data do not allow one to state whether live-born aneuploidy is increased following live-born aneuploid abortions. However, several studies suggest that the risk of live-born trisomy 21 following a trisomic abortus is about 1% (Alberman 1981).

Anatomical Defects of Polygenic/Multifactorial Aetiology

Those first trimester abortuses that do not show chromosomal abnormalities could have undergone fetal demise for genetic aetiologies – Mendelian or polygenic/multifactorial. Technical limitations of studying such populations are formidable. Excellent anatomical studies have been performed by Nishimura et al. (1968; Nishimura 1970) and Opitz (1987). Many anomalies have been observed, but lack of cytogenetic data on dissected specimens makes it impossible to determine the true role of non-cytogenetic mechanisms in embryonic maldevelopment.

One defect that is not likely to be cytogenetic in origin is isolated neural tube defect (NTD). Byrne and Warburton (1986) estimate NTD prevalence to be 1% of abortuses.

Maternal Conditions

Luteal Phase (Progesterone) Deficiency (LPD)

One very plausible explanation for spontaneous abortion is an early pregnancy abnormality resulting from implantation in an unsupportive endometrial environ-ment. The term luteal phase deficiency (LPD) is used to describe an endo-metrium manifesting inadequate progesterone effect. Such an abnormality may theoretically be the result of either inadequate function of the endometrial progesterone, or a low level of progesterone production. In the latter, the corpus luteum may be unable to secrete progesterone in quantities sufficient to maintain the pregnancy until placental secretion becomes self-sustaining (5 weeks post-conception or 7 weeks gestation).

Luteal phase defect is believed by many to be a frequent cause of recurrent pregnancy loss. The phenomenon almost certainly exists but its frequency is quite arguable. Some have estimated LPD to be present in 35% of patients experi-encing recurrent losses (Jones 1976). However, this figure is derived from patients first ascertained on the basis of prior losses and then subjected to endometrial biopsy (Daya et al. 1988). Yet, when regularly menstruating, fertile women with no history of abortions were biopsied in up to 10 serial cycles, the frequency of luteal phase defect proved to be 51.4% in any single cycle and 26.7% in sequential cycles (Davis et al. 1989).

Determining both the frequency as well as validity of LPD is also made difficult by lack of uniform diagnostic criteria. LPD was originally diagnosed on the basis of an endometrial biopsy lagging at least two days behind the actual post-ovulation date, as determined by counting backward from the next menstrual period (assuming 14 days from ovulation to menses). Nuances of histological dating and monthly variations in the menstrual cycle occur, probably accounting for much of the 40% occurrence of LPD in normal women if one relies on only one endometrial biopsy. Even the original endometrial dating by Noyes, Hertig and Rock showed a mean error of 1.81 days in dating (Noyes et al. 1950). This original report suggested that an endometrial biopsy be called "out-of-phase" only if it lags 3 or more days behind the actual post-ovulation date. By way of emphasising this difficulty, 62 endometrial biopsies read by 5 different pathologists resulted in an inter-observer variation that would have altered management in 22%–39% of patients (Scott et al. 1988). When the endometrial biopsy slides were read a second time by the same pathologist, the initial diagnosis was confirmed in only 25% of samples (Li et al. 1989). Therefore, at least two biopsies that are out of phase are considered necessary to make the diagnosis of LPD. It has also been suggested that LPD be diagnosed by correlating histological endometrial dating with a post-ovulation date calculated from the date of the rise in luteal hormone, rather than calculated by counting backwards from the succeeding menses (Li et al. 1987).

Others have suggested that rather than endometrial biopsy one utilises one (Daya and Ward 1988) or more (Wu and Minassian 1987) progesterone concentrations in the luteal phase. Horta et al. (1977) measured progesterone in women with a history of three spontaneous abortions. Of the 15 such women 10 had lower luteal progesterone concentrations than 15 healthy non-pregnant control women; all 10 went on to abort their pregnancies during the first trimester. However, in patients with two or more spontaneous abortions, low progesterone in the luteal phase proved only 71% predictive of a luteal phase defect diagnosed on the basis of an abdominal endometrial biopsy. That the diagnosis be made by observing the length of the elevation of the basal body temperature has been suggested with the proposal that a luteal length of 11 days or less indicates high likelihood of luteal phase defect (Downs and Gibson 1983). A modification of this proposal is that an LH surge–menses interval of less than 10 days be considered diagnostic of LPD (Smith et al. 1984). Progesterone receptors measured in the luteal endometrium have been generally unsuccessful in predicting pathological dating (McRae et al. 1984; Jacobs et al. 1987). One study found lower concentrations of progesterone receptor in the endometrium of women with LPD, but a large overlap with normal women was observed (Spiritos et al. 1985). Another study showed higher concentrations of progesterone receptor accompanied by low serum progesterone in patients with an out-of-phase endometrial biopsy (Saracoglu et al. 1985). However, perturbations in endometrial receptors have not yet been correlated with actual pregnancy loss.

Given such arguable studies concerning diagnostic criteria for LPD, it is hardly surprising that no randomised studies exist to document efficacy of proffered therapeutic regimens, principally progesterone. Although over one hundred published studies have discussed LPD, not a single completed study has been randomised in design with a placebo group. A typical study claiming effective treatment is that of Tho et al. (1979); 23 of 100 women with repetitive spontaneous abortions had "documented" LPDs on the basis of "out-of-phase" endometrial biopsies. All 23 women were treated with progesterone suppositories and 21 completed their pregnancies. The closest approximation to a control group was 37 other women who had no ostensible aetiology for their losses. Of these 37, 22 were treated with "empiric" progesterone; 15 were not. Among the treated women 73% had successful pregnancies compared to 47% of the untreated women. Daya et al. (1988) investigated 65 patients with recurrent abortions, finding 26 patients (40%) to have both two consecutive out-of-phase biopsies and low progesterone levels. All were treated with progesterone, after which the endometrium appeared to be restored to normal. Only three (19%) of 16 subsequent pregnancies aborted. However, there was no control group.

The most convincing data suggesting that LPD is a valid entity are derived from a study of 33 infertile women whose LPD was documented by two out-of-phase biopsies (Daly et al. 1983). Although the study involved women having infertility rather than recurrent abortions, investigators observed no pregnancy losses among the 14 women who conceived after documenting an in-phase endometrial biopsy produced by progesterone treatment. Of the 16 women whose biopsy was not corrected, there were by contrast only 4 pregnancies, all of which ended in spontaneous abortion (Daly et al. 1983).

In conclusion, LPD may or may not be a valid entity. If valid, the entity is surely overdiagnosed. The phenomenon of LPD could also be a secondary effect, the primary defect being an abnormal embryo that cannot trigger the appropriate signal for luteal function. In fact, coexistence of LPD and trisomy 16 has been reported (Saracogla et al. 1985). Alternatively, secretion of follicle stimulating hormone could independently lead both to LPD and to aneuploidy. Cytogenetic data on conceptuses that allegedly abort as result of LPD are badly needed.

Given the controversy, treatment should be instituted only with reticence and only if the diagnosis of LPD is firmly established.

Thyroid Abnormalities

Decreased conception rates clearly occur with overt hypothyroidism or overt hyperthyroidism. However, data implicating subclinical thyroid dysfunction with fetal losses are lacking (Montero et al. 1981). Studies purporting to show a relationship may be questioned on the basis of the arguable diagnostic criteria, and such studies lack proper controls.

Carbohydrate Abnormalities

The large prospective collaborative study conducted by myself and colleagues (Diabetes in Early Pregnancy Study) (Mills et al. 1988) has shown that women whose diabetes is most poorly controlled are at increased risk. In our study metabolic data were gathered from the fifth week of gestation, and information was collected which allowed a variety of confounding variables to be taken into account. Overall, no significant difference in loss rates existed between controls (15.6%) and women with insulin-dependent diabetes mellitus (15.9%). However, subjects whose glycosylated haemoglobin was greater than 4 s.d. above the mean showed highest rates of pregnancy loss (Table 3.4). Miodonik and colleagues (1984, 1985, 1986) have accumulated data consistent with this, as have Greene et al. (1989) in a retrospective analysis. Thus, poorly controlled diabetes mellitus is probably a cause of early pregnancy loss. However, well-controlled and subclinical diabetes should not be considered causes.

Table 3.4. Diabetic control and fetal losses

Initial glycosylated haemoglobin (S.D. from control mean)	N	Pregnancy losses (%)	Mean glycosylated haemoglobin, first trimester	N	Pregnancy losses (%)
<2	137	9.5	<2	137	10.3
2–4	131	14.5	2–4	121	15.2
>4	112	21.4	>4	112	20.2

Relationship of diabetic control of pregnancy losses, as judged by a) initial glycosylated haemoglobin, obtained at 6 or 7 weeks gestations, and b) mean weekly first trimester glycosylated haemoglobin. Derived from data reported of Mills et al. (1988).

Intrauterine Adhesions (Synechiae)

Intrauterine adhesions could interfere with implantation of early embryonic development. Adhesions may follow overzealous curettage of the uterus during the postpartum period, intrauterine surgery (e.g., myomectomy), or endometritis. Curettage accounts for most cases, with adhesions most likely to develop when the procedure is performed 3 or 4 weeks postpartum. Affected individuals are usually suspected because of menstrual abnormalities, but 15%–30% of cases become manifested following repeated abortions. If adhesions are detected in a woman experiencing repetitive losses, lysis of the adhesions under direct hysteroscopic visualisation should be performed. Approximately 50% of subjects conceive after surgery, but the frequency of abortions remains high.

Incomplete Mullerian Fusion and Other Uterine Anomalies

In incomplete uterine fusion, the pregnant uterus may be unable to accommodate the growing fetus, and the placenta may implant on a poorly vascularised septum. First-trimester abortions occurring after ultrasonographic confirmation of a viable pregnancy at 8 or 9 weeks may be plausibly attributed to uterine fusion defects if the latter is present. However, losses occurring at 10 to 12 weeks gestation *without* confirmation of prior viability are statistically more likely to represent missed abortions, fetal demise having occurred prior to 8 weeks gestation.

Uterine fusion defects are more widely accepted as a cause of second-trimester abortions, but still not rigorously studied. The prevalence of abortions in patients with such defects may be as high as 20%–25% (Heinonen et al. 1982). Loss rates may be higher with septate and bicornuate uteri than with unicornuate uteri or uteri didelphys; however, data are sparse, and almost always retrospective.

Women experiencing second-trimester abortions and shown to have a mullerian fusion anomaly probably indeed benefit from uterine reconstruction; however, careful selection is important for optimal results.

Women exposed to diethylstilboestrol in utero are also recognised to be at increased risk for pregnancy loss (Herbst et al. 1989). The aetiology is considered to involve a structurally abnormal (T-shaped) uterus. An 8-year assessment by Ludmir et al. (1990) concluded that "high-risk" obstetric intervention (e.g., weekly examination and tocolysis) did not obviate the potential benefit of reconstruction, fetal survival being the same before and after institution of such a protocol.

Leiomyomas

Uterine leiomyomas are well-circumscribed non-encapsulated benign tumours consisting of smooth muscle and varying amounts of fibrous connective tissue. The lesions are usually multiple. A contribution to pregnancy wastage is plausible but probably uncommon.

The location of leiomyomas is probably more important than their size. Submucous leiomyomas are the type most likely to cause a fetal loss, acting through several potential mechanisms: (1) thinning of the endometrium over the surface of a submucous leiomyoma could predispose to implantation in a poorly decidualised site; (2) rapid growth under the hormonal milieu of pregnancy might compromise blood supply of the leiomyoma, resulting in necrosis ("red degeneration") that in turn leads to uterine contractions and fetal expulsion; (3) large leiomyomas may encroach upon the space required by the developing fetus, thereby leading to premature delivery through mechanisms analogous to those present in incomplete mullerian fusion. Lack of space can also lead to fetal deformations.

Myomectomy may occasionally be warranted for women experiencing repetitive second-trimester abortions. As in incomplete mullerian fusion, it is important to select patients carefully.

Incompetent Cervix

A functionally intact cervix and lower uterine cavity is an obvious necessity for a successful intrauterine pregnancy. Cervical incompetence is characterised by painless dilatation and effacement, usually during the mid-second or early third trimester. Cervical incompetence frequently follows antecedent traumatic events such as surgical dilatation, cervical lacerations, cervical amputations, conisation, or cauterisation. A history of premature cervical dilatation during pregnancy suggests the diagnosis, which is not always easy to verify. Diagnosis may be confirmed in the non-pregnant state if an object of fixed diameter (e.g., No. 8 Hegar dilator) easily traverses the internal cervical os. Ultrasonography readily confirms that dilatation has already occurred, but it is less helpful in identifying women destined to experience premature cervical dilatation.

Various operations for correcting cervical incompetence have been proposed, with success rate approximating 80% (Rock and Jones 1977). At least one study attempted without clear success to determine the value of cerclage in the absence of demonstrable abnormality (Edmonds 1988). It should also be noted that two randomised trials have failed to show a statistically significant positive effect in perinatal outcome in women undergoing cervical cerclage (Lazar and Guegen 1984; Rush et al. 1984). However, the samples were heterogeneous, not limited to those having mid-trimester losses, but also including women having both first-trimester losses as well as any deliveries before 37 weeks. Thus, the power of these studies was diminished.

Infections

Infections are well-known causes of late fetal wastage, and logically could be responsible for early fetal loss as well. Any of several mechanisms could be responsible: (1) intrauterine fetal demise resulting from overwhelming infection; (2) micro-organisms interfering with organogenesis to such an extent that differentiation can no longer proceed; (3) fever *per se*; and (4) teratogenic action of agents used to treat the infection. On the other hand, the question of whether a given infectious agent actually caused the demise, or merely arose after the fetal demise, is unanswered. Lack of knowledge concerning cytogenetic and endocrine status makes it almost impossible to address the above issues in a truly satisfactory fashion.

Micro-organisms claimed to be associated with spontaneous abortion include *Variola*, *Vaccinia*, *Salmonella typhi*, *Vibrio fetus*, *Malaria*, *Cytomegalovirus*, *Brucella*, *Toxoplasmosis*, *Mycoplasma hominis*, *Chlamydia trachomatis*, and *Ureaplasma urealyticum*. However, no data showing relative risks for fetal loss are available for any of them. Antibodies to *Chlamydia trachomatis* are not increased in women having spontaneous abortions (Quinn et al. 1987).

The most solid data relate to *Ureaplasma urealyticum*. Stray-Pedersen et al. (1978) studied 46 women with histories of three or more consecutive losses of unknown aetiology. Endometrial *Ureaplasma* colonisation proved significantly more frequent among women with repetitive abortions (28%) than among female controls (7%). Of 45 women in the former group, 13 harboured *Ureaplasma* in both cervix and endometrium. The 42 women and their husbands were then treated with doxycycline for 11 days, with subsequent cultures showing no *Ureaplasma*, and 19 of the 43 women became pregnant after treatment. Of these 19 women, three experienced another spontaneous abortion and 16 had normal full-term infants. Among 18 women with *Ureaplasma* who were not treated, there were 5 more abortions and 5 full-term pregnancies.

In support of infectious aetiology are claims that empirical antibiotic therapy is of benefit to couples experiencing repetitive spontaneous abortions, thus suggesting infectious aetiology. In a study of pregnancy outcome by Toth et al. (1986), only 10% of patients who were treated with tetracycline for four weeks and who then became pregnant experienced another spontaneous abortion. By contrast, 38% of patients who did not choose to take antibiotics and who later became pregnant had another spontaneous abortion. However, in this study antibiotics were or were not given in accordance to the patients' desires; thus, the validity of the self-selected "control" group is arguable.

Anti-fetal Antibodies

It is obvious that alterations of the immune system could be responsible for fetal wastage. However, the nature of the immunological process responsible for maintaining pregnancy has proved to be complex. Both autoimmune as well as alloimmune factors have been identified as causes of pregnancy losses.

A familiar example of an immunological mechanism causing fetal wastage occurs when an otherwise normal mother produces antibodies against her fetus on the basis of genetic dissimilarities at a given locus. Mid or late gestational fetal loss is well documented in Rh-negative (D-negative) women having anti-D antibodies. A rare but well-documented example involves anti-P antibodies (Levine 1978). Genotypes PP or Pp are most common. However, an occasional female is homozygous pp. If a woman of genotype pp mates with a PP or Pp male, offspring may be Pp. If the mother develops anti-P antibodies, Pp fetuses will be rejected early in gestation. Plasmapheresis may be efficacious (Rock et al. 1985).

Autoimmune Disease

The association between mid-trimester pregnancy loss and certain autoimmune disease is generally accepted (Branch and Ward 1989). Specifically, individuals having lupus anticoagulant (LAC) antibodies and anticardiolipin antibodies have an increased likelihood of fetal wastage. These two antibodies have closely related specificities and could be members of the same family of autoantibodies. Anticardiolipin antibody may be the more sensitive indicator of the two (Lockshin et al. 1985), but it may also be less specific. *In vitro*, LAC is an anticoagulant; *in vivo* it paradoxically increases the likelihood of thrombosis (Gastineau et al. 1985). Lupus anticoagulant (LAC) has been associated with subplacental clotting and fetal losses at all trimesters, as well as with poor reproductive history in general (Elias and Eldor 1984; Harris 1988). Thus, the abortifacient mechanism is presumably decidual. Because only 5%–10% of patients with systemic lupus erythematosus have LAC, individuals with positive antinuclear antibodies (ANA) may or may not have LAC (Exner et al. 1978). Similarly, not all patients with LAC will have SLE. Scott et al. (1987) state that on the basis of their literature survey of 242 untreated women, the frequency of mid-trimester fetal death in women who show LAC or anticardiolipin antibodies is 91%. In their own experience, 83% of 162 prior pregnancies in such women were lost. An increased frequency of other pregnancy complications (e.g., growth retardation, pre-eclampsia) also occurs. Treatment with prednisone and low doses of aspirin may improve outcome (Branch et al. 1985).

The role of LAC and anticardiolipin antibodies in early fetal wastage is less well established. Unander et al. (1987) studied 99 women having three or more abortuses, 68 with no live borns. Increased anticardiolipin antibodies were found in 42. The proportion of antibodies in "primary" and "secondary" aborters was the same, but highest levels of anticardiolipin antibodies were observed in the former. Howard et al. (1987) observed LAC in 9 of 29 women having "three spontaneous miscarriages or stillbirths". Cowchock et al. (1986) observed anticardiolipin antibodies in 13.1% of 61 women with repeated abortuses. The first controlled study was by Petri et al. (1987). Here the frequency of LAC was 9% and anticardiolipin antibodies 11%, neither different from control subjects.

Other evidence for a relationship between autoimmune phenomena and early losses can be cited, but the significance is even more arguable than that of LAC and anticardiolipin antibodies. In the study of Cowchock et al. (1986) the frequency of other antibodies to nuclear antigens (DNA, Ro or SS-A, La, Smith, ribonucleoprotein) was somewhat higher in 61 women with unexplained fetal losses than in 21 women with explained losses (e.g., balanced translocation, uterine anomaly). However, no control subjects were studied. A later study showed a pregnancy loss of 17% in 96 pregnancies in anti-SS-A women; the loss rate was 21% in 235 pregnancies in women without anti-SS-A antibodies (Ramsey-Goldman et al. 1986). Haas et al. (1986) studied anti-sperm antibodies in 109 women "without an immunologic cause for their recurrent abortions". Frequencies of antibodies by tray agglutination test (TAT), sperm immobilisation test (SIT), and ELISA against solubilised sperm and seminal fluid antigens were 2.7%, 8.3%, and 19.3% respectively. No concurrent control group was available.

Finally, claims of increased pregnancy losses in women with endometriosis (Damewood 1989) could be explained on an autoimmune basis, if indeed the association is true.

Alloimmune Disease (Shared Parental Histocompatibility)

Rejection of the fetal allograft by the maternal immune system is prevented by a blocking or suppressive factor that protects the fetus. Blocking antibodies paradoxically seem to develop or to be enhanced by paternal antigens. This has been assumed to be the explanation for the long-standing recognition that pregnant women develop antipaternal antileukocytotic antibodies.

About 20% of women develop such antibodies following their first pregnancy, and about 65% of multiparous women have such antibodies (Weksler et al. 1983; Beard et al. 1983; Gill 1983). These cytotoxic antibodies may or may not be of primary importance, rather alternatively may serve merely as a marker for a more primary phenomenon. Such antibodies, recognised by inhibition of the one-way mixed lymphocyte reaction, are believed to be anti-idiotypic antibodies that interact with maternal lymphocyte antigen receptors.

It follows that maternal–fetal histoincompatibility should enhance pregnancy maintenance. By contrast, greater than expected sharing of histocompatibility antigens (HLA) (or, as preferred by some, trophoblast-like antigens or TLX) (McIntyre et al. 1986; Faulk et al. 1989) between mother and father would be deleterious because fetus and mother would be less likely to differ antigenically. Direct experimental support for a beneficial effect of maternal–fetal incompatibility includes: (1) increased placental size in mouse fetuses that result from matings in which paternally derived histocompatibility antigens differ from maternal antigens; (2) higher implantation frequencies in histoincompatible murine zygotes; and (3) maintenance of genetic polymorphisms at major histocompatibility loci despite over 70 generations of brother–sister matings in rats (Beer and Billingham 1976).

In addition to parental HLA sharing, other circumstantial support for the parental histoincompatibility being beneficial in humans can be cited. Only 16.6% of women with multiple abortions have antipaternal antileukocytoxic antibodies, in contrast to 64% of multiparous women and 20% of primiparous women (Thomas et al. 1985). Similarly, 50% of women with three or more recurrent abortions show no blocking factors, as evidenced by failure to demonstrate a mixed lymphocyte reaction when their lymphocytes are exposed to their spouse's lymphocytes (Beer et al. 1987). Blocking antibodies have been observed in women having successful pregnancies but lacking in those having abortuses (Rocklin et al. 1976, 1982; Stimson et al. 1979; Fitzet and Bousquet 1983).

Not all investigators have observed increased HLA sharing, depressing MLR, or decreased blocking antibodies (Oksenberg et al. 1984). Some couples sharing HLA-DR antigens have shown no spontaneous abortions, despite ten or more pregnancies (Ober et al. 1983). In addition, the critical information of whether the abortus actually inherited the paternal antigen shared by its mother and father is lacking. Antibodies are also absent in some women with successful pregnancy. Moreover, these antibodies develop only late in pregnancy, lack of antibodies therefore probably not reflecting inability to become pregnant per se (Regan and Braude 1987). Sargent et al. (1988), in particular, detected cytotoxic antibodies (T cell and B cell) only rarely in either successful pregnancy (only 1 of 16 cases up to 17 weeks) or unsuccessful pregnancy (abortion) (0 of 9 cases). It is possible that blocking antibodies are the *result* of live births, as opposed to being necessary for pregnancy maintenance.

That some, but not all, couples sharing HLA antigens show deleterious effects could also be explained by postulating that normal pregnancy requires maternal–fetal histocompatibility, not for HLA but rather for another closely linked locus. This hypothesis is not only consistent with HLA antigens failing to be expressed on the trophoblast but is supported as well by direct data. Blocking antibodies said to be present in normal pregnancies but absent in women experiencing spontaneous abortion are directed against neither HLA-A, B, C nor DR (Power et al. 1983). Thus, Faulk and McIntyre believe that immune regulation is stimulated by a series of placental antigens, so-called trophoblast lymphocyte cross-reactive (TLX) antigens (Faulk and McIntyre 1981; Faulk et al. 1989). This group claims to have isolated TLX antigens. They further claim that couples experiencing repetitive spontaneous abortions are more likely to share "TLX antigens" than couples without pregnancy wastage (McIntyre and Faulk, 1983; Faulk et al. 1989).

Although parental antigen sharing of some type can plausibly be expected to lead to repetitive abortion, it is also possible to explain the same data on a non-immunological basis. Closely linked to the mouse histocompatibility (H2) complex is locus T/t. Embryos homozygous for certain alleles at this locus die at various stages of embryogenesis. Whether a T/t-like complex exists in humans is arguable. If it does exist, and if it is linked to HLA on human chromosome 6, histocompatibility between mother and her fetus and (her spouse) for this or another locus could merely secondarily reflect homozygosity for lethal T/t alleles. In fact, evidence for such an effect has been offered by Schacter et al. (1984).

If fetal rejection occurs as a result of diminished fetal–maternal immunological interaction, it follows that immunotherapy to enhance interaction at the few differing loci is plausible. Indeed, pretransplant blood transfusions have been used to decrease allograft rejection after kidney transplantation (Norman et al. 1986). This beneficial effect appears to be due to the lymphocyte-rich fraction ("buffy-coat"). Perhaps blocking factors or suppressor cells are induced. Similarly, immunisation with lymphocytes of the paternal strain greatly increase fetal survival in donkey–horse matings (20% to 65%) (Allen et al. 1986).

These studies served as the experimental basis for human studies in which women lacking blocking antibodies but sharing HLA antigens with their spouse were immunised with either paternal leukocyte (Beer et al. 1981; Takakuwa et al. 1986; Mowbray et al. 1985) or third-party leukocytes (McIntyre and Faulk 1986; Unander and Lindholm 1986). Trophoblast membrane transfusion has also been attempted (McIntyre and Faulk 1986; Johnson et al. 1986).

Potential efficacy of immunotherapy was the subject of exhaustive consideration at a 1987 Royal College of Obstetricians and Gynaecologists symposium (Beard and Sharp 1988), and need not be recounted here in detail. Suffice it to say that few prospective randomised trials are published. Apparent improvement in outcome in the treated group (77% live births) compared to untreated group (37% live births) in the study of Mowbray et al. (1985) is tempered by lower successes in the control group than expected a priori (60%–70%, as reviewed by Simpson and Carson (1992) and Vlaanderen and Treffers (1987). Thus, unwitting selection could exist. Also uncertain is whether pregnancy complications are increased in immunised pregnancies. Resolution awaits multi-centre randomised trials which are currently underway.

Irradiation and Antineoplastic Agents

X-irradiation and antineoplastic agents are accepted abortifacients, but thera-peutic X-rays or chemotherapeutic drugs are administered during pregnancy only to seriously ill women. In diagnostic doses, X-rays have not been proven to cause fetal demise. However, it would be prudent to consider X-rays as a potential confounding variable. Even relatively low levels of anti-metabolites (e.g., methotrexate) might be considered abortifacients (Selevan et al. 1985), consist-ent with successful use of such agents in management of ectopic gestations.

Maternal Health

Cigarette Smoking

Smoking during pregnancy has been positively correlated with spontaneous abortion. Kline et al. (1980) found increased abortion rates in smokers, independent of maternal age and independent of alcohol consumption. Alber-man et al. (1976) also reported that smokers showed a higher (albeit not significantly higher) proportion of abortuses with normal karyotypes, an obser-vation that if verified would suggest that smoking affects the conceptus directly. This would be consistent with data from our group, which show that placental cytotrophoblasts of smokers have more sister chromatid exchanges (SCEs) than non-smokers (Shulman et al. 1991). Our study involved direct analysis of cytotrophoblasts, thus representing assessment of in vivo exposure.

On the other hand, it is possible that smoking and other toxins may exert deleterious effects only on susceptible hosts. In any event, smoking is an important confounding variable in determining fetal loss rates.

Alcohol

Several studies have reported an association between fetal loss and alcohol consumption, making the latter a potential cause. In one study, 616 women experiencing spontaneous abortions were compared with 632 women delivering at 28 gestational weeks or more (Kline et al. 1980). Among women whose pregnancies ended in spontaneous abortion, 17% drank at least twice per week;

8.1% of controls drank similar quantities. After adjusting for potential confounding factors (e.g., smoking, age, prior abortions), the association between alcohol and abortion remained significant. Harlap and Shiono (1980) also found a slightly increased risk of abortion in women who drank in the first trimester. The increase failed to reach statistical significance, but it could not be explained on the basis of smoking, prior abortion, age, or other known risk factors.

Not all studies have implicated alcohol. Halmesmärki (1989) found that alcohol consumption was nearly identical in women who did and did not experience an abortion; 13% of aborters and 11% of control women drank, on average, 3–4 drinks per week. Alcohol consumption was also similar in their spouses. Parazzini et al. (1990) compared Milanese couples with multiple abortuses to 176 women delivered of normal offspring. The relative risk was 0.9 for women reporting one drink per day and 0.8 for those reporting two or more drinks.

Other Environmental Factors

A few chemical agents have been claimed to show an association with fetal losses. These chemicals include anaesthetic gases, arsenic, aniline, benzene, ethylene oxide, formaldehyde and lead (Figa-Talamanaca and Settimi 1984; Barlow and Sullivan 1982). Although many environmental toxicologists accept these agents as proved, evidence is far from convincing at low levels of exposure. Considerable interest followed one study that claimed an association between pregnancy loss and exposure to video display terminals of greater than 20 hours per week (Goldhaber et al. 1988). However, a more rigorous cohort study of female telephone operators who did and did not use VDUs shows no deleterious effects of VDU exposure (Schnorr et al. 1991). The clear consensus, based on other studies as well, is that no such association exists between pregnancy loss and VDU (Blackwell and Chang 1988). Of additional note are studies showing no increased risk for either pregnant laboratory workers (Heidam 1984) or pregnant pharmaceutical industry workers (Taskinen et al. 1984).

Intrauterine Devices and Other Contraceptive Agents

Conception with an intrauterine device (IUD) in situ markedly increases the risk of fetal loss. The presumed pathogenesis is infection. However, exposure to an IUD prior to pregnancy does not increase the risk of fetal loss.

At one time it was believed that use of other contraceptives – before and during pregnancy – was associated with fetal loss. This is now known to be untrue for women who discontinue oral contraceptives before conception (*see* Simpson 1985), as well as those exposed to spermicides prior to or after conception (Mills et al. 1985).

Trauma

Women commonly attribute pregnancy losses to trauma, such as a fall or a blow to the abdomen. However, fetuses are actually well protected from external trauma by intervening maternal structures and amniotic fluid: witness, for example, the relative safety of amniocentesis and chorionic villus sampling.

Psychological Factors

It has been claimed, but not proved, that impaired psychological well-being predisposes to early fetal losses. Neurotic or mentally ill women abort, but whether the frequency of losses is higher than in normal women is unknown. Confounding factors have not been excluded in studies claiming a relationship. A well-known study is that of Stray-Pedersen and colleagues (Stray-Pedersen and Stray-Pedersen 1984, 1988). This group believes there is a beneficial effect for women having experienced repetitive abortions receiving increased attention ("tender-loving-care"), but no specific medical therapy. In their last tabulation, 116 women were more likely (85%) to complete their pregnancy than were 42 women not provided such care (36% success). A deficiency in study design is that only women living "close" to the university were eligible for the increased attention. Women living farther away served as "controls". "Controls" may have unwittingly differed in unknown ways from the experimental group.

This author suspects that any beneficial effect of enhanced psychological well-being is probably either more apparent than real or merely secondary to other factors.

Generalised Effects of Severe Maternal Illness

Almost all debilitating maternal diseases have been implicated in spontaneous abortion. Various pathogenic mechanisms could be invoked, specifically endocrinological, immunological, or infectious. In fact, examples already cited include diabetes mellitus and lupus erythematosus.

Maternal diseases not previously mentioned that may be associated with fetal wastage include Wilson's disease, maternal phenylketonuria, cardiac insufficiency (e.g., cyanotic heart disease), and haematological disorders (e.g., haemoglobinopathies or aplastic anaemia). In fact, any life-threatening disease would be expected to be associated with increased abortion rates. Seriously ill women rarely become pregnant, but in some cases the disease process may deteriorate after onset of pregnancy. Overall, only a small fraction of all fetal losses can be attributable to severe maternal disease. Thus, general probes for maternal health should be sought but detailed disease-by-disease assessment is probably unnecessary.

Of relevance is the well-known maternal age effect in fetal wastage. Women aged 40–44 have approximately twice the likelihood of fetal loss incurred by women two decades younger. Interestingly, this risk holds for both trisomic as well as euploid abortuses (Stein et al. 1980). This is consistent with animal studies showing decreased ability of other animals to retain embryos transferred from young mothers (Biggers 1969). Possible explanations include infections, diminished luteal response, and poorly vascularised endometrium, any of which could be expected to be exacerbated in serious maternal illness.

References

Alberman ED (1981) The abortus as a predictor of future trisomy 21. In: De la Cruz FF, Gerald PS (eds) Trisomy 21 (Down's Syndrome). University Park Press, Baltimore, p. 69

Alberman E, Creasy M, Elliott M, Spicer C (1976) Maternal effects associated with fetal chromosomal anomalies in spontaneous abortions. Br J Obstet Gynaecol 83:621–627

Alfi OS, Chang R, Azen SP (1981) Evidence of genetic control of nondisjunction in man. Am J Hum Genet 32:477–483

Allen WR, Kydd JH, Antczak DF (1986) Successful application of immunotherapy to a model of pregnancy failure in equids. In: Clark DA, Croy BA (eds) Reproductive immunology. Elsevier, New York, p. 253

Angell RR, Aitken JR, van-Look PFGA et al. (1983) Chromosome abormalities in human embryos after in vitro fertilization. Nature 303:336–338

Barlow S, Sullivan FM (1982) Reproductive hazards of industrial chemicals: an evaluation of animal and human data. Academic Press, New York

Beard RW, Sharp F (eds) (1988) Early pregnancy loss: mechanism and treatment. Proceedings of the 18th Study Group of the Royal College of Obstetricians and Gynaecologists. Royal College of Obstetricians and Gynaecologists, London

Beard RW, Braude P, Mowbray JF et al. (1983) Protective antibodies and spontaneous abortion. Lancet 1:1090

Beer AE, Billingham RF (1976) The immunology of mammalian reproduction. Prentice-Hall, Englewood, NJ

Beer AE, Quebbeman JF, Ayers JW et al. (1981) Major histocompatibility complex antigens, maternal and paternal immune responses, and chronic habitual abortions in humans. Am J Obstet Gynecol 141:987–999

Beer AE, Quebbeman JF, Semprini AE (1987) Immunopathological factors contributing to recurrent and spontaneous abortion in humans. In: Bennet MJ, Edmonds DK (eds): Spontaneous and recurrent abortions. Blackwell, Oxford, pp. 90–108

Biggers JD (1969) Problems concerning the uterine causes of embryonic death, with special reference to the effects of aging of the uterus. J Reprod Fertil (Suppl) 8:27–43

Blackwell R, Chang A (1988) Video display terminals and pregnancy. A review. Br J Obstet Gynaecol 95:446–453

Boué A, Gallano P (1973) A collaborative study of the segregation of inherited chromosome structural arrangements in 1356 prenatal diagnosis. Prenat Diag 4:45

Boué J, Boué A, Lazar P (1975) Retrospective and prospective epidemiological studies of 1500 karyotyped spontaneous human abortions. Teratology 12:11–26

Boué J, Phillipe E, Giroud A et al. (1976) Phenotypic expression of lethal chromosomal anomalies in human abortuses. Teratology 14:3–19

Branch DW, Scott JR, Kochenour NK et al. (1985) Obstetric complications associated with the lupus anticoagulant. N Engl J Med 313:1322–1326

Branch DW, Ward K (1989) Autoimmunity and pregnancy loss. Semin Reprod Endocrinol 7:168–179

Byrne J, Warburton D (1986) Neural tube defects in spontaneous abortion. Am J Med Genet 25:327

Carson SA, Simpson JL (1990) Spontaneous abortion. In: Eden RD, Boehm FH (eds) Fetal assessment: physiological, clinical and medico-legal principles. Appleton-Century-Crofts, Norwalk, CT, pp 559–574

Cowchock S, Smith JB, Gocial B (1986) Antibodies to phospholipids and nuclear antigens in patients with repeated abortions. Am J Obstet Gynecol 155:1002–1010

Daly DC, Walters CA, Soto-Albers CE et al. (1983) Endometrial biopsy during treatment of luteal phase defects is predictive of therapeutic outcome. Fertil Steril 40:305–312

Damewood MD (1989) The association of endometriosis and repetitive (early spontaneous abortions. Semin Reprod Endocrinol 7:155–160

Daniels A, Hook EB, Wulf G (1989) Risks of unbalanced progeny at amniocentesis to carriers of chromosome rearrangements: data from United States and Canadian Laboratories. Am J Med Genet 31:14–53

Davis OK, Berkley AS, Cholst IN, Nause GJ, Freedman KS (1989) The indicence of luteal phase defect in normal, fertile women, determined. Fertil Steril 51:582–586

Daya S, Ward S (1988) Diagnostic test properties of serum progesterone in the evaluation of luteal phase defects. Fertil Steril 49:169–170

Daya S, Ward S, Burrows E (1988) Progesterone profiles in luteal phase defect cycles and outcome of progesterone treatment in patients with recurrent spontaneous abortions. Am J Ob Gyn 158:225–232

Downs KA, Gibson M (1983) Basal temperature graph and luteal phase defect. Fertil Steril 40:466–468

Edmonds RF (1988) Use of cervical cerclage in patients with recurrent first trimester abortions. In: Beard RW, Sharp F (eds) Early pregnancy loss: mechanism and treatment. Proceedings of the 18th Study Group of the Royal College of Obstetricians and Gynaecologists. Royal College of Obstetricians and Gynaecologists, London, pp 411–415

Eiben B, Borgmann S, Schubbe I, Hansmann I (1987) A cytogenetic study directly from chorionic villi of 140 spontaneous abortion. Hum Genet 77:137–141

Elias M, Eldor A (1984) Thromboembolism in patients with "lupus" type circulating anticoagulant. Arch Intern Med 1244:510–515

Estop AM, Catala V, Santalo J, Egozcue J (1986) Aneuploidy, maternal age and sexual immaturity. Am J Hum Genet 39(S):A112

Exner T, Richard KA, Kronenberg H (1978) A sensitive test demonstrating LAC and its behavioural patterns. Br J Haematol 40:143–151

Fabricant JD, Schneider EL (1978) Studies on the genetic and immunologic components of the maternal age effect. Devel Biol 66:337–343

Faulk WP, McIntyre JA (1981) Trophoblast survival. Transplantation 32:1–5

Faulk WP, Coulam CB, McIntyre JA (1989) The role of trophoblast antigens in repetitive spontaneous abortion. Semin Reprod Endocrinol 7:182–187

Figa-Talamanaca I, Settimi L (1984) Occupational factors and reproductive outcome. In: Hafez ESE (ed) Spontaneous abortion. MTP Press, Lancaster, pp 61–80

Fitzet D, Bousquet J (1983) Absence of a factor blocking cellular cytotoxicity in the serum of women with recurrent abortion. Br J Obstet Gynaecol 90:453–456

Gastineau DA, Kazimier FJ, Nichols WL, et al. (1985) Lupus anticoagulants: An analysis of the clinical and laboratory features of 219 cases. Am J Hematol 19:265–275

Gerbie AB, Simpson JL (1976) Antenatal detection of genetic disorders. Postgrad Med 59:129–136

Gill TH III (1983) Immunogenetics of spontaneous abortions in humans. Transplantation 35:1–6

Golbus MS (1981) The influence of strain maternal age and method of maturation on mouse oocyte aneuploidy. Cytogenet Cell Genet 31:84–90

Goldhaber MK, Polen MR, Hiatt RA (1988) The risk of miscarriage and birth defects among women who use visual display terminals during pregnancy. Am J Indust Med 13:695–706

Greene MF, Hare JW, Cloherty JP, et al (1989) First trimester hemoglobin A1 and risk for major malformation and spontaneous abortion in diabetic pregnancy. Teratology 39:225–231

Gropp A (1973) Fetal mortality due to aneuploidy and irregular meiotic segregation in the mouse. In: Boué A, Thibault C (eds) Les accidents chromosiques de la reproduction. Paris, INSERM, p 225

Gropp A (1975) Chromosomal animal model of human disease. Fetal trisomy and development failure. In: Berry L, Poswillo DE (eds) Teratology. Springer-Verlag, Berlin, pp 17–35

Guerneri S, Bettio D, Simoni G et al. (1987) Prevalence and distribution of chromosome abnormalities in a sample of first trimester internal abortions. Hum Reprod 2:735–739

Haas GG Jr, Kubota K, Quebbeman JF et al. (1986) Circulating antisperm antibodies in recurrently aborting women. Fertil Steril 45:209–215

Halmesmärki E et al. (1989) Maternal and paternal alcohol consumption and miscarriage. Br J Obstet Gynaecol 96:188–191

Harlap S,, Shiono PH (1980) Alcohol, smoking and incidence of spontaneous abortions in the first and second trimester. Lancet 2:173

Harris EN (1988) Clinical and immunological significance of anti-phospholipid antibodies. In: Beard RW, Sharp F (eds) Early pregnancy loss: mechanism and treatment. Proceedings of the 18th Study Group of the Royal College of Obstetricians and Gynaecologists. Royal College of Obstetricians and Gynaecologists, London, pp 43–60

Hassold T (1980) A cytogenetic study of repeated spontaneous abortions. Am J Hum Genet 32:723–730

Heidam LZ (1984) Spontaneous abortions among laboratory workers: a follow-up study. J Epidemiol Community Health 38:36–41

Heinonen P, Saarikoski S, Pystynen P (1982) Reproductive performance of women with uterine anomalies: An evaluation of 182 cases. Acta Obstet Gynecol Scand 61:157–162

Herbst AL, Senekjian EK, Frey KW (1989) Abortion of pregnancy loss among diethylstilbestrol-exposed women. Semin Reprod Endocrinol 7:124–129

Hertig AT, Rock J (1973) Searching for early human ova. Gyn Investig 4:121–139

Hertig AT, Rock J, Adams EC (1956) Description of human ova within the first 17 days of development. Am J Anat 98:435–493

Hertig AT, Rock J, Adams EC, Menkin MC (1959) Thirty-four fertilized human ova, good, bad and indifferent, recovered from 210 women of known fertility. A study of biologic wastage in early human pregnancy. Pediatrics 25:202–211

Horta JLH, Fernandez JG, DeSoto LB (1977) Direct evidence of luteal insufficiency in women with habitual abortion. Obstet Gynecol 49:705–708

Howard MA, Firkin BG, Healy DL, Choong SC (1987) Lupus anticoagulant in women with multiple spontaneous miscarriage. Am J Hematol 26:175–178

Jacobs MH, Balasch J, Gonzalez-Merlo JM et al. (1987) Endometrial cytosolic and nuclear progesterone receptors in luteal phase deficiency. J Clin Endocrinol Metab 64:472–475

Johnson PM, Chia KV, Risk JM (1986) Immunological question marks in recurrent spontaneous abortion. In: Clark DA, Croy BA (eds) Reproductive immunology. New York, Elsevier, pp 239–245

Jones GS (1976) The luteal phase defect. Fertil Steril 27:351–356

Kline J, Shrout P, Stein ZA et al. (1980) Drinking during pregnancy and spontaneous abortion. Lancet 2:176–180

Lazar P, Gueguen S (1984) Multicentred controlled trials of cervical cerclage in women at moderate risk of preterm delivery. Br J Obstet Gynaecol 91:731–735

Levine P (1978) ABO, P and MN blood group determinants in neoplasm foreign to the host. Semin Oncol 5:25–34

Li TC, Dockery P, Rogers AW, Cooke ID (1989) How precise is histologic dating of endometrium using the standard dating criteria. Fertil Steril 51:759–763

Li TC, Rogers AW, Lenton EA, Dockery P, Cooke I (1987) A comparison between 2 methods of chronological dating of human endometrial biopsies during the luteal phase and their correlation with histological dating. Fertil Steril 48:928–932

Lockshin MD, Druzin ML, Goei S et al. (1985) Antibody to cardiolipin as a predictor of fetal distress or death in pregnant patients with systemic lupus erythematosus. N Engl J Med 313:152–156

Ludmir J, Samuels P, Brooks S, Mennuti M (1990) Pregnancy outcome of patients with uncorrected uterine anomalies managed in high-risk obstetric setting. Obstet Gynecol 73:906

Martin AO, Simpson JL, Deddish RB et al. (1983) Clinical implications of chromosomal inversions. A pericentric inversion in No. 18 segregating in a family ascertaining through an abnormal proband. Am J Perinatol 1:81–88

McIntyre JA, Faulk WP (1983) Recurrent spontaneous abortions in human pregnancy, results of immunogenetic cellular and humoral studies. Am J Reprod Immunol 4:165

McIntyre JA, Faulk WP (1986) Trophoblast antigens in normal and abnormal human pregnancy. Clin Obstet Gynecol 29:976–998

McIntyre JA, Faulk WP, Nichols-Johnson VR et al. (1986) Immunological testing and immunotherapy in recurrent spontaneous abortion. Obstet Gynecol 67:169–172

McRae MA, Blasco L, Lyttle CR (1984) Serum hormones and their receptors in women with normal and inadequate corpus luteum function. Fertil Steril 42:58–63

Michelman HW, Bonhoff A, Mettler L (1986) Chromosome analysis in polypoid human embryos. Hum Reprod 1:243–246

Mills JL, Reed GF, Nugent RP et al. (1985) Are there adverse effects of periconceptional spermicide use? Fertil Steril 43:442–446

Mills JL, Simpson JL, Driscoll SG, et al (1988) Incidence of spontaneous abortion among normal women and insulin-dependent diabetic women whose pregnancies were identified within 21 days of conception. N Engl J Med 319:1617–1623

Miodonik M, Lavin JP, Knowles HC et al. (1984) Spontaneous abortion among insulin dependent diabetic women. Am J Obstet Gynecol 150:372–376

Miodonik M, Mimouni F, Tsang RL et al. (1986) Glycemic control and spontaneous abortion in insulin dependent diabetic women. Obstet Gynecol 68:366–369

Miodonik M, Skillman C, Holroyde JC et al. (1985) Elevated maternal glycohemoglobin in early pregnancy and spontaneous abortion among insulin dependent diabetic women. Am J Obstet Gynecol 153:439–443

Montero M, Collea JV, Frasier D, Mestman J (1981) Successful outcome of pregnancy in women with hypothyroidism. Ann Intern Med 94:31–34

Mowbray JF, Gibbing C, Liddell H et al. (1985) Controlled trial of treatment of recurrent spontaneous abortion by immunization with paternal cells. Lancet 1:941–943

Nishimura H (1970) Incidence of malformations in abortions. In: Fraser FC, McKusick V, Robinson R (eds) Congenital malformation. Proceedings of the 3rd International Conference. Excerpta Medica, Amsterdam, pp 275

Nishimura H, Tokamo K, Tanimura T, Yasuda M (1968) Normal and abnormal development of human embryos: First report of the analysis of 1213 intact embryos. Teratology 1:281

Norman DJ, Barry JM, Fischer S (1986) The beneficial effect of pretransplant third-party blood transfusions on allograft rejection in HLA identical sibling kidney transplants. Transplantation 41:125–126

Noyes RW, Hertig ATR, Rock J (1950) Dating the endometrial biopsy. Fertil Steril 1:3–25

Ober CL, Martin AO, Simpson JL et al. (1983) Shared HLA antigens and reproductive performance among Hutterites. Am J Hum Genet 35:994–1004

Ohno M, Maeda T, Matsunolu A (1991) A cytogenetic study of spontaneous abortion with direct analysis of chorionic villus. Obstet Gynecol 77:394–398

Oksenberg JR, Persitz E, Amar A et al. (1984) Maternal-paternal histocompability: lack of association with habitual abortion. Fertil Steril 42:389–395

Opitz J (1987) The Farber Lecture – Prenatal and perinatal death: the future developmental pathology. Pediatr Pathol 7:363–394

Parazzini F, Bocciolone L, La Vecchia C et al. (1990) Maternal and paternal moderate daily alcohol consumption and unexplained miscarriages. Br J Obstet Gynecol 97:618–622

Petri M, Golbus M, Anderson R et al. (1987) Antinuclear antibody, lupus anticoagulant, and anticardiolipin antibody in women with idiopathic habitual abortion. Arthritis Rheum 30:601–606

Plachot M, Junca AM, Mandelbaum J (1987) Chromosome investigations in early life. II. Human preimplantation embryos. Hum Reprod 2:29–35

Power DA, Mason RJ, Stewart GM et al. (1983) The fetus as an allograft: evidence for protective antibodies to HLA-linked paternal antigens. Lancet 2:701–704

Quinn PA, Petrie M, Barking M et al. (1987) Prevalence of antibody to *Chlamydia trachomatis* in spontaneous abortion and infertility. Am J Obstet Gynecol 156:291–296

Ramsey-Goldman R, Hom D, Deng JS et al. (1986) Anti-SS-A antibodies and fetal outcome in maternal systemic lupus erythematosus. Arthritis Rheum 29:1269–1273

Regan L, Braude PR (1987) Is antipaternal cytotoxic antibody a valid marker in the management of recurrent abortion? Lancet 2:1280

Rock J, Jones HW Jr (1977) The clinical management of the double uterus. Fertil Steril 28:798–806

Rock JA, Shirey RS, Braine HG et al. (1985) Plasmapheresis for the treatment of repeated early pregnancy wastage associated with anti-P. Obstet Gynecol 66:57S–60S

Rocklin RE, Kitzmiller JL, Carpenter CB et al. (1976) Absence of an immunologic blocking factor from the serum of women with chronic abortion. N Engl J Med 295:1209–1213

Rocklin RE, Kitzmiller JL, Garvoy MR (1982) Further characterization of an immunologic blocking factor that develops during pregnancy. Clin Immunol Immunopathol 22:305–315

Rudak E, Dor J, Mashiach S et al. (1985) Chromosome analysis of human oocytes and embryos fertilized in vitro. Ann NY Acad Sci 442:476–486

Rush RW, McPherson K, Jones L et al. (1984) A randomized controlled trial of cervical cerclage in women at high risk of spontaneous preterm delivery. Br J Obstet Gynaecol 91:724–730

Ruzicska P, Cziezel A (1971) Cytogenetic studies on midtrimester abortuses. Humangenetik 10:273–297

Saracoglu OF, Aksel S, Yeoman RR et al. (1985) Endometrial estriadol and progesterone receptors in patients with luteal phase defects and endometriosis. Fertil Steril 43:851–855

Sargent IL, Wilkins T, Redman CWG (1988) Maternal immune responses to the fetus in early pregnancy and recurrent miscarriage. Lancet 11:1099–1104

Schacter B, Weitkamp LR, Johnson WE (1984) Paternal HLA compatibility, fetal wastage, and neural tube defects: evidence for a T/t-like locus in humans. Am J Human Genet 36:1082–1091

Schnorr TM, Grajewski BA, Thornung RW et al. (1991) Videodisplay and the risk of spontaneous abortions. N Engl J Med 324:727–733

Scott JR, Role NS, Branch DW (1987) Immunologic aspects of recurrent abortions and fetal death. Obstet Gynecol 70:645–656

Scott RT, Synder RR, Strickland DM et al. (1988) The effect of interobserver variation in dating endometrial history on the diagnosis of luteal phase defects. Fertil Steril 50:888–892

Selevan SG, Lindbohm M-L, Hornung RW, Hemminki K (1985) A study of occupational exposure to antineoplastic drugs and fetal loss in nurses. N Engl J Med 313:1173–1178

Shulman LP, Elias S, Tharapel AT, Li L, et al. (1992) Sister chromatid exchange frequency in directly-prepared cytotrophoblasts: Demonstration of in vivo DNA damage in pregnancy women who smoke cigarettes. Am J Obstet Gynecol. In Press

Simpson JL (1976) Disorders of sex differentiation: etiology and clinical delineation. Academic Press, New York

Simpson JL (1985) Relationship between congenital anomalies and contraception. Adv Contracept 1:3–30

Simpson JL (1990) Incidence and timing of pregnancy losses: relevance to evaluating safety of early prenatal diagnosis. Am J Med Genet 35:165–173

Simpson JL (1991a) Fetal wastage. In: Gabbe SA, Niebyl JF, Simpson JL (eds) Obstetrics: normal and abnormal pregnancies. 2nd edn. Churchill-Livingston, New York, pp 783–807

Simpson JL (1991b) Aetiology of pregnancy failure. In Chapman M, Grudzinskas G, Chard T (eds) The embryo: normal and abnormal development and growth. Springer-Verlag, London, pp 11–34

Simpson JL, Bombard AT (1987) Chromosomal abnormalities in spontaneous abortions: Frequency, pathology and genetic counselling. In: Edmonds K, Bennet MJ (eds) Spontaneous abortion. Blackwell, London, p 51–76

Simpson JL, Carson SA (1992) Causes of fetal loss. In: Gray R, Leridon L, Spira F (eds) Symposium on biological and demographic determinants of human reproduction. Oxford University Press, Oxford, UK

Simpson JL, Golbus MS (1992) Genetics in Obstetrics and Gynecology. 2nd edn. WB Saunders, Philadelphia

Simpson JL, Tharapel AT (1989) Principles of cytogenetics. In Philip E, Barnes J (eds) Scientific foundations of obstetrics and gynecology. 4th edn. Heinemann Medical Books, London, pp 42–63

Simpson JL, Elias S, Martin AO (1981) Parental chromosomal rearrangements associated with repetitive spontaneous abortions. Fertil Steril 36:584–590

Simpson JL, Meyers CM, Martin AO et al. (1989) Translocations are infrequent among couples having repeated spontaneous abortions but no other abnormal pregnancies. Fertil Steril 51:811–814

Smith SK, Lenton EA, Landgren BM, Cooke ID (1984) The short luteal phase and infertility. Br J Obstet Gynaecol 91:1120–1122

Spiritos NJ, Yurewicz EC, Moghissi KS et al. (1985) Pseudocorpus luteum insufficiency: a study of cytosol progesterone receptors in human endometrium. Obstet Gynecol 65:535–540

Stabile I, Campbell S, Grudzinskas JG (1987) Ultrasonic assessment of complications during first trimester of pregnancy. Lancet 11:1237–1240

Stein Z, Kline J, Susser E et al. (1980) Maternal age and spontaneous abortion. In: Porter IH, Hook EB (eds) Human embryonic and fetal death. Academic Press, New York, pp 107–127

Stimson WH, Strachnan AF, Shepard A (1979) Studies on the maternal immune response to placental antigens: Absence of a blocking factor from the blood of abortion-prone women. Br Obstet Gynaecol 86:41–45

Stray-Pedersen B, Stray-Pedersen S (1984) Etiologic factors and subsequential reproductive performance in 195 couples with a prior history of habitual abortion. Am J Obstet Gynecol 148:140–146

Stray-Pedersen B, Stray-Pedersen S (1988) Recurrent abortion: The role of psychotherapy. In: Beard RW, Sharp F (eds) Early pregnancy loss: mechanism and treatment. Proceedings of the 18th Study Group of the Royal College of Obstetricians and Gynaecologists. Royal College of Obstetricians and Gynaecologists, London, pp 433–440

Stray-Pedersen B, Eng J, Reikvan TM (1978) Uterine T-mycoplasma colonization in reproductive failure. Am J Obstet Gynecol 130:307–311

Sutherland GR, Gardiner AJ, Carter RF (1976) Familial pericentric inversion of chromosome 19 inv (19) (p13q13) with a note on genetic counselling of pericentric inversion carries. Clin Genet 10:53–59

Takakuwa K, Kanazawa K, Takeuchi S (1986) Production of blocking antibodies by vaccination with husband's lymphocytes in unexplained recurrent aborters: The role in successful pregnancy. Am J Reprod Immunol Microbiol 10:1–9

Taskinen H, Lindbohm M-L, Hemminki K (1984) Spontaneous abortions among women working in the pharmaceutical industry. Br J Indust Med 43:199–205

Tho PT, Byrd JR, McDonoough PC (1979) Etiologies and subsequent reproductive performance of 100 couples with recurrent abortions. Fertil Steril 32:389–395

Thomas ML, Harger JH, Wegener DK, et al. (1985) HLA sharing and spontaneous abortion. Am J Obstet Gynecol 151:1053–1058

Toth A, Lesser ML, Brooks-Toth CW et al. (1986) Outcome of subsequent pregnancies following antibiotic therapy after primary or multiple spontaneous abortions. Surg Gynecol Obstet 163:232–250

Unander AM, Lindholm A (1986) Transfusions of leukocyte rich erythrocytes: A successful treatment in selected cases of habitual abortions. Am J Obstet Gynecol 154:516

Unander AM, Norberg R, Hahn L, Arfors L (1987) Anticardiolipin antibodies and complement in ninety-nine women with habitual abortion. Am J Obstet Gynecol 156:114–119

Vlaanderen W, Treffers PE (1987) Prognosis of subsequent pregnancies after recurrent spontaneous abortion in first trimester. Br Med J 295:92–93

Warburton D, Kline J, Stein Z et al. (1980) Cytogenetic abnormalities in spontaneous abortion of recognized conceptions. In: Porter IH, Hatcher NH, Willey AM (eds) Perinatal genetics: diagnosis and treatment. Academic Press, Orlando, pp 23–40

Warburton D, Kline J, Stein Z, et al. (1987) Does the karyotype of a spontaneous abortion predict the karyotype of a subsequent abortion? Evidence from 273 women with two karyotyped spontaneous abortus. Am J Hum Genet 41:465–483

Watt JL, Templeton AA, Messinis I et al. (1987) Trisomy I in an eight-cell human pre-embryo. J Med Genet 24:60–64

Weksler BB, Pett SB, Alsono D et al. (1983) Differential inhibition by aspirin of vascular and platelet prostaglandin synthesis in atherosclerotic patients. N Engl J Med 308:800–805

Wu CH, Minassian SS (1987) Integrated luteal progesterone: an assessment of luteal function. Fertil Steril 48:937–940

Zenzes MT, Belkien L, Bordt J et al. (1985) Cytologic investigation of human in vitro fertilization failures. Fertil Steril 43:883–891

4. Pathology of Spontaneous Abortion

H. Fox

Introduction

Any account of the pathology of spontaneous abortion must suffer from the restraints placed upon the pathologist by the type of material made available for study. In the vast majority of first trimester abortions all that is received in the laboratory is placental tissue and decidua: fetal tissues may or may not be present but it is rather uncommon to receive either an intact fetus or a complete gestational sac. The emphasis of this chapter will, therefore, be on the pathology of the placenta in spontaneous abortion, with little attention being paid to the embryo.

   This approach is in fact optimal when considering the mechanisms of abortion for it is almost certain that the placenta plays a key role both in the maintenance of gestation and in the pathogenesis of early pregnancy failure (Rushton 1988). Thus pregnancy can continue in the absence of an embryo, albeit for only a limited period; the presence of a congenital malformation or a karyotypic abnormality in the fetus does not necessarily lead to pregnancy failure and, perhaps most strikingly, confined placental mosaicism with a diploid cell population in the trophoblast allows for continuing survival, rather than abortion, of cases of fetal trisomy 13 or 18 (Kalousek et al. 1989). Those wishing for a description of embyronic or fetal pathology in spontaneous abortion are referred to other texts in which a full account of this aspect is given (Berry 1980; Rushton 1987; Laurini 1990).

Anatomo-pathological Classification of Material from Abortions

There have been several anatomical (i.e., macroscopic) classifications of abortion material (Mall and Meyer 1921; Geneva Conference 1966; Hertig 1968; Laurini

1990) but the one which has proved most useful in practice is a modification of that of Fujikura et al. (1966). In this, abortion material is classified thus:

I. Incomplete specimen

II. Ruptured empty sac
   a) With cord stump
   b) Without cord stump

III. Intact empty sac

IV. Fetus present
   a) With chorionic sac
      i) Normal non-macerated fetus
      ii) Normal macerated fetus
      iii) Grossly disorganised fetus
      iv) Focal abnormality of fetus
   b) Without chorionic sac
      i) Normal non-macerated fetus
      ii) Normal macerated fetus
      iii) Grossly disorganised fetus
      iv) Focal abnormality of fetus

In this classification the term "focal abnormality" refers to a defect such as spinal bifida whilst the expression "grossly disorganised" is applied to those fetuses which are so ill-formed that they can only be classed as "nodular" or "cylindrical". An "incomplete specimen" is one in which there is no macroscopically recognisable fetus or intact placenta: such specimens may consist solely of placental villous tissue, may contain a mixture of decidua and villous tissue or may comprise only decidua in which there is a placental site reaction i.e., an infiltration of extravillous trophoblastic cells.

Most of the other descriptive categories in this classification are self explanatory though it should be noted that "intact empty sac" and "ruptured empty sac without cord stump" are synonymous with, but are used instead of, "blighted ovum" or "anembryonic pregnancy". The expression "blighted ovum" has been used in many different ways, is open to widely differing interpretations and is, in reality, virtually meaningless. The term "anembryonic pregnancy" is a useful one when referring to a conventional spontaneous abortion but has also been applied, misleadingly, to complete hydatidiform moles and even to choriocarcinomas. It is true that a complete hydatidiform mole is, within the strict usage of the term, a form of abortion as may also be some cases of choriocarcinoma, particularly those which develop *ab initio*. These entities do, however, fall outside the main group of spontaneous abortions and should not be included in any classification of abortion material.

It must be realised that a macroscopic, or anatomical, classification of the type outlined above is useful for descriptive purposes but, with the exception of anembryonic pregnancy and those cases in which the fetus is grossly or focally abnormal, gives little or no indication of the pathogenesis of the abortion. When an intact placenta is present, examination with the naked eye usually reveals little of value. Cord lesions, such as stricture, torsion or true knots, are present in about 3% of abortions (Fox 1978; Rushton 1988) but the site of cord insertion is of no relevance. Retroplacental haematomas are moderately common in placentas from spontaneous abortions, being noted in about 10% of cases: these are, however, usually marginally situated and clearly of recent origin and there must be considerable doubt as to whether such lesions are a primary or secondary phenomenon. A massive subchorial thrombus (Breus' mole) is found in a small proportion of placentas from abortuses but the significance, if any, of this lesion is unknown. A macroscopic finding which is noted with some frequency in abortion material is "placental floor infarction" (Benirschke and Driscoll 1967; Rushton 1984, 1987): in this condition there is marked thickening of the basal plate of the placenta because of deposition of fibrin which may envelop the basal villi and decrease the height of the intervillous space: it is almost certain that maternal floor infarction is a post-mortem change and that this lesion plays no role in the aetiology of early pregnancy loss.

Perhaps the most important macroscopic finding in placentas from cases of abortion is the finding of vesicular villi scattered throughout an otherwise normal villous population: this is virtually diagnostic of a partial hydatidiform mole and thus strongly suggestive of fetal triploidy.

Histological Classification of Material from Abortions

Because the material received in the laboratory from cases of spontaneous abortion usually consists only of placental villous tissue and decidua it is clear that any logical classification of abortion material must be histologically based, this being emphasised by the lack of useful information gleaned from macroscopic examination.

There have been many proposed histological classifications of placental tissue from cases of early pregnancy failure but most of these have been based on the belief that it is possible to correlate placental villous morphology either with specific chromosomal abnormalities or, less ambitiously, with an abnormal, as opposed to a normal, karyotype (Philippe and Boué 1969; Philippe 1973; Honore et al. 1976: Geisler and Kleinebrecht 1978; Gocke et al. 1982, 1985: Muntefering et al 1988; Rockelein et al. 1989). These claims have been examined by Rehder et al. (1989) who correlated cytogenetic data with placental morphology in 200 cases of spontaneous abortion: they divided the placentas into five groups, one of which was equivalent to a partial hydatidiform mole and one to a hydropic abortion, the other three groups comprising placentas showing varying degrees of hydropic and post-mortem change. There was an 80% incidence of chromosomal abnormalities amongst the partial hydatidiform moles but an approximately 50%–65% incidence of such anomalies in all of the other four groups. They concluded that, with the probable exception of fetal triploidy, it was not possible to identify any morphological criteria to allow for either the diagnosis or the exclusion of a chromosomal abnormality of any type.

Minguillon et al. (1989), as a result of a rather similar study, also concluded that the predictive value, in terms of recognising a chromosomal abnormality, of placental villous histology, is inadequate and, indeed, no higher than would be anticipated by mere chance. Novak et al. (1988) came to the same conclusion and were of the opinion that, with the exception of triploidy, villous structure was an inaccurate and insensitive indicator of an abnormal karyotype.

It is clear that in these studies the authors have been reasonably confident of

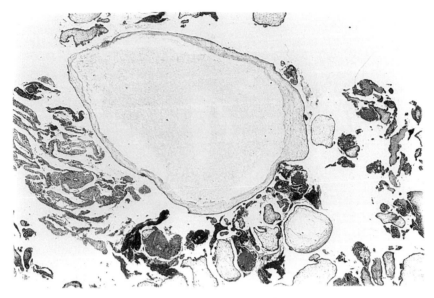

Fig. 4.1. A partial hydatidiform mole. This field shows the typical mixture of small villi of normal configuration and a large vesicular villus (H. & E. × 18.5).

their ability to identify, on histological grounds, a fetal triploidy. This is because in such gestations the placenta has the appearance of a partial hydatidiform mole, a specific histological entity. It cannot be assumed, however, that the diagnosis of a partial hydatidiform mole is always easy or that a partial mole always indicates a fetal triploidy. In a partial mole, villi showing vesicular change are intermingled with villi of normal size (Fig. 4.1); fetal vessels are usually present in both the vesicular and the normally-sized villi. The vesicular villi frequently show central cistern formation and have an irregular contour with deep indentations, or fjords (Fig 4.2): if these indentations are cut in cross section they may be seen within the villi as so-called "trophoblastic inclusions". A degree of atypical villous tropho-blastic proliferation is always present though this is usually focal and rarely as marked as that seen in complete moles. From this description it would appear that partial hydatidiform moles are easy to recognise but in fact there is considerable interobserver difference between pathologists in the diagnosis of this entity.

It was originally thought that the partial hydatidiform mole was always associated with a fetal triploidy (Lawler et al. 1982) with the extra complement of chromosomes being of paternal origin (Jacobs et al. 1982). More recently, however, a number of diploid partial moles have been described in both cytogenetic and flow cytometry studies (Teng and Ballon 1984: Ohama et al. 1986; Hemming et al. 1987; Davis et al. 1987; van Oven et al. 1989) whilst tetraploid partial moles have also been described (Surti et al. 1986; Lage et al. 1989).

It would appear, therefore, that an accurate histological classification of placental villous morphology in spontaneous abortions, in terms of normal and abnormal karyotypes, is not attainable. Rushton (1981, 1987, 1988) has proposed

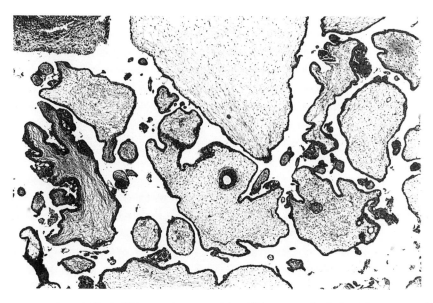

Fig. 4.2. A partial hydatidiform mole; many of the villi have a markedly irregular contour with deep indentations (H. & E. × 37).

a more realistic classification of abortion material, though again based largely upon placental morphology. His classification may, after excluding partial moles, be paraphrased along the following lines:

Group 1. A considerable proportion of the villi show hydropic change

Group 2. Some villi are hydropic but most show post mortem changes such as stromal fibrosis and sclerosis of the villous fetal vessels.

Group 3. The villi show no evidence of hydropic or post mortem change and are of normal appearance for the length of the gestational period

Rushton has emphasised that each of these groups is, in terms of the aetiology of the abortion, heterogeneous and that the appearances reflect more the stage of gestation at which the pregnancy failed than any other specific factor. Nevertheless, it would be reasonable to assume that placentas from Group 1 are either from cases of very early fetal death or from gestations in which an embryo has failed to develop: the hydropic villi are avascular, swollen, oedematous, rounded and have a covering mantle of attenuated trophoblast (Fig. 4.3), these appearances probably being due to a failure of fetal villous vascularisation. It could be assumed that in such cases the factor leading to pregnancy failure is more likely to be intrinsic to the fetus than to lie in the maternal environment and that a fetal karyotypic abnormality is statistically the most likely cause. In Group 2 cases the placental changes typify those characteristically found after fetal death and cessation of the fetal villous circulation, namely villi of approximately normal size for the length of the period of gestation but showing sclerosis of their fetal vessels and fibrosis of their stroma (Fig. 4.4). It is clear in these cases that fetal death

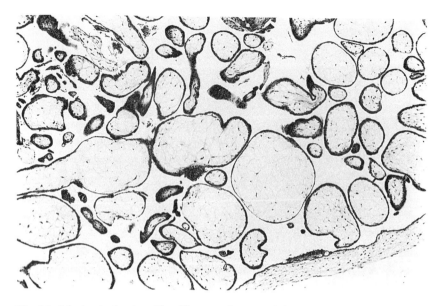

Fig. 4.3. A hydropic abortion. The villi are swollen, rounded and covered by an attenuated mantle of trophoblast (H. & E. × 47).

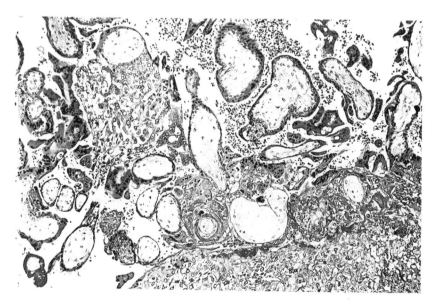

Fig. 4.4. Spontaneous abortion. The stroma in many of the villi has undergone fibrosis consequent upon fetal death: there is also sclerosis of many of the fetal villous vessels (H. & E. × 93).

preceded the abortion, the fetus having been dead for some time before the pregnancy terminated. It is therefore probable, but not certain, that in this Group also the primary factor leading to pregnancy failure was fetal rather than maternal in origin. Finally, in Group 3 cases, which are usually from abortions occurring later in gestation than the other two groups, the normal appearance of the placenta (Fig. 4.5) indicates that the fetus was either alive at the time of abortion or had died only very shortly before abortion occurred. In this group it appears reasonable to postulate that the pregnancy failed because of a fault in the maternal environment rather than because of any fetal abnormality.

The reasoning behind Rushton's histological classification is impeccable; but how useful is this approach in practice? Any morphological classification of abortion material is probably only of real value in recurrent abortions and it is probable that most cases of repetitive pregnancy failure are due to maternal rather than fetal factors. A valid morphological classification of abortion material should, therefore, tend to identify those apparently sporadic cases of abortion which are likely to recur and should reveal a different pattern in sporadic and recurrent pregnancy failures. Houwert-de Jong and his colleagues (Houwert-de Jong 1989; Houwert-de Jong et al. 1990a) have used Rushton's classification to examine placental material from cases of both sporadic and recurrent abortion: they found that the pattern of placental changes was identical in these two groups and that, furthermore, they could not correlate the histo-pathological findings with the outcome of subsequent pregnancies. Studies such as these require further confirmation but they do tend to indicate that the currently employed histological classifications of abortion material are unlikely to be of any great value in the study and management of cases of recurrent abortion.

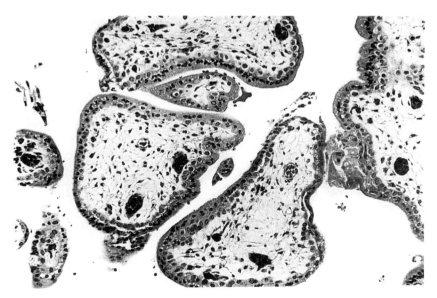

Fig. 4.5. Spontaneous abortion. The villi are fully normal for the length of the period of gestation. The villi contain patent fetal vessels in which fetal red blood cells are present. There is no evidence of hydropic or post mortem change (H. & E. × 186).

Specific Pathological Abnormalities in Abortion

Infection

A wide range of maternal infections are considered to be a causal factor in abortion (Charles and Larsen 1990), prominent amongst these being toxoplasmosis, rubella, syphilis, listerosis, cytomegalovirus and herpesvirus. These organisms are thought to reach the feto-placental unit either from the maternal blood stream or from an infective focus in the endometrium and the pathological hallmark of an infection via this route is a villitis, i.e. an inflammatory process within placental villous tissue (Fox 1978; Russell 1987). In practice, villitis is very rarely encountered in abortion material and in humans, in contrast to animals, blood-borne infections do not appear to be an important factor in early pregnancy loss.

Infection may, of course, also reach the conceptus by ascent via the birth canal, such infections resulting in a chorioamnionitis (inflammation of the membranes). Some cases of chorioamnionitis may be a consequence of streptococcal colonisation of the vagina (McDonald et al. 1989; Mattoras et al. 1989) but most are probably due either to organisms normally commensal in the vagina or to mixed faecal bacteria. It is certainly possible that a chorioamnionitis may initiate an abortion, probably by causing rupture of the membranes, and it is therefore of note that whilst inflammation of the membranes is a rather uncommon finding in placentas from early pregnancy loss it is present in nearly a third of cases of abortion in the early weeks of the second trimester (Rushton 1987, 1988). The actual mechanism by which a chorioamnionitis causes membrane rupture is still not fully clear but it has been suggested that it is due to release and collagenases from the neutrophil polymorphonuclear leucocytes infiltrating the membranes (Naeye 1987). It is also possible that the enzymes released from infiltrating inflammatory cells act in concert with bacterial proteases to weaken the membranes (Schoonmaker et al. 1989) whilst the possibility that interleukin-1-alpha, derived from infiltrating leucocytes, stimulates local tissue synthesis of collagenases has also been entertained (Katsura 1989). Before accepting uncritically the role of chorioamnionitis in the aetiology of abortion it is, however, necessary to bear in mind the possibility that in some cases the membranous infection may be secondary to cervical incompetence.

Placental Ischaemia and Inadequate Placentation

Both Rushton (1987, 1988) and Laurini (1990) have identified a sub-group of first and early second trimester abortions in which they believe that there is evidence of uteroplacental ischaemia, the placentas from these cases showing areas of infarction, accelerated villous maturation and excess syncytial knot formation. Rushton (1988) has suggested that some of these aborted cases may represent latent cases of pre-eclampsia which terminate before the disease becomes clinically manifest in the mother.

When evaluating this claim it is necessary to consider the patho-physiological basis of uteroplacental ischaemia in pregnancies complicated by pre-eclampsia. It is now well established that during the process of placentation the spiral arteries of the placental bed undergo a physiological change, being converted into uteroplacental vessels by extravillous cytotrophoblastic cells which stream out from the tips of anchoring villi into the lumina of the spiral arteries. Here, these cells destroy and replace the vascular endothelium and then invade the arterial wall where they destroy the medial muscular and elastic tissue, this being replaced by fibrinoid material. This results in the thick walled spiral arteries being converted into flaccid, sac-like uteroplacental vessels which can passively dilate to accommodate the greatly increased maternal blood flow required for fetal oxygenation and growth as gestation progresses. The process of trophoblastic invasion of the spiral arteries is accomplished in two stages: in the first stage, which is complete by the end of the first trimester, the intradecidual segments of the spiral arteries are invaded by cytotrophoblast whilst in the second stage, which occurs between the 14th and 20th week of gestation, the trophoblastic cells migrate into the intramyometrial segments of these vessels. It is now clear that in women destined to develop pre-eclampsia there is, during early pregnancy, a partial failure of this process of placentation. This failure has two components: firstly, in a normal pregnancy all the spiral arteries in the placental bed are invaded by trophoblast but in pregnancies destined to be complicated by pre-eclampsia this process occurs in only a proportion of these vessels, a significant proportion of the placental bed arteries showing no evidence of physiological change (Khong et al. 1986). Secondly, in those arteries which are invaded by extravillous trophoblast only the first of the two stages takes place and there is no progression into the intramyometrial segments of the spiral arteries (Robertson et al. 1967, 1975).

There have recently been reports that in a proportion of spontaneous abortions there is markedly inadequate invasion by extravillous trophoblast of the intra-decidual portion of the spiral arteries of the placental bed (Khong et al. 1987; Michel et al. 1990). It was suggested that in such cases the inadequate placentation led to placental ischaemia and abortion: these findings would appear, at first sight, to lend credence to Rushton's (1988) hypothesis that these may be cases of latent pre-eclampsia.

There must, however, be considerable doubt if the placenta could actually suffer ischaemia at this early stage of gestation as a result of inadequate maternal blood flow, for there are good grounds for believing that there is little, if any, significant blood flow through the utero-placental vessels during the first trimester (Hustin et al. 1988: Schaaps and Hustin 1988).

An alternative view of the significance of inadequate placentation in early pregnancy has been proffered by Hustin et al. (1990) who have confirmed that in a high proportion of spontaneous abortions there is markedly decreased tropho-blastic invasion of the spiral arteries of the placental bed: their interpretation of this finding is, however, radically different to the conventional view. They argue that one of the functions of the plugging of the spiral arteries by intravascular cytotrophoblast is to restrict maternal blood flow into the intervillous space in early pregnancy. They postulate, therefore, that the absence of trophoblastic plugging allows a free entry of maternal blood into the intervillous space at an unduly early stage in gestation and that this causes disruption of the trophoblastic shell and subsequent abortion.

Immunological Factors

The possibility that immunological factors may be involved in abortion, particularly recurrent abortions, has recently been somewhat sceptically discussed by Houwert-de Jong et al. (1990b). Nevertheless the belief that some cases of spontaneous abortion may represent a form of graft rejection is still widely canvassed and it is worth noting here that no histological features suggestive of a classical graft rejection phenomenon have ever been noted in placentas from cases of either sporadic or recurrent abortion.

It has recently been suggested that the morphological hallmark of an immunological reaction within placental tissue is the presence within villi of macrophages which stain positively for Class II (HLA–DR) antigens of the major histocompatibility complex, these activated macrophages also reacting positively with monoclonal antibodies to HLA–DP and HLA–DO (Labarrere et al. 1989, 1990). Lesions of this type appear, however, to be found to some extent in all placentas and there is currently no evidence that they occur more extensively in placentas from cases of early pregnancy loss.

It is now known that the decidua has an immunosuppressive function, though the cells responsible for this suppressive activity have not as yet been fully identified (Bulmer and Ritson 1988). There have, however, been reports that the numbers of large granulated lymphocytes in the decidua are reduced in many cases of spontaneous abortion (Clark et al. 1987; Clark 1988; Michel et al. 1989, 1990) and it has been suggested that this may result in a loss of decidual immunosuppressive activity and thus allow for an immune attack on the conceptus. There is, however, no evidence that the large granular lymphocytes contribute to decidual immunosuppressive function (Bulmer and Ritson 1988).

Anti-phospholipid Antibodies

The presence in a woman's serum of anti-phospholipid autoantibody, also often known as "lupus anticoagulant", is associated with a high incidence of both venous and arterial thrombotic episodes and with recurrent fetal loss, often during the first trimester (Harris 1988). It is commonly thought that fetal death in these cases is a consequence of thrombosis of uteroplacental vessels and extensive infarction of the placenta (Carreras et al. 1981; De Wolf et al. 1982; Derue et al. 1985). This has, however, not been a universal finding and in some studies of abortion associated with the presence of anti-phospholipid antibodies, placental infarction was not a feature (Lockshin et al. 1985, 1987).

Congenital Uterine Abnormalities

A conventional view is that congenital abnormalities of the uterus are associated with a high incidence of spontaneous abortion (Bennett 1987) and therefore the pathology of these uterine abnormalities should be considered in this chapter. However, a recent critical review of the role played by congenital uterine abnormalities concluded that there is no sound patho-physiological basis for the assumed causal relationship between such anomalies and abortion and that the statistical association between the two entities is weak and partly explicable by patient selection (Treffers 1990).

Conclusions

Any consideration of the pathology of spontaneous abortion must inevitably lead to the conclusion that morphological studies have relatively little to offer, at the moment, to our understanding of the aetiology or pathogenesis of early pregnancy loss.

Histological examination of aborted material does not provide information of any predictive value, in terms of subsequent pregnancies, and does not allow for discrimination between sporadic and recurrent abortions.

Too much of the literature on the pathology of spontaneous abortion confuses cause and effect. Thus it is obvious that an abnormal fetal karyotype is associated unduly frequently with early pregnancy failure: what is not clear is why an abnormal chromosomal constitution leads to pregnancy loss or why only a proportion of such cases abort, some proceeding to term. Confined placental mosaicism may offer an explanation for some examples of this phenomenon but will not serve to explain the high abortion rate of malformed, but chromosomally normal, embryos.

There remains the possibility, still to be adequately explored, that the common factor to all cases of early pregnancy loss consequent upon a fetal abnormality is inadequate placentation and that the pathogenesis of the abortion in such cases is premature entry of maternal blood into the intervillous space. However, this would still leave unexplained the mechanism responsible for abortion of a normal fetus.

Acknowledgement.   All the figures are reproduced from Buckley and Fox (1989) *Biopsy Pathology of the Endometrium*, Chapman and Hall, London, by kind permission of the publishers.

References

Benirschke K, Driscoll SG (1967) The pathology of the human placenta. Springer-Verlag, Berlin Heidelberg New York

Bennett SJ (1987) Congenital abnormalities of the fundus. In: Bennett MJ, Edmonds DK (eds) Spontaneous and recurrent abortion. Blackwell, Oxford, pp 109–129

Berry CL (1980) The examination of embryonic and fetal material in diagnostic histopathology laboratories. J Clin Pathol 33:317–326

Bulmer JN, Ritson A (1988) The decidua in early pregnancy. In: Beard RW, Sharp F (eds) Early pregnancy loss; mechanisms and treatment. Springer-Verlag, London, pp 171–180

Carreras LO, Defreyn G, Machin SJ et al. (1981) Arterial thrombosis, intrauterine death and the "lupus" antocoagulant: detection of immunoglobulin interfering with prostacyclin formation. Lancet 1:244–246

Charles D, Larsen B (1990) Spontaneous abortion as a result of infection. In: Huisjes HJ, Lind T (eds) Early pregnancy failure. Churchill Livingstone, Edinburgh, pp 161–176

Clark DA (1988) Host immunoregulatory mechanisms and the success of the conceptus fertilised in vivo and in vitro. In: Beard RW, Sharp F (eds) Early pregnancy loss: mechanisms and treatment. Springer-Verlag, London pp 215–227

Clark DA, Moybray J, Underwood J, Liddell H (1987) Histopathologic alterations in the decidua of spontaneous human abortion: loss of cells with large cytoplasmic granules. Am J Reprod Immunol Microbiol 13:19–22

Davis JR, Kerrigan DP, Way DM, Weiner SA (1987) Partial hydatidiform moles: deoxyribonucleic acid content and course. Am J Obstet Gynecol 157:969–973

Derue DJ, Englert HJ, Harris EN et al. (1985) Fetal loss in systemic lupus: association with anti-cardiolipin antibodies. J Obstet Gynaecol 5:207–209

De Wolf F, Carreras LO, Moerman P, Vermylen J, van Assche A, Renaer M (1982) Decidual vasculopathy and extensive placental infarction in a patient with thromboembolic accidents, recurrent fetal loss, and a lupus anticoagulant. Am J Obstet Gynecol 142:829–834

Fox H (1978) Pathology of the placenta. Saunders, Philadelphia

Fujikura J, Froehlich LA, Driscoll SG (1966) A simplified anatomic classification of abortions. Am J Obstet Gynecol 95:902–905

Geisler K, Kleinebrecht J (1978) Cytogenetic and histologic analysis of spontaneous abortion. Hum Genet 45:239–251

Geneva Conference (1966) Standardisation of procedures for chromosome studies in abortion. Cytogenetics 5:361–393

Gocke H, Muradow I, Cremer H (1982) Morphologische und zytogenetische Befunde bei Fruhaborten Ver Dtsch Ges Pathol 66:141–146

Gocke H, Schwanitz G, Muradow I, Zerres K (1985) Pathomorphologie und Genetik iin der Fruhschwangerschaft. Pathologe 6:249–259

Harris EN (1988) Clinical and immunological significance of anti-phospholipid antibodies. In: Beard RW, Sharp F (eds) Early pregnancy loss: mechanisms and treatment. Springer-Verlag, London, pp 43–60

Hemming JD, Quirke P, Womack C, Wells M, Elston CW, Bird CC (1987) Diagnosis of molar pregnancy and persistent trophoblastic disease. J Clin Pathol 40:615–620

Hertig AT (1968) Human trophoblast. Thomas, Springfield, Illinois

Honore LH, Dill FJ, Poland BJ (1976) Placental morphology in spontaneous human abortions with normal and abnormal karotypes. Teratology 14:151–166

Houwert-de Jong MH (1989) Habitual abortion: views and fact-finding. Thesis, University of Utrecht

Houwert-de Jong MH, Bruinse HW, Eskes TKAB, Mantingh A, Termijtelen A, Kooyman CD (1990a) Early recurrent miscarriage; histology of conception products. Br J Obstet Gynaecol 97:533–535

Houwert-de Jong MH, Bruinse HW, Termijtelen A (1990b) The immunology of normal pregnancy and recurrent abortion. In: Huisjes HJ, Lind T (eds) Early pregnancy failure. Churchill Livingstone, Edinburgh, pp 27–38

Hustin J, Schaaps JP, Lambotte R (1988) Anatomical studies of the utero-placental vascularization in the first trimester of pregnancy. Trophoblast Res 3:49–60

Hustin J, Jauniaux E, Schaaps JP (1990) Histological study of the materno-embryonic interface in spontaneous abortion. Placenta 11:477–486

Jacobs PA, Szulman AE, Fumkhouser J, Matsuura R, Wilson CC (1982) Human triploidy: relationship between paternal origin of additional haploid complement and development of partial hydatidiform mole. Ann Hum Genet 46:225–231

Kalousek DK, Barrett IJ, McGillivray BC (1989) Placental mosaicism and intrauterine survival of trisomies 13 and 18. Am J Hum Genet 44; 338–343

Katsura M (1989) Effect of human recombinant interleukin-I-alpha on glycosaminoglycan and collagen metabolism in cultured human chorionic cells. Acta Obstet Gynaec Jap 41:1943–1950

Khong TY, De Wolf F, Robertson WB, Brosens I (1986) Inadequate maternal vascular response to placentation in pregnancies complicated by pre-eclampsia and by small for gestational age infants. Br J Obstet Gynaecol 93:1049–1059

Khong TY, Liddell HS, Robertson WB (1987) Defective haemochorial placentation as a cause of miscarriage: a preliminary study. Br J Obstet Gynaecol 94:649–655

Labarrere CA, Faulk WF, McIntyre JA (1989) Villitis in normal human term placentae: frequency of the lesion determined by monoclonal antibody to HLA-DR antigen. J Reprod Immunol Microbiol 16:127–135

Labarrere CA, McIntyre JA, Faulk WP (1990) Immunohistologic evidence that villitis in human normal term placentas is an immunologic lesion. Am J Obstet Gynecol 162:515–522

Lage JM, Weinberg DS, Yavner DL, Bieber FR (1989) The biology of tetraploid hydatidiform moles: histopathology, cytogenetics and flow cytometry. Hum Pathol 20:419–425

Laurini RN (1990) Abortion from a morphological viewpoint. In: Huisjes HJ, Lind T (eds) Early pregnancy failure. Churchill Livingstone, Edinburgh, pp 79–113

Lawler SD, Fisher RA, Pickhall VJ, Povey S, Evans MW (1982) Genetic studies on hydatidiform moles. 1. The origin of partial moles. Cancer Genet Cytogenet 5:309–320

Lockshin MD, Druzin ML, Goei S et al. (1985) Antibody to cardiolipin as a predictor of fetal distress or death in pregnant patients with systemic lupus erythematosus. N Engl J Med 313:152–156

Lockshin MD, Quamar T, Druzin ML, Goei S (1987) Antibody to cardiolipin, lupus anticoagulant, and fetal death. J Rheumatol 14:259–262

Mall FP, Meyer AW (1921) Studies on abortuses: a study of pathologic ova in the Carnegie embryological collection. Contrib Embryol Carnegie Inst Washington 12:1–364

Matorras R, Garcia-Perea A, Omenaca F, Usandizaga JA, Nieto A, Herruzo R (1989) Group B streptococcus and premature rupture of the membranes and premature delivery. Gynecol Obstet Invest 27:14–18

McDonald H, Vignerwaran R, O'Loughlin JA (1989) Group B streptococcal colonization and preterm labour. Aust N Z J Obstet Gynaecol 29:291–293

Michel M, Underwood J, Clarke DA, Mowbray JF, Beard RW (1989) Histologic and immunologic study of uterine biopsy tissue of women with incipient abortion. Am J Obstet 161, 409–414

Michel MZ, Khong TY, Clark DA, Beard RW (1990) A morphological and immunological study of human placental bed biopsies in miscarriage. Br J Obstet Gynaecol 97:984–988

Minguillon C, Eiben B, Bahr-Porsch S, Vogel M, Hansmann H (1989) The predictive value of chorionic villus histology for identifying chromosomally normal and abnormal spontaneous abortions. Hum Genet 82:373–376

Muntefering R, Dallenbach-Hellweg G, Ratschek M (1988) Pathologische-anatomische Befunde bei der gestorten Fruhschwangerschaft. Gynakologie 21:262–272

Naeye RL (1987) Functionally important disorders of the placenta, umbilical cord and fetal membranes. Hum Pathol 18:681–691

Novak R, Agamonalis D, Dasu S et al. (1988) Histological analysis of placental tissue in first trimester abortions. Paediat Path 8:477–482

Ohama K, Ueda K, Okamoto M, Takemata M, Fujiwara A (1986) Cytogenetic and clinicopathological studies of partial moles. Obstet Gynecol 68:259–262

Philippe E (1973) Morphologie et morphometrie des placentas d'aberration chromosomique fetale. Rev Fr Gynecol Obstet 68:645–649

Philippe E, Boué J (1969) Le placenta dan les aberrations chromosomique fetales. Ann Anat Pathol 14:249–266

Rehder H, Coerdt W, Eggers R, Klink F, Schwinger E (1989) Is there a correlation between morphological and cytogenetic findings in placental tissue from early missed abortions? Hum Genet 82:377–385

Robertson WB, Brosens I, Dixon HG (1967) The pathological response of the vessels of the placental bed in hypertensive pregnancy. J Pathol Bacteriol 85:581–592

Robertson WB, Brosens I, Dixon HG (1975) Uteroplacental vascular pathology. Eur J Obstet Gynecol Reprod Biol 5:47–65

Rockelein G, Schroder J, Ulmer R (1989) Korrelation von Karotyp und Plazentamorphologie beim Fruhabort. Pathologe 10:306–314

Rushton DI (1981) Examination of products of conception from previable human pregnancies. J Clin Pathol 34:819–835

Rushton DI (1984) The classification and mechanisms of spontaneous abortion. Perspect Pediatr Pathol 8:269–287

Rushton DI (1987) Pathology of abortion. In: Fox H (ed) Haines and Taylor: Obstetrical and gynaecological pathology, 3rd edn. Churchill Livingstone, Edinburgh, pp 1117–1148

Rushton DI (1988) Placental pathology in spontaneous miscarriage. In: Beard RW, Sharp F (eds) Early pregnancy loss: mechanisms and treatment. Springer-Verlag, London, pp 149–157

Russell P (1987) Infections of the placental villi (villitis). In: Fox H (ed) Haines and Taylor: Obstetrical and gynaecological pathology, 3rd edn. Churchill Livingstone, Edinburgh, pp 1014–1029

Schaaps JP, Hustin J (1988) Dynamic imaging of the utero-placental border in the first trimester of human pregnancy. Trophoblast Res 3:37–45

Schoonmaker JN, Lavellin DW, Lunt B, McGregor GA (1989) Bacteria and inflammatory cells reduce chorioamniotic membrane integrity and tensile strength. Obstet Gynecol 74:590–596

Surti U, Szulman AE, Wagner K, Leppert M, O'Brien SJ (1986) Tetraploid partial hydatidiform
    moles: two cases with a triple paternal contribution and a 92,XXXY karotype. Hum Genet 72:15–
    21
Teng NMM, Ballon SC (1984) Partial hydatidiform mole with diploid karotype: report of three cases.
    Am J Obstet Gynecol 150:961–965
Treffers PE (1990) Uterine causes of early pregnancy failure – a critical evaluation. In: Huisjes HJ,
    Lind T (eds) Early pregnancy failure. Churchill Livingstone, Edinburgh, pp 114–147
van Oven MW, Schoots CJF, Oosterhuis JW, Klef JF, Dam-Metring A, Huisjes HJ (1989) The use of
    DNA flow cytometry in the diagnosis of triploidy in human abortions. Hum Pathol 20:238–240

5. Ultrasound Diagnosis of Spontaneous Miscarriage

Isabel Stabile and S. C. Campbell

Introduction

Since neither the extent and duration of bleeding nor the presence or absence of lower abdominal pain in the first trimester are reliable indicators of pregnancy outcome (Stabile 1988), attention has turned to biophysical and biochemical means of evaluating early human pregnancy. This chapter will describe the role of biophysical tools such as transabdominal ultrasound (TAS), transvaginal ultrasound (TVS) and doppler ultrasound in answering the following questions: am I pregnant? is my pregnancy normal? when is my baby due? will I miscarry? is my baby normal?

Am I Pregnant?

Pregnancy can be detected biochemically using rapid, sensitive human chorionic gonadotrophin (hCG) assays following implantation of the blastocyst. Controversy surrounds the acceptable cut-off limit for the diagnosis of pregnancy on quantitative hCG measurements. Following in vitro Fertilisation and Embryo Transfer (IVF–ET), implantation is generally diagnosed at an hCG level of 10 IU/l. However a substantial number of these early pregnancies will subsequently abort (Grudzinskas and Chard 1991). In clinical practice it is, therefore, customary to base the diagnosis of pregnancy on a single hCG level greater than 25 IU/l, or a lower level which doubles within 3 days (Jones et al. 1983). Whatever the cut-off used, the clinician interpreting the result should be aware of the type of assay used to measure hCG (radioimmunoassay, immunofluorometric assay, enzyme linked monoclonal antibody assay, chemiluminescent assay etc) as well as its detection limit. Although a negative qualitative hCG test (the type most commonly used to diagnose pregnancy at home), with a detection limit of say 50 IU/l will miss a number of very early pregnancies, more sensitive tests are widely available.

Pregnancy can be diagnosed ultrasonically by demonstrating an intrauterine gestational sac (Fig. 5.1). This is consistently possible using transabdominal ultrasound (TAS) from 6 weeks amenorrhoea onwards, although high resolution scanners are reportedly capable of visualising a sac one week earlier. Yeh et al. (1986) reported finding focal echogenic thickening of the endometrium as early as 3.5 weeks from the last menstrual period (LMP) using TAS. This finding has not been reproduced by others. Recent improvements in ultrasound technology allow the consistent demonstration of a gestational sac within the uterus from 4.5 weeks onwards using transvaginal sonography (TVS) (Bernaschek et al. 1988). In this respect it is important to note the distinction between consistent observation of a specific feature (the discriminatory level) and the earliest detection of that same feature (the threshold level). This difference accounts for the variation in reported times at which ultrasound features are visualised with TVS. For example, Bernaschek et al. (1988) reported that an intrauterine gestational sac (mean diameter of 2 mm) was identified in only 2 of 8 patients at hCG values between 50 and 280 IU/l (2nd IS) two days after the missed period (the threshold level). It was only at hCG levels greater than 300 IU/l that a gestational sac was always seen (discriminatory level). This author feels that each ultrasound department must determine its own threshold and discriminatory levels, based on the experience of their staff, resolution of their equipment and audit of their results.

Is My Pregnancy Normal?

The answer to this question involves the sonographic evaluation of two points: a) is the pregnancy intrauterine? and b) is the pregnancy viable? These will be addressed in turn.

Once pregnancy is suspected it is important to differentiate between a true intrauterine gestational sac and the pseudogestational sac that results from the decidual response of the uterus to an ectopic pregnancy. Several ultrasound parameters have been proposed to allow this distinction to be made with confidence. Although these were first described using TAS they are equally applicable to use with TVS in the situation when information about hCG is unavailable or simply qualitative in nature.

Characteristically, the early intrauterine gestational sac is eccentrically located within the uterine cavity and is surrounded by an asymmetrical trophoblast ring (Fig. 5.1). This asymmetry distinguishes normal pregnancy from ectopic gestation and from hormone-induced changes associated with the normal menstrual cycle. At this stage the normal sac has two layers which represent the decidua capsularis and parietalis. This double echogenic wall appearance is reportedly missing in the pseudosac of ectopic pregnancy (Bradley et al. 1982). Although dramatic, this double decidual sign is not consistently seen in early pregnancy, and at least in one study was also noted in one-third of patients with ectopic pregnancy (Nyberg et al. 1988).

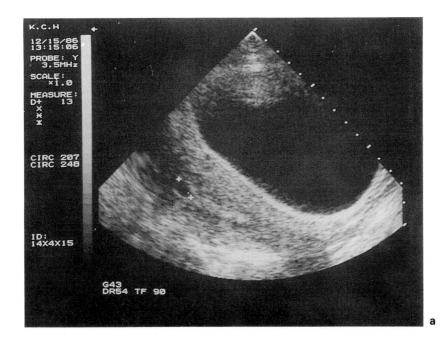

a

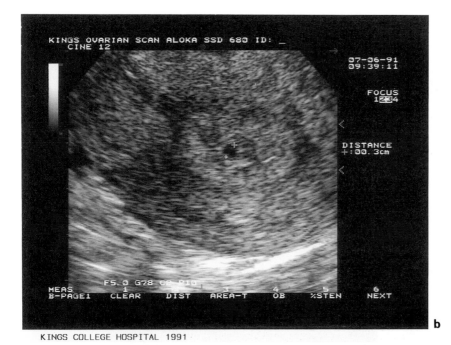

b

Fig. 5.1a,b. Intrauterine gestational sac. **a** Visualised by TAS at 6 weeks from LMP. **b** TVS at 5 weeks from LMP. It is surrounded by an asymmetrical trophoblast ring.

Sonographic identification of the yolk sac confirms the presence of an intrauterine pregnancy even before a living embryo is detected. It is, in fact, the first structure to be seen normally within the gestational sac, appearing as a spherical structure a few millimetres in diameter. It is visible with TAS in all normal gestational sacs of mean diameter exceeding 20 mm (which corresponds to 7 weeks amenorrhea). TVS allows earlier identification of the yolk sac, typically when the mean gestational sac diameter is larger than 8 mm (Levi et al. 1988) or 10 mm (Cacciatore et al. 1990). Although the presence of a yolk sac may be critical in differentiating an early intrauterine sac from a pseudosac (decidual cast), its presence does not guarantee that the intrauterine pregnancy is normal (vide infra).

On a technical note, it should be emphasised that careful inspection of the entire sac contents may be required in order to demonstrate the yolk sac, as it is often found near the periphery of the sac. Moreover as the early embryo lies very close to the yolk sac at this stage of development, care should be taken to avoid including this structure in the measurement of crown–rump length (CRL), an error which could alter the measurement (and hence estimation of menstrual age) by more than 50% (Fig. 5.2).

In view of the important role of the primary yolk sac in transfer of nutrients prior to establishment of the placental circulation, the association between defects in yolk sac development and poor pregnancy outcome is theoretically obvious. Several studies have addressed the potential value of abnormal yolk sac biometry and morphology in predicting embyronic demise (Pedersen et al. 1984; Green and Hobbins 1988; Harris et al. 1988; Ferrazzi et al. 1988; Reece et al.

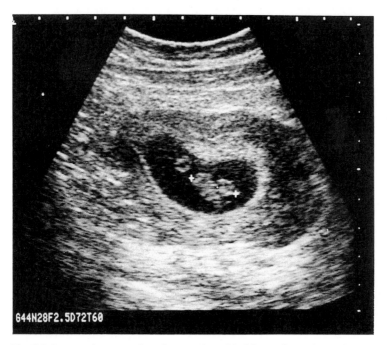

644N28F2.5D72T60

Fig. 5.2. Intrauterine sac at 6 weeks gestation with 6.9-mm size embryo, demonstrating blood flow.

1988). The size of the yolk sac alone appears to be a poor predictor of embryonic viability, which is perhaps not surprising since the structure measured ultrasonically represents the secondary yolk sac (Table 5.1). Unlike the primary yolk sac this is essentially non-functional. Absence of a yolk sac in the presence of an embryo does not indicate poor prognosis (Ferrazzi et al. 1988), whereas its calcification has been associated with intrauterine demise in the first trimester (Harris et al. 1988).

Table 5.1. Summary of time line of embryonic development correlated with TVS appearance

Days from LMP	Embryological event	Ultrasound appearance
14	Ovulation	
14–15	Fertilisation	
20	Blastocyst stage	
20–23	Implantation	
23	Primary yolk sac	
27–28	Secondary yolk sac	
30	Trilaminar disc embryo	Earliest detectable gestational sac mean diameter 2 mm
33–35	Circulation begins	Consistently detectable gestational sac
38–40		Earliest embryonic heart activity and yolk sac detected
46		Consistent detection of cardiac action

The embryological changes that occur during the first trimester of pregnancy (Moore 1982) are correlated with ultrasound appearance in Table 5.1. Using TVS it is possible to identify an embryo with a CRL as small as 1–3 mm, depending on the resolution of the equipment used (Fig. 5.3). The corresponding figure for TAS is 5–6 mm (6 weeks' gestation). Using TAS, cardiac activity can be identified even before the embryo is clearly seen, by careful examination of the yolk sac region (Cadkin and McAlpin 1984). Using TVS, Bree et al. (1989) consistently demonstrated cardiac activity in all pregnancies beyond 40 days from the LMP in patients with reliable dates. In the elegant longitudinal study of Cacciatore et al. (1990) in which ovulation was based on LH timing, TVS reliably detected an intrauterine sac by 33 days gestation, a yolk sac by 38 days and embryonic echoes with a visible heart motion by 43 days. However since reliable dates are not a consistent feature in the obstetric population and since detection of the LH surge is not, as yet, routine practice, it is probably best to consider the smallest embryo size at which cardiac activity can consistently and reliably be determined using TVS. Rempen (1990) has determined the value of TVS (using a 5 MHz transducer) in identifying the embryonic heart action in 363 normal singleton pregnancies. The earliest recorded cardiac activity in this study occurred at 40 days from the LMP, at a mean gestational sac diameter of 9.3 mm, an hCG level of 6700 IU/l (First IRP) and a CRL of 2 mm. However, these parameters cannot be used consistently to diagnose viability sonographically as their identification is operator- and equipment-dependent. Rather it is important to determine the earliest consistent detection of the cardiac action (threshold value). In this well-designed study this occurred at a menstrual age of 46 days, a CRL of 3 mm, a mean gestational sac diameter of 18.3 mm and an hCG level greater than 47171

IU/l (first IRP). The author also emphasised the ease with which it is possible to miss such early embryos altogether, as they typically appear as echogenic structures adjacent to the yolk sac in the periphery of the gestational sac. Moreover, while embryos smaller than 5 mm may have visible cardiac activity, in the study of Pennel et al. (1990), one-third of embryos (subsequently shown to be normal) with a CRL less than 5 mm did not demonstrate cardiac activity. Similar results were reported by Levi et al. (1990).

Therefore the diagnosis of embryonic demise (missed abortion as it used to be called) should not be made by TVS in embryos measuring less than 5 mm without a visible heart beat. On a technical note, there is a device used by ultrasound manufacturers which averages adjacent frames. It is recommended that if cardiac activity is not identified, the frame-averaging mode be switched off and the frame rate increased to avoid missing the cardiac action while utilising TVS. Those clinicians who continue to rely on TAS should note that, provided high resolution equipment gives images of good technical quality, it should always be possible to see the cardiac action whenever an embryo is visualised.

When Is My Baby Due?

The important landmarks of embryonic development in the first trimester of pregnancy such as the gestational sac, the yolk sac and the embryo itself can be identified using high resolution TVS from 1 to 3 mm in size onwards (Fig. 5.1 to 5.3). At this stage there is minimal biological variation in the size of these structures, which explains why menstrual age can be determined most accurately during the first trimester. The close association between gestational sac size and hCG levels is presumably related to the fact that they are both products of trophoblastic activity. This relationship is the basis for the ability of both biophysical and biochemical measurements to accurately determine gestational age in early pregnancy (Klopper and Ahmed 1985).

Gestational sacs less than 10 mm in diameter are typically circular, although later they become ellipsoid. One advantage of expressing gestational sac dimensions in terms of diameter rather than volume (which entails taking three measurements perpendicular to each other along the internal border of the sac) is that it is not always possible to see structures in two planes at right angles using TVS. Moreover the sac diameter increases linearly with gestational age, unlike the exponential rise of the gestational sac volume (Robinson 1975a). The use of TVS avoids compression and distortion of the sac inherent in the full bladder technique. However errors can easily be introduced using either technique by sloppy operators who fail consistently to measure from the interface between the inner sac wall and the chorionic fluid. A small error in taking a small measurement is more significant than the same error over a larger dimension.

Once an embryonic pole can be identified it should be measured three times and the average value compared to published data to estimate the duration of pregnancy. Although the early nomograms were derived using static B scanners (Robinson and Fleming 1975), there is a remarkable correlation between measurements taken using static and dynamic (real time) scanners in the same patients (Adam et al. 1979), as well as between transabdominal and transvaginal

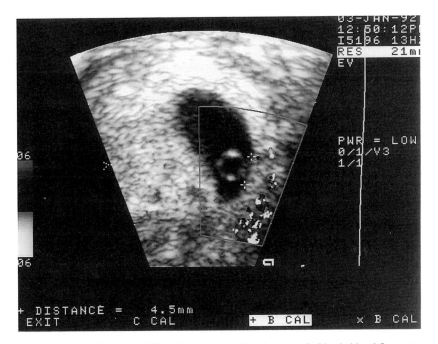

Fig. 5.3. Intrauterine sac at 5.5 weeks gestation, showing a trophoblastic blood flow pattern.

equipment. However because the resolution of TAS is limited, the early CRL charts (still widely used today) are available only from 6 weeks and 2 days onwards (CRL of 6 mm). Clinicians wishing to date pregnancies from measurements smaller than this will have to await full length publication of nomograms using transvaginal equipment (Lasser et al. 1990).

Evans (1991) has recently pointed out another limitation of the original studies of CRL measurements in the first trimester, namely that they were based upon the LMP in normal menstrual cycles. He and others (MacGregor et al. 1987) have demonstrated a 2–4 day difference between CRL observations based upon ovulation timing in infertility patients and those based upon the LMP. Population differences, selection bias in the original studies and the fertility status of the women included in the most recent studies may partly account for this variation. It is also possible that accurate recollection of the LMP was limited in the original studies. In fact, Hertz et al. (1978) have documented that less than a quarter of all pregnancies have a reliable LMP as defined by certain dates and both regular and normal menses. Those clinicians looking after pregnancies resulting from assisted conception should be reassured by the observation that although ovulation induction with human menopausal gonadotrophin has been shown to slow gestational sac growth (Mayden et al. 1986), this is not the case for embryonic growth (MacGregor et al. 1987; Cacciatore et al. 1990; Evans 1991). These pregnancies can be dated accurately using Evans' charts.

One final point concerns the variability of the menstrual age estimate. This is generally expressed at ±2 standard deviations which therefore applies to 95% of the normal population. It follows that 5% of normal embryos will have measurements above or below this range. In practical terms, both gestational sac dimensions and embryonic CRL measurements are accurate to within ± one week, provided care has been taken to obtain the measurements in a reliable and reproducible manner.

Will I Miscarry?

In our study of several hundred women presenting with vaginal bleeding with or without lower abdominal pain, a single ultrasound examination confirmed that the pregnancy had already failed in nearly 50% of women (Stabile et al. 1987). Of the remaining live intrauterine pregnancies, 97% proceeded uneventfully. Similarly, in an apparently normal population the observation of embryonic life in utero (between 9 and 11 weeks amenorrhea) was associated with normal progress and outcome in all but 2% of women (McKensie et al. 1988). It has been demonstrated that the earlier the diagnosis of pregnancy is made, the greater is the incidence of pregnancy failure (Grudzinskas and Chard 1991). Thus, although the improved resolution of TVS allows us consistently to demonstrate embryonic viability at a CRL of greater than 5 mm, it does not follow that 98% of these pregnancies will have normal outcome. The extent of this difference is highlighted by the work of Rosen et al. (1990) who attempted to evaluate prognosis on the basis of early observation of embryonic viability using TVS in previously infertile couples in whom the exact date of ovulation (± 1 day) was known. Of the 293 patients in this series in whom the embyronic cardiac activity was eventually demonstrated, a total of 33 (11.3%) subsequently miscarried. When subdivided according to when the cardiac motion was observed in relation to ovulation, 13 of these abortions occurred after cardiac motion was observed at 4 weeks after ovulation (i.e., 6 weeks from the LMP), while 20 occurred after cardiac motion was observed 5 weeks after ovulation. It is unclear why the appearance of the embryonic heart action 4 weeks after ovulation should be a better prognostic sign than the same observation one week later. Confirmation of these interesting results is awaited.

The earliest description of ultrasound findings in patients destined to miscarry included a low ratio of amniotic sac to embryo and cervical incompetence (Robinson 1975b). These observations have been expanded by several authors to include intrauterine haematomata, double gestational sacs, low lying placenta, uterine abnormalities, fetal growth delay and early bradycardia.

Intrauterine Haematomata

Mantoni and Pedersen (1981) were the first to report the observation of intrauterine haematomata in women with viable pregnancies between 12 and 20 weeks gestation (Fig. 5.4). Subsequent reports have confirmed these findings (Goldstein et al. 1983; Jouppila 1983; Ylostalo et al. 1984; Stabile et al. 1987;

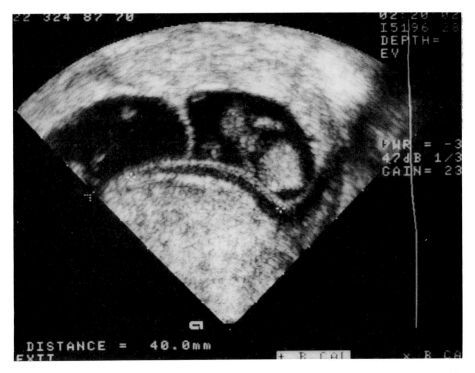

Fig. 5.4. TAS showing subchorionic haematoma (+—+) between the membranes and uterine wall in 10-week-old twin pregnancy which continued uneventfully.

Pedersen and Mantoni 1990). The underlying mechanism is thought to be placental separation with blood appearing as an echo-free space between the membranes and the uterine wall (subchorionic haematoma). Retroplacental clots have been described between the placenta and the myometrium and pre-placental clots between the placenta and the amniotic membrane (Nyberg et al. 1987).

We have recently reported on 624 women with threatened miscarriage, 5.4% of whom had an intrauterine haematoma (less than 16 ml in volume) noted ultrasonically. In each case this decreased in size as the patients experienced repeated episodes of bleeding (Stabile et al. 1989b). Twenty of the 22 haematomata (91%) visualised were subchorionic, and 2 (9%) were retroplacental. None of these women subsequently miscarried. Levels of hCG and other trophoblastic products (Schwangerschaftsprotein 1 (SP1) and pregnancy-associated plasma protein A (PAPP-A)) were not significantly different in women with or without haematomata. We originally thought that our observations concerning the inocuous nature of intrauterine haematomata were probably related to their relatively small size. However Pedersen and Mantoni (1990) have recently confirmed these findings on a series of 23 patients with haematomata ranging from 50 to 150 ml in volume. Only one patient miscarried and two had a pre-term delivery, confirming that even large haematomata do not seem to represent serious threat to the pregnancy.

Double Gestational Sacs

The true incidence of twinning in the first trimester of normal pregnancy is unknown. Early ultrasound studies in spontaneous and clomiphene-induced cycles revealed that approximately 65% of twins diagnosed in the first trimester resulted in singleton pregnancies at the time of delivery (Schneider et al. 1979). Thus emerged the concept of the vanishing twin. Dickey et al. (1990) have determined that the proportion of twin gestational sacs which deliver at term following induction of ovulation with clomiphene is identical to that in spontaneous cycles. It has been proposed that when empty, the second sac may not be a true gestational sac at all (i.e., not a concomitant anembryonic pregnancy), but rather a variant of normal wherein blood accumulates at the site of implantation, thus mimicking another sac. Which of these theories is correct awaits prospective evaluation of normal pregnancies examined serially from conception onwards using TVS and followed up until spontaneous abortion or delivery occur. Apart from difficulty in distinguishing ultrasonically between double sacs (noted in 3.9% of our study group with threatened miscarriage and a live embryo (Stabile et al. 1987)) and the haematomata described above, there is general agreement that the finding of an additional apparently abnormal sac is a common benign observation in women with first trimester bleeding.

Low Lying Placenta

Among women scanned during the first and second trimesters of pregnancy 7% were noted to have a low lying placenta in one study (Varma 1981). Not surprisingly these women were three times more likely to experience frequent episodes of vaginal bleeding than the control group with a normally situated placenta. In addition, the incidence of spontaneous abortion was twice as high as in the controls (16% versus 8%). These observations have been confirmed by Mantoni (1985) who suggested that the higher abortion rate in these women was probably related to the unfavourable site of placentation.

Low Ratio of Amniotic Sac to Embryo

The rare abnormality of a low ratio of amniotic sac to embryo (Fig. 5.5) has been described by several authors (Robinson 1975b; Mantoni 1985; Stabile et al. 1987), all of whom reported poor prognosis for the pregnancy. Chow and Vengadasalam (1986) have implicated maternal infection with cytomegalovirus as a possible underlying factor although the pathophysiology of this abnormality is as yet undetermined. Over a 5-year period, Bromley et al. (1991) retrospectively identified 16 women with small sac size, which they defined as a difference between mean sac diameter and CRL of less than 5 mm. All but one of these women (94%) subsequently aborted at an unspecified time in the pregnancy. Only 5 of the 16 women underwent ultrasound scanning because of vaginal bleeding. This raises the question of how best to identify this group of women (in

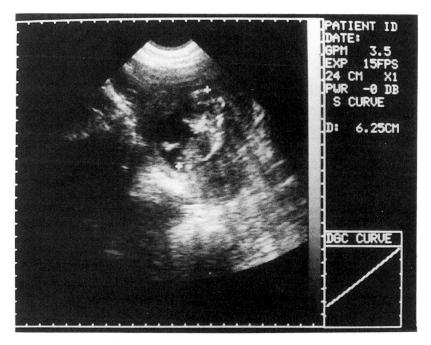

Fig. 5.5. TAS showing crumpled embryo (2.5 cm) surrounded by reduced amniotic fluid volume.

whom the prognosis for pregnancy outcome is so poor) in those centres that do not practise routine ultrasound scanning.

Uterine Abnormalities

Although easily identified ultrasonically, as a group uterine abnormalities are an uncommon cause of early pregnancy wastage. They include fibroids, congenital defects such as bicornuate uterus and partial or complete dilatation of the endocervical canal. Apart from abortion, complications include antepartum haemorrhage and premature rupture of membranes. This is discussed in greater detail in Chap 3.

Embryonic Growth Delay

The first suggestion that women with threatened miscarriage and smaller than normal embryos are less likely to have a successful outcome of pregnancy came from Denmark (Mantoni and Pedersen 1982). Similar observations have been made in diabetic pregnancies (Pedersen et al. 1984). Benacerraf (1988) has documented a case of first trimester growth retardation associated with triploidy. Clearly this observation can only be identified in that subgroup of women with good menstrual data upon which to base the duration of pregnancy, or those in whom serial measurements in the first trimester are available.

Early Bradycardia

Several studies have analysed the embryonic heart rate in early pregnancy, the earliest report being that of Robinson and Shaw-Dunn (1973). The embryonic heart rate increases from a mean of 110 ± 8 at 5 weeks to a maximum of 170 ± 6 at 9 weeks, falling thereafter to approximately 160 ± 14 by the end of the first trimester (Rempen 1990). The normal slower heart rate between 5 to 8 weeks may be due to immaturity of the sino-atrial node or possibly the atrial pacemaker itself may be slower at this stage in pregnancy (Shenker et al. 1986). Thus early in the first trimester the embryonic and maternal heart rates may be very similar and care must be taken not to confuse the two. Laboda et al. (1989) reported that 5 of 9 embryos which subsequently aborted had a heart rate below 85 beats per minute when examined between 6 and 8.5 weeks. Unfortunately the authors did not specify whether the remainder of the ultrasound examination was entirely normal; neither was morphological or chromosomal examination of the abortuses reported.

The appearance and development of embryonic cardiac activity was studied by Schats et al. (1990a) in 47 women whose pregnancies were established by IVF-ET. The advantage of studying IVF pregnancies is that some of the variables in estimating menstrual age such as time of ovulation and embryo transfer are known. In this series there were 7 embryos (6 pregnancies) with abnormal heart rate patterns between 25 and 42 days after oocyte recovery, all of which aborted in the first trimester. An abnormal chromosome pattern was noted in 2 of the 5 abortuses from which embryonic karyotyping was feasible. An abnormal embryonic heart rate pattern was subsequently reported in a case of Down's syndrome (Schats et al. 1990b).

Is My Baby Normal?

Fetal anatomy is generally explored ultrasonically in the second trimester, at the time of the routine booking scan. Improvements in ultrasound technology now make it possible for defects in development to be identified in the first trimester using TVS (Timor Tritsch et al. 1988). Gross discrepancy between menstrual dates and CRL size may be the first and sometimes only indicator of embryonic abnormality in the first trimester. By contrast, many abnormal fetuses may appear entirely normal when examined ultrasonically at this time. Controversy surrounds the earliest time at which specific diagnoses can confidently be made ultrasonically. Until such time as these are defined, a follow-up examination is indicated in the majority of cases in the second trimester. Finally it is important for the ultrasonographer to understand normal embryological development to avoid mistaking physiological events (e.g., anterior wall herniation at 8 to 12 weeks) for abnormalities.

Specific Complications of Early Pregnancy

In this section we shall consider the sonographic diagnosis of early embryonic demise (missed abortion), anembryonic pregnancy and complete and incomplete abortion with particular emphasis on the role of TVS in making the diagnosis of a non-viable pregnancy. Clinically it is impossible to distinguish between these subgroups of pregnancy failure. Although it may be argued that the distinction is irrelevant, since management is identical in each case, there are epidemiological and aetiological reasons for classifying a failed pregnancy into one or other of these groups.

Early Embryonic Demise

The advantages and limitations of TVS with respect to the identification of the embryonic heart action have already been described. Provided the embryo is larger than 5 mm (approximately 6 weeks menstrual age), TVS can confidently be used to identify the heart action, which if absent is diagnostic of embryonic demise. Using high resolution TAS, the equivalent embryonic size is 6 mm, although difficulty may be encountered in distinguishing a hydatidiform mole from early embryonic demise (Fig. 5.6) and vice versa (Stabile et al. 1989a).

The diagnosis of embryonic demise was made in only 8% of our study group of several hundred women with threatened miscarriage (Stabile et al. 1987). This figure is lower than previously published data (Mantoni 1985), perhaps because our study design included unselected consecutive patients with threatened miscarriage, with histological confirmation of the diagnosis in each case. A

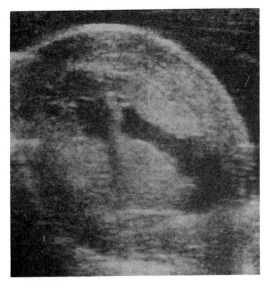

Fig. 5.6. TAS showing enlarged uterus containing irregular echogenic areas and cystic spaces. A hydatidiform mole was diagnosed.

similar study (Schaaps and Soyeur 1989) using TVS in women without threatened miscarriage identified this condition in 22% of the study group (n=127). It is interesting to note that one-third of the women with embryonic demise in our study had had one or more previous miscarriages (Stabile et al. 1989a), confirming the observation of Regan et al. (1989) that, for some unknown reason, the outcome of a woman's first pregnancy seems to affect her future reproductive performance.

Anembryonic Pregnancy

The sonographic diagnosis of anembryonic pregnancy was originally based on the absence of embryonic echoes within a gestational sac large enough for such structures to be visible, independent of clinical or menstrual data (Fig. 5.7). Robinson (1975b) defined the critical sac volume as 2.5 ml, equivalent to a mean diameter of 1.7 cm. This definition is still a practical one, the novelty being that improved resolution confers upon TVS the advantage of being able to identify embryonic echoes at an earlier stage in gestation. The elegant study of deCrespigny (1988) defined the minimum mean sac diameter at which embryonic cardiac activity was always seen using a 5 MHz vaginal transducer. Cardiac activity was not demonstrated in 42 of 171 patients with a mean sac diameter of 1–1.5 cm. In 10 (24%) of these, the embryo was subsequently shown to be alive. All remaining patients with mean sac diameters greater than 1.6 cm without cardiac activity were subsequently shown to have a failed pregnancy. Using a 6.5 MHz transducer, Levi et al. (1988) reported that a sac greater than or equal to 0.8 cm in

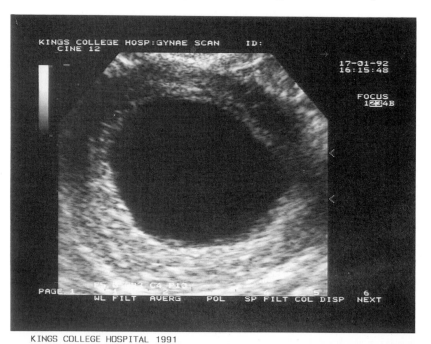

KINGS COLLEGE HOSPITAL 1991

Fig. 5.7. Anembryonic pregnancy: gestational sac volume of 3 ml without embryonic echoes.

size (mean diameter) without a yolk sac or a sac greater than 1.6 cm without an embryo was diagnostic of a non-viable pregnancy. The authors also noted that the presence of a yolk sac within a gestational sac greater than 0.8 cm in diameter did not in itself guarantee a normal pregnancy, as 5 patients with this feature were eventually diagnosed as having a non-viable pregnancy. Cacciatore et al. (1990) demonstrated that the yolk sac and embryonic heart action were always detected when the average diameter of the gestational sac exceeded 1.0 and 1.8 cm respectively. These authors feel that the sonographic criteria for the diagnosis of anembryonic pregnancy should be sufficiently stringent to allow a pregnancy to be terminated without fear of error. While not wishing to prolong maternal anxiety unecessarily, it is advocated that a broad margin of error be adopted before reporting a non-viable pregnancy. Provided both operator and equipment are technically adequate, a mean gestational sac diameter greater than 1.5 cm (using TVS) or 1.7 cm (using TAS) should be identified before diagnosing this form of pregnancy failure (deCrespigny 1988).

Evidence is accumulating from biochemical (Stabile et al. 1989c), sonographic (Pirrone et al. 1990) and pathological studies (Meegdes et al. 1988) that apparently empty gestational sacs actually contained an embryo at one time which subsequently was resorbed. Prospective studies of apparently normal pregnancies examined serially with TVS will be necessary to confirm or refute this hypothesis. If this proves to be the case, then early embryonic demise (missed abortion) and anembryonic pregnancy can probably be considered an extension of the same process, the time elapsing between arrest of embryonic development and clinical presentation determining the sonographic features (Stabile 1991).

Complete and Incomplete Abortion

The ultrasonic appearance of thick irregular echoes in the midline of the uterine cavity is not diagnostic of retained products of conception (incomplete abortion), as blood clot may look remarkably similar (Robinson 1972). Conversely, the finding of a well-defined regular endometrial line excluded this diagnosis in our study (Stabile et al. 1989a). Complete and incomplete abortion was identified in 14% of patients with vaginal bleeding presenting at 7 to 8 weeks, 31% at 10 weeks, 36% at 11 weeks and 5% at 12 weeks, confirming that the majority of pregnancies that fail do so between 10 and 11 weeks menstrual age (Fig. 5.8). The value of ultrasound scanning in the diagnosis of complete abortion awaits a larger study. The ideal way to manage these patients is to refer them to an early pregnancy assessment unit, which has been shown to improve the quality of care and result in considerable savings in financial and staff resources (Bigrigg and Read 1991).

Doppler Ultrasound in the Diagnosis of Pregnancy Failure

Pregnancy is associated with marked haemodynamic changes, substantial increase in uterine blood flow resulting from the sharp rise in maternal cardiac

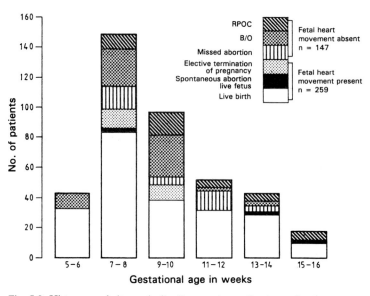

Fig. 5.8. Histogram of ultrasonically diagnosed complications of early pregnancy.

output in the first trimester. The doppler ultrasound technique has been applied to the measurement of uterine blood flow impedance both in non-pregnant women (Matta et al. 1988) and in the early stages of pregnancy (Deutinger et al. 1988; Schaaps and Soyeur 1989; Stabile et al. 1989d; den Ouden et al. 1990). Diastolic blood flow in the uterine circulation increases progressively starting in the first trimester. This has been demonstrated using the transabdominal approach (Stabile et al. 1988), the transvaginal approach (Deutinger et al. 1988) as well as with colour flow mapping (Jaffe and Warsoff 1991). This presumably reflects the fall in peripheral resistance, which is thought to result from unplugging of the spiral arteries by invading villous trophoblast (Pijenborg et al. 1980).

Early studies in the first trimester using pulsed wave doppler were limited by the fact that only vessels large enough to be seen could be sampled, if reproducible results were to be obtained. Because of this limitation, most first trimester studies examined vessels located beneath the placenta. Difficulty in reproducibly obtaining blood velocity waveforms from precisely the same vessel is reflected in the wide normal ranges reported both in early pregnancy (Stabile et al. 1988; Thaler et al. 1990) and in non-pregnant women (Farquhar et al. 1989). Surprisingly wide ranges of pulsatility index values in the uterine arteries were also reported by Steer et al. (1990) using transvaginal colour flow imaging in the luteal phase of non-pregnant women.

We (Stabile et al. 1989d) and others (Mehalek et al. 1989; Jauniaux et al. 1991) have recently investigated differences in blood velocity waveforms obtained at several different points along the arterial tree leading to the placental bed in normal first trimester pregnancy. In our study, waveforms were obtained three times by the same observer at the level of the cervix (uterine artery), just within the myometrium (arcuate artery or branch thereof), at the base of the chorion frondosum and at the opposite side under the chorion laeve. In every case, a gradual decline in the impedance to flow was noted, the Resistance Index (RI) falling from 0.6 to 0.85 at the level of the uterine artery to values 50% of this at the chorion frondosum (Fig. 5.9). The RI was consistently higher on the non-placental side as defined by the chorion laeve. This and other studies have demonstrated that waveforms obtained from just within the myometrium (arcuate artery) differ from those obtained both upstream (uterine artery) and downstream (intervillous space) from this point. Moreover, intervillous flow is characteristically non-pulsatile, unlike that in the spiral, radial, arcuate and uterine vessels. Similar results were obtained recently by Jurkovic et al. (1991) with the benefit of transvaginal colour doppler equipment. This normal gradation in blood flow must be considered physiological and is probably a reflection of trophoblast invasion of the spiral artery at the implantation site as well as branching in the circulation with increased total cross sectional area (Figs. 5.10, 5.11).

Schaaps and Soyeur (1989) studied normal early pregnancies uncomplicated by threatened miscarriage. They found no evidence of doppler signals from the trophoblastic ring (intervillous space). Jauniaux et al. (1991) have reported a continuous intervillous flow pattern around 14 weeks, which they postulate corresponds to complete dislocation of the trophoblast plugs, thus allowing uninhibited circulation in the entire intervillous space. By contrast, Schaaps and Soyeur (1989) always obtained pulsatile signals from the peritrophoblastic area in

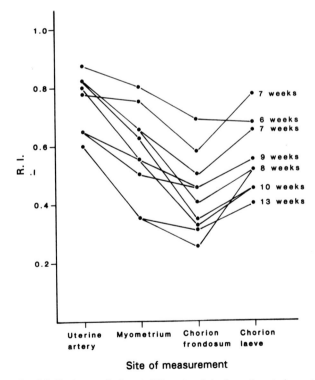

Fig. 5.9. Resistance Index at different points along the uterine arterial tree in early pregnancy.

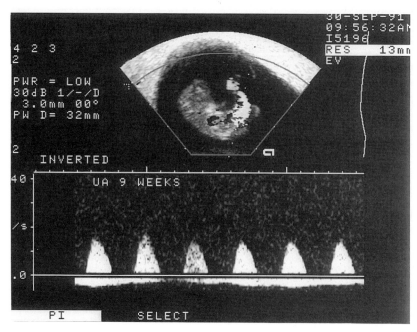

Fig. 5.10. Diagram of blood velocity waveforms obtained from the umbilical circulation at 9 weeks gestation.

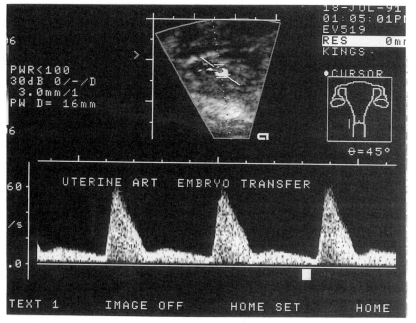

Fig. 5.11a

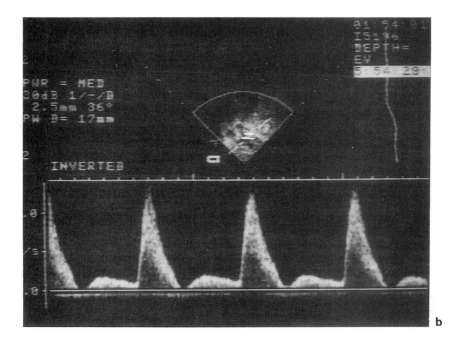

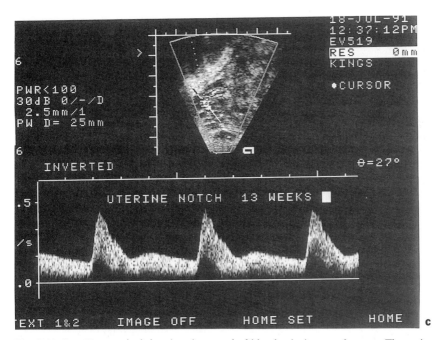

Fig. 5.11a,b,c. Transvaginal doppler ultrasound of blood velocity waveforms. **a** The main uterine artery (7 weeks). **b** Uteroplacental vessels near the base of the placental plate (12 weeks). **c** The intervillous space (13 weeks).

uncomplicated pregnancies. When cardiac activity was absent (embryonic demise), intervillous flow at the level of attachment of the umbilical cord was consistently observed. Studies such as these have improved our understanding of the physiology of early pregnancy and have also served to highlight the importance of carefully defining the site from which measurements are obtained when using pulsed wave duplex systems.

Attention has recently turned to whether this research tool can be put to practical use in the clinical setting of threatened abortion or suspected ectopic pregnancy. Doppler studies were performed (Stabile et al. 1990a) in the first trimester in 10 women with pregnancies which had failed, or subsequently did so, due to anembryonic pregnancy (n=4), embryonic demise (n=1), subsequent spontaneous abortion of a live fetus (n=2) and ectopic pregnancy (n=3). Blood velocity waveforms were obtained just within the myometrium three times by the same observer (within observer CV of 5%). There was no apparent difference in the values for RI in the 10 patients with failed pregnancy, as compared with the control group of 111 women with normal intrauterine pregnancy. However the three ectopic pregnancies studied, in all of whom a live embryo was seen, had significantly higher RI values (Stabile et al. 1990b). By far the largest study, however, on pulsed doppler evaluation of ectopic pregnancy is that of Taylor et al. (1989). High velocity flow was noted in 38 of 70 (54%) patients who subsequently proved to have an ectopic pregnancy. There were 9 women with vascular adnexal masses, in whom luteal flow was thought to represent flow from the ectopic placenta (false positives). The authors proposed that absence of detectable flow in almost half the patients with ectopic pregnancy may have been the result of demise of the ectopic gestation. This is consistent with the observation of detectable flow in each of our 3 patients with a viable ectopic pregnancy (Stabile et al. 1990b).

Colour flow imaging using a transvaginal transducer should eliminate the problem of false-positive results, except in the rare situation of ovarian pregnancy. Indeed, Jurkovic et al. (1992) have studied 19 women with ectopic pregnancy (3 with a live embryo) and 33 women with an intrauterine pregnancy using TVS with colour flow. They found no significant difference between impedance to flow in the uterine or spiral arteries or the corpora lutea. They concluded that peak flow velocity in the uterine arteries reflects a decreased blood supply to ectopic pregnancies.

In conclusion, although the use of this non-invasive technique has improved our understanding of the development of the uteroplacental circulation in normal early pregnancy, it does not appear to offer the clinician additional information relating to the diagnosis of non-viable gestation, with the possible exception of ectopic pregnancy.

References

Adam AH, Robinson HP, Dunlop C (1979) A comparison of crown rump length measurements using a real time scanner in the antenatal clinic and a conventional B scanner. Br J Obstet Gynaecol 86:521–524

Bernaschek G, Rudelstorfer R, Csaicsich P (1988) Vaginal sonography versus serum hCG in early detection of pregnancy. Am J Obstet Gynecol 158:608–612

Benacerraf BR (1988) Intrauterine growth retardation in the first trimester associated with triploidy. J Ultrasound Med 7:153–155

Bigrigg MQ, Read MD (1991) Management of women referred to early pregnancy assessment unit: care and cost effectiveness. Br Med J 302:577–579

Bradley WG, Fiske CE, Filly RA (1982) The double sac sign of early intrauterine pregnancy: use in exlcusion of ectopic pregnancy. Radiol 143:223–226

Bree RL, Edwards M, Bohm-Velez M, Beyler S, Roberts J, Mendelson AB (1989) Transvaginal sonography in the evaluation of normal early pregnancy: correlation with hCG level. AJR 153:75–79

Bromley B, Harlow BL, Laboda LA, Benacerraf BR (1991) Small sac size in the first trimester: a predictor of poor fetal outcome. Radiol 178:375–377

Cacciatore B, Tiitinen A, Stenman UH, Ylostalo P (1990) Normal early pregnancy: serum hCG levels and vaginal ultrasonography findings. Br J Obstet Gynaecol 97:899–903

Cadkin AV, McAlpin RT (1984) Detection of fetal cardiac activity between 41 and 43 days of gestation. J Ultrasound Med 3:499–503

Chilcote WS, Asokan S (1977) Evaluation of first trimester pregnancy by ultrasound. Clin Obstet Gynecol 20:253–264

Chow KK, Vengadasalam D (1986) The predictive value of routine ultrasound in the clinical measurement of early pregnancy wastage. 12th World Congress on Fertility and Sterility, Singapore (Abstract), p 624

deCrespigny L (1988) Early diagnosis of pregnancy failure with transvaginal ultrasound. Am J Obstet Gynecol 159:408–409

den Ouden M, Cohen-Overbeek TE, Wladimiroff JW (1990) Uterine and fetal umbilical artery flow velocity waveforms in normal first trimester pregnancies. Br J Obstet Gynaecol 97:716–719

Deutinger J, Rudelstorfer R, Bernaschek G (1988) Vaginosonographic velicometry of both main uterine arteries by visual vessel recognition and pulsed doppler method during pregnancy. Am J Obstet Gynecol 159:1072–1076

Dickey RP, Olar TT, Curole DN, Taylor SN, Rye PH, Matulich EM (1990) The probability of multiple births when multiple gestational sacs or viable embryos are diagnosed at first trimester ultrasound. Hum Reprod 5:880–882

Evans J (1991) Fetal crown rump length values in the first trimester based upon ovulation timing using the luteenizing hormone surge. Br J Obstet Gynaecol 98:45–51

Ferrazzi E, Brambati B, Lanzani A, Oldrini A, Stripparo L, Guerneri S, Makowski EL (1988) The yolk sac in early pregnancy failure. Am J Obstet Gynecol 158:137–142

Farquhar CM, Rae T, Thomas DC, Wadsworth J, Beard RW (1989) Doppler ultrasound in the non pregnant pelvis. J Ultrasound Med 8:451–457

Goldstein SR, Subramanyan BR, Raghavendra BN, Horii SC, Hilton S (1983) Subchorionic bleeding in threatened abortion. AJR 141:975–978

Green JJ, Hobbins JC (1988) Abdominal ultrasound examination of the first trimester fetus. Am J Obstet Gynecol 159:165–167

Grudzinskas JG, Chard T (1991) Endocrinology and metabolism in early pregnancy. In: Chapman M, Grudzinskas JG, Chard T (eds) The embryo. Normal and abnormal development and growth. Springer-Verlag, London, pp 195–207

Harris RD, Vincent LM, Askin FB (1988) Yolk sac calcification: a sonographic finding associated with intrauterine embryonic demise in the first trimester. Radiol 166:109–110

Hertz RH, Sokol RJ, Knoke JD, Rosen MG, Chik L, Hirsch VJ (1978) Clinical estimation of gestational age: rules for avoiding preterm delivery. Am J Obstet Gynecol 139:500–506

Jaffe R, Warsoff SL (1991) Transvaginal colour doppler imaging in the assessment of uteroplacental blood flow in the normal first trimester pregnancy. Am J Obstet Gynecol 164:781–785

Jauniaux E, Jurkovic D, Campbell S (1991) In vivo investigations of the anatomy and the physiology of early human placental circulations. Ultrasound Obstet Gynaecol 1:435–445

Jones HW, Acosta AA, Andrews MC et al. (1983) What is pregnancy? A question for in vitro fertilization. Fertil Steril 40:728–733

Jouppila P (1983) Clinical consequences after ultrasonic diagnosis of intrauterine haematoma in threatened abortion. J Clin Ultrasound 13:107–111

Jurkovic D, Jauniaux E, Kurjak A, Hustin J, Campbell S, Nicolaides KH (1991) Transvaginal color doppler assessment of the uteroplacental circulation in early pregnancy. Obstet Gynecol 77:365–369

Jurkovic D, Bourne TH, Jauniaux E, Campbell S, Collins WP (1992) Transvaginal colour doppler study of blood flow in ectopic pregnancies. Am J Obstet Gynecol, In Press.

Klopper A, Ahmed AG (1985) New applications for the assay of placental proteins. Placenta 6:173–184

Laboda LA, Estroff JA, Benacerraf BR (1989) First trimester bradycardia: a sign of impending fetal loss. J Ultrasound Med 8:561–563

Lasser D, Vollebergh J, Peisner DB, Sharma S, Timor-Tritsch IE (1990) First trimester fetal biometry using high frequency transvaginal ultrasound. Abstract #1114 Proceedings 34th Annual Convention of the American Institute for Ultrasound in Medicine, JUM 9:S41

Levi CS, Lyons EA, Lindsay DJ (1988) Early diagnosis of non viable pregnancy with endovaginal ultrasound. Radiol 167:383–385

Levi CS, Lyons EA, Zheng XH, Lindsay DJ, Holt SC (1990) Endovaginal ultrasound demonstration of cardiac activity in embryos of less than 5 mm in crown rump length. Radiol 176:71–74

MacGregor SN, Tamura RK, Sabbagha RE, Minogue JP, Gibson ME, Hoffman DI (1987) Underestimation of gestational age by conventional crown rump length dating curves. Obstet Gynecol 70:344–348

Mantoni M, Pedersen JF (1981) Intrauterine haematomata. An ultrasound study of threatened abortion. Br J Obstet Gynaecol 88:47–51

Mantoni M, Pedersen JF (1982) Fetal growth delay in threatened abortion: an ultrasound study. Br J Obstet Gynaecol 89:525–527

Mantoni M (1985) Ultrasound signs in threatened abortion and their prognostic significance. Obstet Gynecol 65:471–475

Matta W, Stabile I, Shaw B, Campbell S (1988) Doppler assessment of uterine blood flow changes in patients with fibroids receiving the LHRH agonist buserelin. Fertil Steril 49:1083–1085

Mayden KL, Confino E, Miller CE, Friberg J, Gleicher N (1986) Decreased gestational sac volumes in pregnancies induced by human menopausal gonadotrophin. Fertil Steril 45:879–882

McKensie WE, Holmes DS, Newton JR (1988) Spontaneous abortion rate in ultrasonographically viable pregnancies. Obstet Gynecol 71:81–83

Meegdes BHLM, Ingenhoes R, Peeters LLH, Exalto N (1988) Early pregnancy wastage: relationship between chorionic vascularisation and embryonic development. Fertil Steril 49:216–219

Mehalek KE, Rosenberg J, Berkowitz GS, Chitkara U, Berkowitz RL (1989) Umbilical and uterine artery flow velocity waveforms: Effect of sampling site on doppler ratios. J Ultrasound Med 8:171–176

Moore KL (1982) The developing human: clinically oriented embryology, 3rd edn. WB Saunders, Philadelphia

Nyberg D, Mack L, Benedetti T (1987) Placental abruption and placental hemorrhage. Correlation of sonographic findings with fetal outcome. Radiol 164:357–359

Nyberg DA, Mack LA, Harvey D, Wang K (1988) Value of the yolk sac in evaluating early pregnancies. J Ultrasound Med 7:129–135

Pedersen JF, Molsted-Pedersen L, Mortensen HB (1984) Fetal growth delay and maternal haemoglobin Alc in early diabetic pregnancy. Obstet Gynecol 64:351–354

Pedersen JF, Mantoni M (1990) Large intrauterine haematomata in threatened miscarriage. Frequency and clinical consequences. Br J Obstet Gynaecol 97:75–77

Pennell RG, Needleman L, Pajak T, Baltarowich O, Vilaro M, Goldbeg BB, Kurtz AB (1990) Prospective comparison of vaginal and abdominal sonography in normal early pregnancy. J Ultrasound Med 10:63–67

Pijenborg R, Dixon G, Robertson WB, Brosens I (1980) Trophoblast invasion of human decidua from 8 to 18 weeks of pregnancy. Placenta 1:3–19

Pirrone E, Monteagudo A, Timor Tritsch IE (1990) Does blighted ovum really exist? Abstract #1116 Proceedings 34th Annual Convention of the American Institute for Ultrasound in Medicine, JUM 9:S41

Reece EA, Scioscia AL, Pinter E, Hobbins JC, Green J, Mahoney MJ, Naftolin F (1988) Prognostic significance of the human yolk sac assessed by ultrasonography. Am J Obstet Gynecol 159:1191–1194

Regan L, Braude PR, Trembath PL (1989) Influence of past reproductive performance on risk of spontaneous abortion. Br Med J 299:541–545

Rempen A (1990) Diagnosis of viability in early pregnancy with vaginal sonography. J Ultrasound Med 9:711–716

Robinson HP (1972) Sonar in the management of abortion. J Obstet Gynaecol Br Cwlth 79:90–94

Robinson HP, Shaw-Dunn J (1973) Fetal heart rates as determined by sonar in early pregnancy. J Obstet Gynaecol Br Cwlth 80:805–809

Robinson HP (1975a) Gestational sac volumes as determined by sonar in the first trimester of pregnancy. Br J Obstet Gynaecol 82:100–107

Robinson HP (1975b) The diagnosis of early pregnancy failure by sonar. Br J Obstet Gynaecol 82:849–857

Robinson HP, Fleming JE (1975) A critical evaluation of sonar crown rump length measurements. Br J Obstet Gynaecol 82:702–707

Rosen GF, Silva PD, Patrizio P, Asch RH, Yee B (1990) Predicting pregnancy outcome by the observation of a gestational sac or of early fetal cardiac motion with transvaginal ultrasonography. Fertil Steril 54:260–265

Schaaps JP, Soyeur D (1989) Pulsed doppler on a vaginal probe: Necessity, convenience or luxury? J Ultrasound Med 8:315–320

Schats R, Jansen CAM Wladimiroff JW (1990a) Embryonic heart activity: appearance and development in early human pregnancy. Br J Obstet Gynaecol 97:989–994

Schats R, Jansen CAM, Wladimiroff JW (1990b) Abnormal embryonic heart rate pattern in early pregnancy associated with Down's syndrome. Hum Reprod 5:877–879

Schneider L, Bessis R, Simonnet T (1979) The frequency of ovular resorption during the first trimester of twin pregnancy. Acta Genet Med Gemellol 28:271–272

Shenker L, Astle C, Reed K (1986) Embryonic heart rates before the seventh week of pregnancy. J Reprod Med 31:333–336

Stabile I (1988) Pregnancy associated plasma protein A in complications of early pregnancy with particular reference to ectopic gestation. Ph.D. Thesis, University of London

Stabile I (1991) Anembryonic pregnancy. In: Chapman M, Grudzinskas JG, Chard T (eds.) The embryo. Normal and abnormal development and growth. Springer-Verlag, London, pp 35–43

Stabile I, Campbell S, Grudzinskas (1987) Ultrasonic assessment of complications during first trimester of pregnancy. Lancet ii:1237–1240

Stabile I, Bilardo C, Panella M, Campbell S, Grudzinskas JG (1988) Doppler measurement of uterine blood flow in the first trimester of normal and complicated pregnancies. Troph Res 3:301–307

Stabile I, Campbell S, Grudzinskas (1989a) Ultrasound and circulating placental protein measurements in complications of early pregnancy. Br J Obstet Gynaecol 96:1182–1191

Stabile I, Campbell S, Grudzinskas (1989b) Threatened miscarriage and intrauterine hematomas: Sonographic and biochemical studies. J Ultrasound Med 8:289–292

Stabile I, Olajide F, Chard T, Grudzinskas JG (1989c) Maternal serum alphafetoprotein levels in anembryonic pregnancy. Hum Reprod 4:204–205

Stabile I, Campbell S, Grudzinskas (1989d) Doppler assessed uteroplacental blood flow impedance in the first trimester: physiological variation with site of measurement. J Obstet Gynaecol 9:177–179

Stabile I, Campbell S, Grudzinskas (1990a) Doppler assessed uteroplacental blood flow in normal and failed first trimester pregnancy. In: Echocardiography: A review of cardiovascular ultrasound 6:353–356

Stabile I, Grudzinskas JG, Campbell S (1990b) Doppler ultrasonographic evaluation of abnormal pregnancies in the first trimester. J Clin Ultrasound 18:497–501

Steer CV, Campbell S, Pampiglione JS, Kingsland CR, Mason BA, Collins WP (1990) Transvaginal colour flow imaging of the uterine arteries during the ovarian and menstrual cycles. Hum Reprod 5:391–395

Taylor KJW, Ramos IM, Feyock AL, Snower DP, Carter D, Shapiro BS, Meyer WR, deCherney AH (1989) Ectopic pregnancy: duplex doppler evaluation. Radiol 173:93–97

Thaler I, Manor D, Itskovitz J, Rottem S, Levit N, Timor-Tritsch IE, Brandes JM (1990) Changes in uterine blood flow during human pregnancy. Am J Obstet Gynecol 162:121–125

Timor Tritsch IE, Rottem S, Thaler I (1988) Review of transvaginal sonography: a description with clinical application. Ultrasound Quarterly 8:1–34

Varma TR (1981) The implication of a low implantation of the placenta detected by ultrasonography in early pregnancy. Acta Obstet Gynecol Scand 60:265–268

Yeh HC, Goodman JD, Carr L, Rabinowitz JG (1986) Intradecidual sign: an ultrasound criterion of early intrauterine pregnancy. Radiol 161:463–467

Ylostalo P, Ammala P, Seppala M (1984) Intrauterine haematoma and placental protein 5 in patients with uterine bleeding during pregnancy. Br J Obstet Gynaecol 91:353–356

.

6. Assessment of Early Pregnancy: Measurement of Fetoplacental Hormones and Proteins

J. G. Grudzinskas and T. Chard

The human fetus and placenta, and the surrounding maternal endometrium, secrete a wide range of products which may be "specific" in the sense that they are present in much higher levels than in non-pregnant women. The products (Table 6.1) appear in maternal blood, urine and amniotic fluid. Their measurement in these sites provides useful biological and clinical information on the state of a pregnancy (Chard and Klopper 1982; Chard and Grudzinskas 1987; Grudzinskas et al. 1988). This chapter deals with the clinical biochemistry of these substances in the first trimester.

Table 1. Major fetal trophoblast and decidual proteins identified in early pregnancy

Fetal
Alphafetoprotein (AFP)
Fetal antigen 1 (FA–1)
Fetal antigen 2 (FA–2)

Trophoblast
Human chorionic gonadotrophin (hCG)
Schwangerschaftsprotein 1 (SP1)
Human placental lactogen (hPL)
Pregnancy-associated plasma protein A (PAPP–A)
Placental protein 5 (PP5)

Decidual or endometrial
Insulin-like growth factor binding protein (IGF–BP; α-1 PEG; PP12; α-1 PAMG)
Progesterone-dependent endometrial protein (PEP; α-2 PEG; PP14; α-2 CMG; α-2 PAMG; AUP)

Diagnosis of Pregnancy

Early diagnosis of pregnancy typically depends on the detection of human chorionic gonadotrophin (hCG) in maternal urine, or 1–2 days earlier in blood as the test becomes positive shortly after the time of implantation. Claims for earlier detection of human pregnancy by measurement of an "early pregnancy factor" have not been substantiated (Chard and Grudzinskas 1987). As highly specific and sensitive immunometric assays have shown the ubiquitous nature of hCG at low concentrations (<15 IU/l), in clinical practice a single estimation of hCG should only be considered definitive if it is greater than 25 IU/l or if a lower level of hCG is seen to increase twofold at an interval of 3 days (Jones et al. 1983). When hCG has been administered therapeutically, estimations should be delayed until clearance of the exogenous hCG has occurred, i.e., a delay of up to 14 days. Under these circumstances assays for other placental proteins such as Schwangerschaftsprotein (SP1) (Grudzinskas et al. 1977) may be appropriate. Other proteins associated with pregnancy, such as human placental lactogen (hPL), pregnancy-associated plasma protein A (PAPP-A) and placental protein 5 (PP5), are not candidates for diagnostic tests since the rise in maternal blood cannot be easily identified until after 6 weeks of amenorrhoea. Finally, positive hCG values found immediately after implantation should be interpreted with care as at this stage many pregnancies may be diagnosed which subsequently abort (Chard 1991).

Normal Pregnancy

Chorionic gonadotrophin and other trophoblast products might be produced by the blastocyst prior to implantation. However, significant amounts are secreted into the maternal circulation only after the trophoblast makes direct contact with maternal synthesis in the course of implantation. There is no obvious trigger for the synthesis of hCG, or for compounds such as SP1, PAPP-A, hPL and PP5. Production of these substances appears to be a function of the trophoblast with no obvious control or feedback mechanisms of the type which are usually seen in adult endocrinology.

The trends in blood levels of SP1 seem to parallel the growth rate curve of functioning trophoblast (Grudzinskas et al. 1977) (Fig. 6.1). The synthesis of SP1, at least in the earlier weeks of pregnancy, is independent of the presence of an embryo as it is found in women with hydatidiform mole, and of the site of implantation as it is found in women with ectopic gestation. In normal pregnancy the doubling times for hCG and SP1 are equivalent: the concentrations of both double in 2–3 days in the first 6 weeks of pregnancy. The disappearance rate of SP1 and hCG after removal of trophoblast tissues is also similar (40–60 h). Blood levels of both hPL and PP5 increase as pregnancy advances, and have a relationship to functioning placental mass. PAPP-A can be detected in maternal blood 28 days after fertilisation, which is too late for use as an early diagnostic test for pregnancy (Chemnitz et al. 1986) (Fig. 6.2). PAPP-A levels increase throughout pregnancy with a doubling time of 4.9 days during the first trimester; the disappearance rate after removal of the placenta is several days (Sinosich 1985).

In the first 6 weeks of gestation the majority of steroid hormones (oestrogen and progesterone) required for the maintenance of the pregnancy is provided by the corpus luteum. Thereafter most steroid production is derived from the

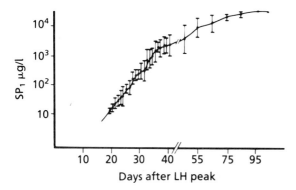

Fig. 6.1. Mean serum SP1 levels in nine women in the first trimester of normal pregnancy. (From Lenton et al. 1981, by permission from Acta Obstetrica et Gynecologica Scandinavica.)

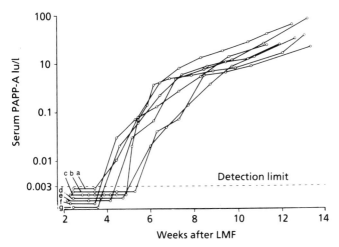

Fig. 6.2. Serum PAPP-A levels in seven women in the first trimester of normal pregnancy. (From Chemnitz et al. 1986, by permission from British Journal of Obstetrics and Gynaecology.)

fetoplacental unit. The production of AFP by embryonal endodermal tissues (principally the yolk sac) is reflected by an increase in circulating levels during the first trimester; increasing concentrations of AFP are detected in maternal blood after 10 weeks gestation (Olajide et al. 1989). Secretion of proteins of endo-metrial origin parallels the morphological changes in this tissue (Bell 1988). Placental protein 14, also known as progesterone-dependent endometrial pro-tein, which is derived from the glandular epithelium of the endometrium, has a pattern of blood levels in early pregnancy which bears a resemblance to hCG. By contrast, insulin-like growth factor binding protein (IGF-BP1; PP12), which originates in stromal cells of the gestational endometrium reaches peak levels in the second trimester (Wang et al. 1991).

Control of Synthesis and Secretion

The mechanisms which control the production of placental proteins are poorly understood; uteroplacental perfusion plays a major role, influencing synthesis and secretion by short-short feedback or mass action. Nevertheless, there may be effects from the ovary, the embryo and endometrium. Up to 6 weeks of gestation the ovary provides steroid support for the pregnancy. It also secretes a molecule (possibly relaxin) which is responsible for endometrial secretion of PP14. Thus, in donor pregnancies in women without ovaries (e.g., Turner's syndrome) the dramatic increase of PP14 levels seen in a normal pregnancy is largely absent (Critchley et al. 1990).

An embryo may not be essential, as evidenced by placental protein secretion in blighted ovum and hydatidiform mole. The exact site of implantation and the interaction between the trophoblast and gestational endometrium may also not be important factors for the normal secretion of the substances considered here, at least in the earliest days of pregnancy. Circulating placental proteins are consistently present in ectopic pregnancy, but often at concentrations lower than those observed in a normal pregnancy of the same gestation. The difference is particularly striking in the case of PAPP-A (reviewed by Stabile et al. (1988b)). There are also significant changes in placental protein synthesis in aneuploid pregnancies (see below) but the precise mechanism of these changes is uncertain (Chard and Grudzinskas 1991). In rare pregnancies there is total absence of a particular placental protein, due to gene deletion. This has been described for hPL, SP1, placental sulphatase, and PAPP-A. In the latter case the deficiency has been associated with the Cornelia de Lange syndrome in the child (Westergaard et al. 1983). In the case of hPL and SP1 deficiencies there is no obvious abnormality in either the mother or the child.

The control of endometrial protein synthesis is a combination of increased bulk of the tissue of origin (endometrial glands in the case of PP14; endometrial stroma in the case of IGF-BP1) and other factors. It was originally considered that progesterone was the main factor controlling PP14 synthesis. However, this now seems unlikely (Howell et al. 1989), although an ovarian factor is of undoubted importance (Critchley et al. 1990).

Early Pregnancy Failure

If a woman wishes to become pregnant, her chances of producing a viable offspring in any one ovarian cycle is approximately 25%. There have been many estimates of the frequency of early pregnancy failure, several based on studies on the transient appearance of hCG in association with a potentially fertile cycle.

Estimates of the incidence of this phenomenon vary from 8 to 55% (for review see Chard 1991).

Threatened and Spontaneous Miscarriage

Maternal blood levels of proteins and hormones of fetal, trophoblastic and maternal origin have been used to predict the outcome in women with vaginal bleeding in early pregnancy (Niven et al. 1972; Salem et al. 1984). In general, concentrations of placental products are reduced in association with threatened miscarriage in which the outcome is fetal loss, but normal in cases in which the pregnancy proceeds. As a clinical predictive tool, measurement of these compounds may be unnecessary if fetal life can be demonstrated by ultrasound (Stabile et al. 1987). Nevertheless, a proportion of patients in whom fetal heart action has been demonstrated will spontaneously abort. We have described blood levels of hPL, SP1, PAPP-A, progesterone, oestradiol, AFP and pregnancy-zone protein (PZP) in 108 women in whom the history and clinical findings were diagnostic of threatened abortion (Westergaard et al. 1985). Eleven patients showed a fetal heart action until miscarriage occurred. In this group, the predictive value of an abnormal level in the sample obtained at presentation was greatest for PAPP-A. All 11 women who had evidence of a live fetus but subsequently miscarried had depressed PAPP-A levels. The levels of the other substances generally remained within the normal limits.

Consequently it is possible to conclude: (1) if fetal heart action is not evident ultrasonically after 7 weeks gestation (gestational sac volumes >3 ml) then depressed levels of fetoplacental products will not provide any additional information; (2) spontaneous miscarriage after the detection of fetal heart action is extremely uncommon; in this small group the levels of hormones and proteins will be in the normal range, with the exception of low levels of PAPP-A.

Studies of women with apparently normal pregnancies at 6–10 weeks gestation (awaiting chorionic villus sampling for chromosomal abnormalities) have revealed depressed levels of serum AFP, PAPP-A, and to a lesser degree hCG, within 2–3 weeks of spontaneous miscarriage (Brambati, Grudzinskas and Chard, personal observations). Many of these fetuses may have had an abnormal karyotype: measurement of hormones and proteins in the first trimester may identify this particular group as do similar measurements in the second trimester (Wald et al. 1988).

Anembryonic Pregnancy

In some cases of miscarriage an embryo cannot be found. This condition can be diagnosed ultrasonically if a fetus is not apparent in a gestational sac of greater than 3 ml (7 weeks gestation) (Stabile et al. 1989). Levels of placental hormones and proteins are low or normal. Serum AFP levels are within the normal range in many patients with this condition, suggesting that an embryo has been present at some stage and that the term anembryonic pregnancy is in fact a misnomer (Stabile et al. 1989).

Mean blood levels of hCG have also been shown to be depressed at 4 weeks gestation in a group of patients studied prospectively at a subfertility clinic who subsequently were shown to have "blighted ovum"; mean levels of maternal PAPP-A, oestradiol and progesterone fell some 3 weeks later (Yovich et al. 1986). Regardless of the pathogenesis of this condition these findings confirm that a deviation from the normal rise in blood levels of hCG is highly suggestive of failed pregnancy at a time before ultrasound can provide useful information (i.e., in the absence of fetal heart action).

Ectopic Pregnancy

The principal value of biochemical tests in this condition, especially hCG, is to alert the clinician to the possibility of a pregnancy-related disorder, and to exclude such a disorder if a negative result (i.e., <25 IU/l) is obtained (Seppala et al. 1980). Stabile and her colleagues (1988a) have reported a sensitivity of 100% for estimations of hCG used in conjunction with abdominal ultrasound to make the diagnosis. Quantitative estimations of hCG may also be of some value, since depressed levels are commonly seen in ectopic gestation; in conjunction with ultrasonic examination, hCG can often distinguish between normal or failed intrauterine pregnancy and ectopic gestation (Pittaway et al. 1985). The use of a discriminatory zone for hCG together with ultrasound can also be useful. If levels of hCG are greater than 6500 IU/l, ultrasound examination should reveal the presence of a live embryo in utero; if this is not the case, failed pregnancy, in particular ectopic gestation, should be considered (Kadar 1983; Rottem and Timor-Tritsch 1988).

Similar findings have been reported with SP1 and PAPP-A, secretion of PAPP-A being more severely compromised (Chemnitz et al. 1984; Sinosich 1985). In one study PAPP-A levels were depressed in all 17 women with ectopic gestation, with PAPP-A being detected in only two women (Sinosich 1985). Stabile and her colleagues (1987) examined 60 women with proven ectopic pregnancy: circulating PAPP-A was detected in only 30 and levels were low in 24 women (Fig. 6.3). Levels of IGF-BP1 (PP12) were normal in this group (Stabile et al. 1990).

Westergaard and his colleagues (1988) noted depressed levels of progesterone, oestradiol and PP14 in the same group of women. They concluded that it was not possible to distinguish between failed intrauterine pregnancy and ectopic gestation by the measurement of serum hormones and proteins, but that it was possible to exclude ectopic pregnancy by these measurements. At the time of presentation the detection of hCG would alert the clinician to the possibility of a pregnancy-related condition. The finding of normal levels of progesterone or PAPP-A or PP14 would indicate a normal intrauterine pregnancy (Stabile et al. 1988c).

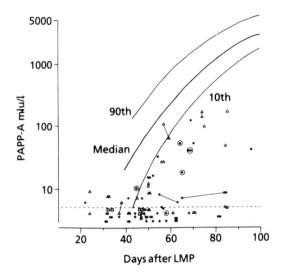

Fig. 6.3. Circulating PAPP-A levels in 60 women with ectopic gestation in relation to the normal range. The encircled symbols indicate that fetal tissue was identified. (From Stabile et al. 1988c, by permission from Springer-Verlag.)

Trophoblastic Disease

Trophoblast tissue in hydatidiform mole retains its ability to synthesise hormones and proteins; the capacity is reduced for hPL and steroids, but greater for hCG.

The risk of choriocarcinoma is higher in women with very high levels of hCG in gestational trophoblast tumours. In untreated hydatidiform mole, Tsakok et al. (1983) have noted reduced levels of PAPP-A prior to treatment and elevated levels of SP1 and PP5 (Fig. 6.4). High SP1 levels were found in a proportion of patients who developed subsequent malignant disease. Than and colleagues (1988) observed high serum concentrations of PP14 in patients prior to treatment for hydatidiform mole, falling rapidly after evacuation. Circulating PP14 was not seen in women with choriocarcinoma. In women with choriocarcinoma, serum SP1 levels are usually lower than in benign disease and circulating PP5 cannot be detected (Lee et al. 1981, 1982).

Prenatal Diagnosis: Chorionic Villus Sampling

Brambati and colleagues (1991) have made detailed studies on women scheduled for chorionic villus sampling (CVS) for diagnosis of chromosome abnormalities. Some of these patients miscarried spontaneously before the procedure, some after, while others had an ongoing pregnancy. Those who miscarried before CVS generally had lower levels of AFP, PAPP-A and hCG (Brambati, Chard, Grudzinskas, unpublished data). In most of these cases the fetus generally showed an abnormal karyotype. In 25 women with pregnancies complicated by aneuploidy which proceeded beyond 9 weeks, circulating SP1, PAPP-A and AFP

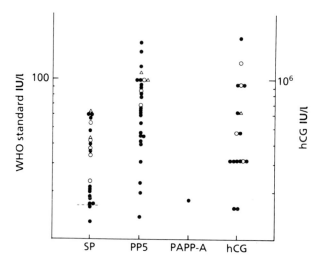

Fig. 6.4. Serum SP1, PP5, PAPP-A and hCG levels in 31 women with gestational trophoblastic disease before treatment: hydatidiform mole; choriocarcinoma, O = lung metastases, = - - - 16.5 IU/l WHO standard 78/610. Levels of SP1, PP5, PAPP-A <IU/l or hCG <100000 IU/l not shown. (From Tsakok et al. 1983, by permission from British Journal of Obstetrics and Gynaecology.)

levels were depressed in 50% of women when measured between 6 and 9 weeks of gestation. By contrast, serum progesterone and hCG levels were greater than the 5th centile of the normal range. The sensitivity of depressed AFP and SP1 levels was greatest for Down's syndrome (Brambati et al. 1991).

It is well-known that maternal serum AFP levels can show a substantial rise following invasive procedures in early pregnancy, notably amniocentesis (Chard et al. 1976), and surgical (Naik et al. 1988), or medical (Chard et al. 1990) termination. A similar phenomenon is seen after CVS (Knott et al. 1988; Ward et al. 1985). Ward et al. (1985) examined serum levels of AFP, hCG, SP1 and PAPP-A before and 6 h after chorionic villus sampling in 20 women. In the majority of cases AFP levels rose after sampling. Depressed or elevated pre-operative levels of AFP, hCG and PAPP-A were associated with fetal anomalies and pregnancy loss in 7 of the 11 pregnancies which did not progress. The two highest levels of hCG were seen in pregnancies in which the fetus was homozygous for α- or β-thalassaemia. Similar findings have been made for hPL and SP1 in pregnancies complicated by hydrops fetalis in late pregnancy (Bellman et al. 1980). There is no significant change in proteins and hormones of placental origin following CVS (Ward et al. 1985).

Conclusions

Detection of hCG is still the mainstay of the diagnosis of early pregnancy. When used in conjunction with ultrasound it can provide useful clinical information in the first 12 weeks of pregnancy.

After detection of the fetal heart at 6–7 weeks gestation, spontaneous miscarriage is uncommon. In some women with apparently normal pregnancies, but who will miscarry within a few weeks, depressed levels of hCG and PAPP-A have been reported. In women presenting with vaginal bleeding after 7 weeks gestation, if the fetal heart is seen, only PAPP-A estimations may predict the small group who will subsequently miscarry.

In women with suspected ectopic pregnancy detection of hCG confirms a pregnancy-related disorder. High serum levels of progesterone or PP14 may exclude this condition, while depressed levels of PAPP-A increase the likelihood of the diagnosis.

The identification of secretory proteins of the endometrium and decidua which can be measured in maternal blood suggests that IGF-BPI and PP14 are active rather than passive participants in reproductive function. However, the fact that pregnancy may proceed normally in the absence of any rise in PP14 concentrations suggests that this molecule does not have an essential role in the maintenance of an early pregnancy (Critchley et al. 1990). Since the endometrium produces proteins and hormones which act both locally and systemically, it is possible to consider this tissue as an endocrine organ. The ability to measure these substances, in particular IGF-BP1 and PP14, may provide both a non-invasive test of endometrial function in the assessment of fertility and an index of endometrial and decidual function in the earliest days of pregnancy.

Many fetuses in pregnancies which will fail in the first trimester have an abnormal karyotype. It is possible the hormone and protein measurements at this time may identify these particular patients as is the case in the second trimester.

References

Bell SC (1988) Synthesis and secretion of proteins by the endometrium and decidua. In: Chapman MG, Grudzinskas JG, Chard T (eds) Implantations. Springer-Verlag, London, pp 95–108

Bellman O, Tebbe J, Lang N, Baur MP (1980) Determination of SP1 and hPL for predicting perinatal asphyxia. In: Klopper A, Genazzani A, Crosignani PG (eds) The human placenta: proteins and hormones. Academic Press, London, pp 99–108

Brambati B, Lanzani A, Tului L (1991) Ultrasound and biochemical assessments of first trimester pregnancy. In: Chapman M, Grudzinskas JG, Chard T (eds) The embryo. Springer-Verlag, London, pp 181–194

Chard T (1991) Frequency of implantation of early pregnancy loss in natural cycles. In: Baillière's Clinical Obstetrics and Gynaecology. Baillière-Tindall, London, vol 5, pp 179–189

Chard T, Grudzinskas JG (1987) Early pregnancy factor. Biol Res Preg 8:53–56

Chard T, Grudzinskas JG (1991) The endocrinology of the fetoplacental unit in the second trimester of pregnancy. In: Chapman M, Grudzinskas JG, Chard T (eds) The embryo. Springer-Verlag, London, pp 209–226

Chard T, Klopper A (1982) Placental function tests. Springer-Verlag, Berlin

Chard T, Kitau MJ, Ledward R, Coltart T, Embury S, Seller MJ (1976) Elevated levels of maternal plasma alpha-fetoprotein after amniocentesis. Br J Obstet Gynaec 83:33–34

Chard T, Olajide F, Kitau M (1990) Changes in circulating alphafetoprotein following administration of mifepristone in first trimester pregnancy. Br J Obstet Gynaec 97:1030–1032

Chemnitz J, Folkersen J, Teisner B (1986) Comparison of different antibody preparations against pregnancy-associated plasma protein A (PAPP-A) for use in localisation and immunoassay studies. Br J Obstet Gynaec 93:111–118

Chemnitz J, Tornehave D, Teisner B, Poulsen HK, Westergaard JG (1984) The localisation of pregnancy proteins (hPL, SP1 and PAPP-A) in intra- and extrauterine pregnancies. Placenta 5:489–494

Critchley HOD, Chard T, Lieberman BA, Buckley CH, Anderson DC (1990) Serum PP14 levels in a patient with Turner's syndrome pregnancy after frozen embryo transfer. Hum Reprod 5:250–254

Grudzinskas JG, Gordon YB, Jeffrey D, Chard T (1977) Specific and sensitive determination of pregnancy specific beta-1 glycoprotein by radioimmunoassay. Lancet i:333–335

Grudzinskas JG, Stabile I, Campbell S (1988) Early pregnancy failure: biochemical and biophysical assessment. In: Beard RW, Sharp F (eds) Early pregnancy loss: mechanisms and treatment. RCOG, London, pp 183–190

Howell RJS, Olajide F, Telsner B, Grudzinskas JG, Chard T (1989) Circulating levels of placental protein 14 and progesterone following mifepristone (RU38486) and gemeprost for termination of first trimester pregnancy. Fertil Steril 52:66–68

Jones HW, Acosta AA, Andrews MC et al. (1983) What is pregnancy? A question for in vitro fertilisation. Fertil Steril 40:728–733

Kadar N (1983) Ectopic pregnancy. In: Studd J (ed) Progress in obstetrics and gynaecology, Vol 3. Edinburgh. Churchill Livingstone, pp 305–323

Knott PD, Chan B, Ward RHT, Chard T, Grudzinskas JG, Petrou M, Modell B (1988) Changes in circulating alphafetoprotein and human chorionic gonadotrophin following chorionic villus sampling. Eur J Obstet Gynec Reprod Biol 27:277–281

Lee JN, Salem HT, Al-Ani ATM, Chard T (1981) Circulating concentrations of specific proteins (human chorionic gonadotrophin, pregnancy-specific beta-1 glycoprotein and placental protein 5) in untreated gestation trophoblastic tumours. Am J Obstet Gynec 39:702–704

Lee JN, Salem HT, Chard T, Huang SC, Ouyang PC (1982) Circulating placental proteins (hCG, SP1 and PP5) in trophoblastic disease. Br J Obstet Gynaec 89:69–72

Lenton EA, Grudzinskas JG, Gordon YB, Chard T, Cooke LD (1981) Pregnancy specific β, glycoprotein and chorionic gonadotrophin in early pregnancy. Acta Obstet Gynecol Scand 60:489–492

Naik K, Kitau M, Setchell ME, Chard T (1988) The incidence of fetomaternal haemorrhage following elective termination of first trimester pregnancy. Europ J Obstet Gynec Reprod Biol 27:355–357

Niven PAR, Landon J, Chard T (1972) Placental lactogen levels as a guide to outcome of threatened abortion. Br Med J iii:799–801

Olajide F, Kitau MJ, Chard (1989) Maternal serum AFP levels in the first trimester of pregnancy. Europ J Obstet Gynec Reprod Biol 30:123–128

Pittaway DE, Wentz AC, Maxon WS, Herbert C, Daniell HJ, Fleischer AC (1985) The efficacy of early pregnancy monitoring with serial chorionic gonadotrophin determinations and realtime ultrasonography in an infertile population. Fertil Steril 44:190–194

Rottem S, Timor-Tritsch IE (1988) In: Timor-Tritsch IE, Rottem S (eds) Transvaginal ultrasonography. Heinemann Medical Books, London, pp 125–142

Salem HT, Ghaneimah SA, Shaaban MM, Chard T (1984) Prognostic value of biochemical tests in the assessment of fetal outcome in threatened abortion. Br J Obstet Gynaec 91:382–385

Seppala M, Rantaa T, Tontti K, Stenman UH, Chard T (1980) Use of a rapid hCG-beta-subunit radioimmunoassay in acute gynaecological emergencies. Lancet i:165–166

Sinosich MJ (1985) Biological role of pregnancy-associated plasma protein A in human reproduction. In Bischof P, Klopper A (eds) Proteins of the placenta. Karger, Basel, pp. 158–184

Stabile I, Grudzinskas JG, Campbell S (1987) Ultrasonic assessment of complications during first trimester of pregnancy. Lancet ii:1237–1240

Stabile I, Campbell S, Grudzinskas JG (1988a) Can ultrasound reliably diagnose ectopic pregnancy? Br J Obstet Gynaec 95:1247–1252

Stabile I, Grudzinskas JG, Chard T (1988b) Clinical applications of pregnancy protein estimations with particular reference to pregnancy-associated plasma protein A (PAPP-A). Obstet Gynec Surv 43:73–82

Stabile I, Westergaard JG, Grudzinskas JG (1988c) Ectopic pregnancy: diagnostic aspects. In: Chapman MG, Grudzinskas JG, Chard T (eds) Implantation: biological and clinical aspects. Springer-Verlag, London, pp 229–238

Stabile I, Olajide F, Grudzinskas JG (1989) Maternal serum alphafetoprotein levels in anembryonic pregnancy. Hum Reprod 4:204–205

Stabile I, Teisner B, Chard T, Grudzinskas JG (1990) Circulating levels of placental protein 12 in ectopic pregnancy. Arch Gynec Obstet 247:149–153

Than GN, Tatra G, Szabo DG, Osaba K, Bohutt E (1988) Beta lactoglobulin homologue placental protein 14 (PP14) in serum of patients with trophoblastic disease and non-trophoblastic gynaecological pregnancy. Arch Gynaec 243:131–137

Tsakok FTM, Koh M, Ratnam SS et al. (1983) Pregnancy associated proteins in trophoblastic disease. Br J Obstet Gynaec 90;483–486

Wald MJ, Cuckle HS, Densem W, Nanchahal K, Royston P, Chard T et al. (1988) Maternal screening for Down's syndrome in early pregnancy. Br Med J ii:883–887

Wang HS, Perry LA, Kanisius J, Iles RK, Holly JMP, Chard T (1991) Purification and assay of insulin-like growth factor-binding protein-1: measurement of circulating levels throughout pregnancy. J Endocrinol 128:161–168

Ward RHT, Grudzinskas JG, Bolton AE et al. (1985) Fetoplacental products as a prognostic guide following chorionic villus sampling. In: Fraccaro M, Simoni G, Brambati B (eds) First trimester diagnosis. Springer-Verlag, Berlin, pp 73–76

Westergaard JG, Chemnitz J, Teisner B et al. (1983) Pregnancy-associated plasma protein A – A possible marker in the classification and diagnosis of Cornelia de Lange syndrome. Prenat Diag 3:225–232

Westergaard JG, Teisner B, Sinosich MJ, Masden LT, Grudzinskas JG (1985) Does ultrasound examination render biochemical tests obsolete in the prediction of early pregnancy failure. Br J Obstet Gynaec 92:77–83

Westergaard JG, Teisner B, Stabile I, Grudzinskas JG (1988) Ectopic pregnancy: diagnostic: aspects. In: Tomoda S, Mizutani S, Narita O, Klopper A (eds) Endometrial and placental proteins: basis concepts and clinical applications. International Science Publishers, The Netherlands, pp 615–622

Yovich JL, McColin JC, Willcox DL, Grudzinskas JG, Bolton AE (1986) The prognostic value of beta hCG, PAPP-A, oestradiol and progesterone in early human pregnancies and the effect of medroxy progesterone acetate. Aust NZ J Obstet Gynaec 26:59–64

7. The Aetiology and Management of Recurrent Miscarriage

Lesley Regan

Introduction

The term "recurrent miscarriage" implies that repeated episodes of early pregnancy loss have a unique cause but this need not be so. A single underlying cause is likely in a proportion of women only, since sporadic miscarriage is the commonest complication of pregnancy and approximately 25% of all women who become pregnant will experience one or more pregnancy losses (Warburton and Fraser 1964). The distinction between recurrent abortions from a single persisting cause and repeated abortions from different causes is difficult. However, there do seem to be factors distinguishing some women with repeated abortion from others, suggesting that in addition to random causes, in a proportion of cases specific components are involved and that "recurrent miscarriage" is a distinct clinical entity.

The clinical management of patients presenting with recurrent miscarriage presents the patient and her doctor with a distressing and frustrating dilemma. There are inconsistencies in the terminology used and an absence of generally accepted figures for the number of individuals affected. The aetiology must be multifactorial, since the clinical presentation is so variable, ranging from early occult failures of implantation to overt miscarriages in the first and second trimester of pregnancy. But even after careful investigation a cause can only be identified in a minority of cases, hence treatment is usually empirical. The results of such treatment regimens are necessarily inconclusive.

In this account primary recurrent spontaneous abortion will be defined as the consecutive loss of three pregnancies before 20 weeks gestation and secondary recurrent spontaneous abortion as the consecutive loss of three pregnancies after the delivery of a live child.

Incidence

The incidence of recurrent miscarriage in the population has not been precisely determined. It has been estimated that the problem affects up to 0.5% of all couples (Javert 1957; Stenchever 1980), but the definition of recurrent miscarriage is not always comparable. Some authors have studied only those couples with three or more spontaneous abortions (Glass and Golbus 1978; Stray-Pedersen and Stray-Pedersen 1984), whereas others have included couples with two pregnancy losses (Tho et al. 1979; Byrd et al. 1977; Poland et al. 1977; Harger et al. 1983; Fitzsimmons et al. 1983).

If it is assumed that the incidence of spontaneous abortion in any pregnancy is 15%, and that the risk of abortion is the same for all couples, the statistical risk of a woman experiencing two successive abortions should be 2% and the chance of three successive abortions should be 0.34% (Huisjes 1984), which is not dissimilar to the empirical figure of 0.5% quoted earlier. Observed frequencies appear to be higher (0.8%–1%) (Alberman 1988) suggesting that in a proportion of cases there may be a persistent cause, and that some couples are at increased risk. Evidence supporting this argument is derived from two sources. The first is that the risk of a subsequent abortion increases with the number of previous abortions experienced, or with characteristics of the index abortion such as karyotype, gestation or morphology. The second is evidence from studies demonstrating that the reproductive characteristics of "repeaters" and "non-repeaters" differ significantly. For example, a history of premature deliveries, low birthweight infants, episodes of subfertility and a family history of miscarriage is found commonly among women experiencing recurrent miscarriages (Strobino et al. 1986; Regan 1989) and confers a poor prognosis for future pregnancy outcome.

The Risk of Recurrence

The literature is replete with studies attempting to quantify a woman's risk of miscarriage after her first, second, third or subsequent pregnancy loss. The results vary widely because they are directly dependent on the population sample studied and the method of data analysis employed. A retrospective hospital-based study design in which a declared pregnancy forms the basis for recruitment has the advantage of accumulating large amounts of data quickly. However, such a study will only include pregnancies that have reached the gestational age required for entry and are likely to under-represent the contribution of early miscarriages. The much cited study of Warburton and Fraser (1964) attempted to minimise this bias by excluding the recruitment pregnancy of over 2000 women referred to a medical genetics unit after the delivery of a live-born child, and considering for analysis only previous pregnancies. This study concluded that the risk of a further abortion after one, two or three previous abortions was 23.7%, 26.2% and 32.2% respectively. However, these figures included all women who had experienced previous abortions, whether or not a successful pregnancy had intervened and since recruitment was dependent on the woman having achieved a viable pregnancy, "abortion-only" sequences were selected out.

Similar risk figures were later reported by Naylor and Warburton (1979) who analysed 14 000 pregnancy histories and took into consideration both the number of previous abortions and the sequence of abortions and live births. Although the overall risk of abortion after three or more abortions was 33.3%, amongst the 51 histories with three consecutive abortions the risk of a further abortion was 45%. Those retrospective studies which considered women with three consecutive abortions, have recorded higher recurrence risk figures (Macnaughton (1964)– 58%; Poland et al. (1977)–47%). Moreover the risk of a further abortion was higher in women who had never had a successful pregnancy (primary aborters) than in those who had achieved a viable pregnancy in the past (secondary aborters). In a review of all the available studies, the risk of miscarriage following three previous pregnancy losses varied from 20%–70% (Regan 1988). This disparity has important clinical implications, since the prognosis for future pregnancy outcome is not clear.

The ideal study recruits non-pregnant women of reproductive age and prospectively observes their subsequent pregnancies. Prospective studies that recruit patients who are already pregnant are strongly influenced by the special interests of the clinician to whom they are referred. Further bias may be introduced either by the exclusion of early abortions not requiring medical intervention, or alternatively by exaggerating the incidence of loss, unless women who present with symptoms of threatened miscarriage or who abort within a short interval after entry to the study are excluded.

The Cambridge early pregnancy loss study was designed to exclude most of these biases and had three aims: (1) to determine the incidence of miscarriage in a well-documented population recruited before pregnancy; (2) to identify factors predisposing to miscarriage; and (3) to assess the risk of recurrent miscarriage (Regan et al. 1989). The prospective study design ensured that all early clinical abortions were reported and since all women in this catchment area received antenatal care at a single hospital, complete data collection for all the study recruits was achieved. The overall incidence of early loss of pregnancy in this study was 12% (50/407 pregnancies). No significant associations between the risk of spontaneous abortion and social class, smoking habit, drug ingestion, contraceptive usage, previous termination of pregnancy or past medical history were found. Most importantly, this study demonstrated that a woman's risk of miscarriage can be quantified by examining her past obstetric history, the single most important predictive factor being a previous miscarriage. A summary of the results is shown in Table 7.1, which documents the percentage risk of abortion categorised by reproductive history. This table should be useful in counselling patients who have miscarried recently. The risk of abortion for those women who had only ever aborted was noted to increase cumulatively as the number of abortions increased from one (20%) to two (28%) and reached 43% after three consecutive pregnancy losses.

In conclusion there is an increased risk of abortion after a previous abortion, although the likelihood of a successful pregnancy following three previous abortions is approximately 60%, which leads many clinicians to question whether the implementation of any treatment is justifiable. However, expectant management for the patient who has undergone repeated pregnancy losses is rarely acceptable, and the doctor is frequently pushed into investigating and implement-

Table 7.1. Effect of reproductive history upon the risk of miscarriage (n=407)

History	No. of patients miscarrying	Total no. of patients	% Risk of miscarriage in study pregnancy
Last pregnancy miscarried	40	214	19
Only miscarriages in past	24	98	24
Only pregnancy miscarried	12	59	20
Last pregnancy successful	5	95	5
All pregnancies successful	3	73	4
Only pregnancy successful	3	62	5
Previous termination of pregnancy	2	32	6
Primigravidae	4	87	5

ing treatment in a patient for whom no cause for the repeated losses can be demonstrated, and it may be argued, has been statistically unlucky. This point has been illustrated repeatedly over the last couple of decades by the public demand for any proposed "new" treatment option, a factor which frequently prevents the completion of adequately controlled clinical trials.

Aetiology of Recurrent Miscarriage

The relative importance of genetic, anatomical, infective, endocrine and immunological abnormalities in the aetiology of recurrent miscarriage has proved difficult to establish. In most series, small patient numbers have prevented statistical analysis and frequently reflect the bias of the clinicians concerned. The following section therefore attempts to put forward the evidence for and against the various causes of recurrent abortion and emphasises the lack of data available in several areas.

Genetic Causes

In addition to the established contribution that chromosomal abnormalities of the fetus make to sporadic miscarriage, they are also a cause of recurrent miscarriage. They may be due to recurrent aneuploidy or parental chromosome abnormalities (Verp and Simpson 1985). The risk of spontaneous abortion increases with the number of previous abortions and the magnitude of risk is affected by the karyotype of the abortion. Couples who have a chromosomally normal abortion typically have had more previous abortions and fetal losses (Hassold et al. 1980). They also run a higher risk of having another abortion than couples having an abortion with abnormal karyotype (Boué et al. 1975; Lauritsen 1976). These observations suggest that chromosomally normal abortions are less random than abnormal ones. Studies in which two consecutive abortuses have been karyotyped have shown a trend towards both abortuses being karyotypically normal or both karyotypically abnormal (Kajii and Ferrier 1978; Lauritsen 1976; Simpson and Bombard 1987), although the type of abnormality need not be the same (Boué and Boué 1973).

Balanced translocations are usually detected when cytogenic studies are performed in couples who have repeated abortions or a live-born child with a congenital malformation (Sachs et al. 1985; Adamoli et al. 1986). Overall, the frequency of balanced translocations in couples with a history of two or more abortions is about 3%–5% (Simpson et al. 1981), but the prevalence in couples with a history heavily weighted with congenital defects can be as high as 30% (Byrd et al. 1977; Stenchever et al. 1977). Couples whose abortions have all occurred in the first trimester of pregnancy have an increased frequency of balanced translocations when compared to couples with second trimester losses (Schwartz and Palmer 1983). Women are twice as likely as men to show a translocation, since structural abnormalities of chromosomes in males may be associated with sterility (Lippman-Hand and Vekemans 1983; Simpson and Bombard 1987). If chromosomal variants are included, the incidence of chromosomal abnormalities in couples with repeated abortions increases to 5%–10% (Simpson 1980; Schwartz and Palmer 1983; Campana et al. 1986). Pericentric inversions occur in about 1% of the population and are usually considered to be a normal variant. The frequency of inversions among couples with recurrent abortion varies from normal (Simpson et al. 1981) to 4%–5% (Tibiletti et al. 1981).

Anatomical Causes

The incidence of all congenital uterine anomalies in women with recurrent abortion varies from 0.1% to 10% while prevalence in the general female population has been estimated at 1% (Stoot 1978). Most authors conclude that only a minority of women with uterine anomalies experience reproductive difficulties (Glass and Golbus 1978, and reviewed by Bennett 1987). Hence, the majority of congenital uterine anomalies will remain unrecognised, most women with recognised anomalies will have successful pregnancies while those in whom the diagnosis of both uterine anomaly and pregnancy wastage have been made can achieve successful pregnancies without any treatment.

Historically, uterine anomalies were associated with late second trimester pregnancy losses. Later reports of an increased risk of early miscarriages in this group has led to the presumption that the presence of a relatively avascular septum predisposes to a failure of implantation or early pregnancy development (Rock and Zacur 1983; Buttram and Gibbons 1979; Stray-Pedersen and Stray-Pedersen 1984). For similar reasons uterine fibroids have been implicated as a cause of recurrent miscarriage, although objective data concerning the relationship between this common gynaecological problem and reproductive outcome is lacking.

Cervical incompetence is believed to be strongly associated with recurrent spontaneous abortion and may account for one in five cases of late abortion (McDonald 1980). However, the diagnosis of an incompetent cervix is rarely sought in women who have not had pregnancy losses or have not been pregnant. A weakness in the sphincter at the internal cervical os may be congenital, but is more usually acquired following dilatation and curettage, cone biopsy or lacerations at the time of a previous delivery. In the series of 269 cases reported by McDonald (1980) fewer than 2% of the cases occurred in non-parous women without demonstrable aetiological factors.

Infective Causes

For a micro-organism to cause recurrent pregnancy loss, it must persist for long periods and produce minimal symptoms to escape diagnosis and treatment. Numerous studies have implicated various infectious agents in the aetiology of recurrent abortion, but these data remain inconclusive since in all available reports the number of genital organisms cultured has been limited and adequate control groups have not been used.

Viral infections during pregnancy are extremely common. In the majority of cases the fetus is left unharmed and the pregnancy continues normally (Waterson 1979). Well known exceptions to this rule are rubella and cytomegalovirus (CMV) infections. However, since maternal rubella antibody production (from primary infection or immunisation) protects against subsequent fetal infection, recurrent pregnancy losses from rubella would not be expected and have not been reported (Watts and Eschenbach 1988). CMV is the most common viral infection transmitted to the fetus, rarely producing an asymptomatic secondary viraemia, during the latent phase of infection. Recurrent in-utero infections have been reported (Stagno et al. 1982), although it is difficult to differentiate between infected tissue and contamination from asymptomatic cervical infection. Viraemia and consequent in-utero infection of the fetus do not occur with latent or recurrent genital herpes infection. In-utero transmission of human immunodeficiency virus (HIV) is known to occur but at the present time insufficient data exist to link this virus with an increased risk of sporadic or recurrent abortion.

Chronic vaginal carriage of *Listeria* has not been well documented and proof that listeriosis is a cause of recurrent abortion in humans awaits controlled study. A subgroup of patients may be at risk of recurrent losses due to reinfection with *Chlamydia trachomatis* (secondary to sexual exposure), but since *Chlamydia* is found so commonly in the cervix it is doubtful whether cervical or fetal tissue cultures from women with recurrent abortion will provide evidence of an aetiologic role for this organism (Watts and Eschenbach 1988). The high prevalence and low virulence of genital *Mycoplasma* infections has led to the suggestion that they may cause chronic endometritis and recurrent pregnancy loss (Horne et al. 1974). Syphilis is a proven cause of recurrent pregnancy loss, and can be easily diagnosed and treated. Its contribution to recurrent abortion in developed countries where widespread serologic screening is performed is small.

Although toxoplasmosis is frequently cited as a possible cause of recurrent abortion, fetal infection with *Toxoplasma gondii* occurs only when the mother acquires her primary infection during gestation (Desmonts and Couvreur 1974). There is no evidence that latent *Toxoplasma* infection causes congenital infection or abortion except in the rare situation of an immuno-incompetent mother experiencing reactivation (Lee 1988).

Chronic Maternal Disorders, Drugs and Environmental Pollutants

For some maternal diseases an association with recurrent abortion has been presumed because the causal factors are likely to be present in all of the woman's pregnancies. Thyroid dysfunction is a commonly quoted but unsubstantiated cause of both sporadic and recurrent miscarriage (Harger et al. 1983; Stray-Pedersen and Stray-Pedersen 1984). Diabetic women with good metabolic control are no more likely to miscarry than non-diabetic women (Kalter 1987; Mills et al. 1988) but diabetic women with high glycosylated haemoglobin concentrations in the first trimester are at significantly higher risk (Miodovnik et al. 1988). There is no objective evidence to support the view that epilepsy is a cause of recurrent miscarriage. Patients with Wilson's disease (disturbed hepatic copper metabolism) invariably abort their pregnancies although the causal mechanism is not understood. When treated with penicillamine, which is not teratogenic, the pregnancy usually proceeds normally. Although Wilson's disease is rare, a serum caeruloplasmin measurement in unexplained cases of recurrent abortion may be indicated (Klee 1979).

Women who drink alcohol regularly and heavily have a higher incidence of recurrent abortion (Sokol et al. 1980). Although these women tend to be cigarette smokers, in a prospective study designed to assess smoking and drinking habits in pregnancy independently, the effect of alcohol on the incidence of recurrent miscarriage was much stronger than that of smoking (Harlap and Schiono 1980). Use of the oral contraceptive pill does not influence the risk of sporadic or recurrent abortion (Risch et al. 1988). The claims that female anaesthetists and women working with video display terminals are at increased risk of miscarriage have not been confirmed (Blackwell and Chang 1988; Bryant and Love 1989).

Endocrine Causes

The possibility that an endocrine abnormality is the underlying cause of many cases of recurrent miscarriage has always been attractive. The majority of studies have emphasised the importance of progesterone secretion during the luteal phase and in early pregnancy. Indeed inadequate luteal function, however it is defined, has been reported to occur in 23%–60% of patients with recurrent miscarriage (reviewed by Fritz 1988), but despite this common presentation, no consensus about its underlying mechanism, diagnosis or treatment exists.

More recently, advances in assisted fertility treatment have highlighted the fact that endocrine events before ovulation, may be important determinants of the successful outcome of pregnancy. In particular, high levels of luteinising hormone (LH) during the period of follicular development have been shown to exert an adverse effect upon the fertility and pregnancy outcome of patients undergoing treatment for infertility (Stranger and Yovich 1985; Howles et al. 1986; Punnonen et al. 1988). That a history of relative infertility (particularly ovulatory defects) confers a poor prognosis for subsequent pregnancy outcome and is present in some 30% of women with recurrent miscarriage (Strobino et al. 1986; Regan 1989) raises the possibility that infertility and miscarriage (both sporadic and recurrent) may represent two ends of a spectrum of disease, both of which start with an abnormality in follicular development.

The impact of high follicular phase LH levels in women with regular spontaneous menstrual cycles has recently been investigated prospectively in a field study of 193 women all of whom were planning to conceive (Regan et al. 1990. Hypersecretion of LH before conception was associated with a significant impairment of fertility and a striking increase in the rate of miscarriage. In the women who conceived with a "normal" pre-pregnancy LH value, the incidence of miscarriage was 12%, consistent with the rate of sporadic miscarriage in the general population (Regan et al. 1989; Wilcox et al. 1988). In the women with elevated day-8 serum LH concentrations (over 10 IU/l, as measured by radioimmunoassay, using MRC 68/40 reference preparation and polyclonal F87 anti-LH antiserum) the incidence of miscarriage was 65%. The adverse effect of a high follicular phase LH measurement was seen not only in primigravidae, but also in women with previously successful pregnancies and those whose obstetric history included miscarriages. Among the 30 patients with recurrent abortion in the study, the rate of miscarriage in those with a "normal" prepregnancy LH level was 7%, but in the "high" LH group the miscarriage rate rose to 67%.

Although these preliminary results may provide us with the most powerful predictive test for miscarriage presently available, the underlying mechanism is unclear. It may be a secondary association, signalling the presence of polycystic ovaries (PCO), the commonest cause of consistently elevated follicular phase LH levels. Using ultrasound criteria for diagnosis, the incidence of polycystic ovaries is 23% in the general population (Polson et al. 1988) rising to 80% in women with a history of recurrent miscarriage (Sagle et al. 1988). However, it would seem more likely that it is the hypersecretion of LH (rather than the presence of ultrasound-detected PCO themselves) which is the critical factor, since studies of patients undergoing treatment for PCO have demonstrated that the incidence of refractory infertility and of miscarriage are significantly higher in those PCO patients with elevated follicular phase serum LH concentrations (Homburg et al. 1988; Conway et al. 1989). It may be that the raised levels of LH exert an adverse effect on ovarian function, possibly by triggering a premature steroidogenic switch to progesterone or testosterone production. In a recent study, mean follicular phase serum testosterone levels were significantly higher in those recurrent miscarriage patients who had raised follicular phase LH levels when compared to a control group of patients with normal LH levels. However serum progesterone levels were normal in the follicular and luteal phases of both study and control patients (Watson et al. 1991). Another hypothesis is that the hypersecretion of LH exerts an adverse effect upon the endometrium. Interestingly, hCG/LH binding sites have been demonstrated recently in the non-pregnant uterus and decidua, which must raise the possibility that LH has a direct regulatory function in these tissues (Reshef et al. 1990). Endometrial lymphoid cells undergo cyclical changes in proliferation indicating that their function may be hormonally regulated (King and Loke 1990).

Alternatively, the adverse effect may be exerted directly on oocytes. Conditions for producing a normal embryo are dependent on the specific interval between completion of the first meiotic division of the oocyte and its fertilisation (Baker 1982). If the interval is extended (either by premature exposure of oocytes to high LH concentrations, the ovulatory stimulus (Hunter et al. 1976) or by delay of insemination (Austin 1982)), the premature completion of meiosis results in the ovulation of a physiologically aged egg. Such oocytes, if fertilised, may produce embryos of low viability with a higher tendency to abort, perhaps also recurrently (Jacobs and Homburg 1990).

Immunological Causes

Considerable attention has been paid to the possibility of immunologically mediated miscarriage. The subject is addressed elsewhere in this volume and hence only a brief summary of the impact of auto-immune and allo-immune disorders in the aetiology of recurrent miscarriage will be included here.

The most common auto-immune disorder found in women of childbearing years is systemic lupus erythematosus (SLE). Sporadic and recurrent abortion, intrauterine growth retardation and pre-term labour are well recognised complications of the disorder. The serum of women with repeated fetal losses may contain a number of auto-antibodies, but considerable evidence points to the two antiphospholipid antibodies (anticardiolipin and lupus anticoagulant) as having the greatest influence upon fetal loss (Lockwood et al. 1986; Lubbe and Liggins 1985, 1988; Cowchock et al. 1986; Tincani et al. 1987). These antiphospholipid antibodies are thought to inhibit prostacyclin production, with a resultant increase in levels of thromboxane, causing thrombosis of placental vessels which leads to placental infarction and fetal death. Fetal loss can occur at any stage in pregnancy, but mostly in the first trimester (Derue et al. 1985; Branch et al. 1985), with a trend for progressively earlier losses to occur in the same patient (Lubbe et al. 1984).

It is now recognised that some women without overt connective tissue disease carry antiphospholipid antibodies, and may present with recurrent pregnancy losses. Although some of these patients develop clinical signs of SLE at a later date, many have no manifestations of auto-immune disease when not pregnant. Women with anticardiolipin antibodies are more likely to have second trimester secondary losses, whereas those with antinuclear antibodies are prone to primary recurrent miscarriage in the first or second trimesters (Cowchock et al. 1986).

The notion that some women miscarry recurrently because of an allo-immune aberration, which prevents them from mounting the appropriate protective response towards their genetically dissimilar conceptus, has also been explored. Couples who suffer repeated abortions have been reported to share more HLA antigens than do couples with normal pregnancies. It is possible that increased sharing of HLA alleles between partners could lead to the inheritance of recessive lethal genes which are incompatible with fetal development (Thomas et al. 1985; Gill 1986). The immunological interpretation of increased HLA sharing is that compatibility results in maternal hyporesponsiveness to paternal antigens and a failure to generate the appropriate protective response to maintain the pregnancy. However, it has not been possible to correlate materno-fetal histocompatibility with pregnancy outcome (Jazwinska et al. 1987). The hypothesis of increased HLA sharing has been critically reviewed (Adinolphi 1986) and challenged by data from Christiansen et al. (1989) demonstrating that HLA sharing among recurrently aborting couples with and without auto-immune aberrations was not different.

Investigation and Management

A wide range of diagnostic tests have been used to identify genetic, anatomical, infective, endocrine and immunological causes of recurrent miscarriage. However, even after exhaustive investigation a significant number of patients remain in whom no aetiology can be found. A proportion of these women must surely have miscarried recurrently due to random causes. However, because of investigative bias some patients included in this "unknown" category in one study may be classified alternatively in others (Stray-Pedersen and Stray-Pedersen

1984; Parazzini et al. 1988). Furthermore, the possible benefits of therapeutic regimes are based on the results of investigations adopted by individual clinics. The subsequent pregnancy outcome of women receiving treatment for an "identified" cause is often (wrongly) compared to the expectant management offered to those patients in the "unknown" aetiology group (Tho et al. 1979; Stray-Pedersen and Stray-Pedersen 1984).

Obtaining a detailed, directed patient history is the cornerstone of management, and provides the clinician with a rationale for investigative tests and possible therapeutic regimens. For example, ultrasound details of a previous pregnancy may reveal that a pregnancy which allegedly miscarried at 18 weeks gestation by menstrual dating actually failed in the first trimester. Establishing that the woman has experienced delay in conceiving must raise the possibility of an underlying endocrine abnormality common to both her sub-fertility and early pregnancy losses. Most importantly, the use of investigations which cannot be translated into a practical management option cause patient distress and cannot be justified.

Genetic. When repeated abortions are being investigated, peripheral blood karyotyping should be performed on both partners. Whenever an abnormality is documented, prompt referral for genetic counselling will provide the couple with information regarding the future risk of miscarriage and ensure that they are aware of the importance and implications of prenatal diagnosis in a subsequent ongoing pregnancy. Although financial restrictions usually dictate that cytogenetic studies are only initiated after three pregnancy losses, the incidence of balanced translocations is increased significantly in couples with a history of two abortions and in couples with one normal live child in addition to their miscarriages. The geneticist is frequently able to allay much anxiety, since the prognosis is not always as gloomy as the patient fears. For example, amniocentesis surveillance demonstrates that the risk of a fetus with an unbalanced translocation in couples carrying a balanced reciprocal translocation is 12%, far less than the theoretical risk of 50%, since natural selection via early abortion occurs. Recurrence risks vary in different Robertsonian translocations. In the most common (involving chromosomes 14 and 21), amniocentesis data reveal that only 10%–15% of the viable offspring of balanced carriers have trisomy 21, whereas theoretically, one-third of the viable offspring should have trisomy 21 and 50% of all gametes should be lethal (Boué and Gallano 1984). If a Robertsonian translocation involves homologous chromosomes the prognosis is hopeless. The only live borns are abnormal (trisomy 13 or 21) and all other conceptions miscarry spontaneously. Couples with this type of translocation should be informed about embryo transfer techniques, artificial insemination or sterilisation. The finding of a chromosomal inversion is usually not clinically significant.

Wherever possible, cytogenetic analysis of abortus material from couples with repeated abortion should be performed irrespective of the parental karyotype, since the findings may influence the advice offered to the couple for management of a future pregnancy. Some couples have an increased risk of abortion because they produce chromosomally abnormal gametes, not as a result of translocation but presumably because of an increased tendency to non-disjunction, either inherited or induced environmentally. Identification of these individuals permits antenatal diagnosis in subsequent pregnancies and conversely, among those couples whose abortuses are chromosomally normal, a search for non-genetic,

Mendelian or polygenic causes is required. Perhaps most importantly, the finding of a fetal chromosomal abnormality in products of conception may, paradoxically, be the only measure of comfort that can be offered to a grieving couple.

Anatomical. The diagnosis of congenital uterine anomalies relies on the clinician's index of suspicion. The presence of a uterine septum can be sought at the time of evacuation of retained products of conception. Hysterosalpingography (HSG) or hysteroscopy should be performed if an abnormality is suspected, together with laparoscopy to inspect the external aspect of the uterus and adnexae. The use of ultrasound in experienced hands is a useful non-invasive screening procedure for congenital abnormalities. Remarkable pregnancy success rates have been reported following surgical reconstruction of the bicorunate or septate uterus (reviewed by Stoot 1978). However, metroplasty is complicated by the formation of pelvic adhesions and a significant number of women never conceive again after this type of surgery. In two independent reviews of the literature (Huisjes 1984; Bennett 1987) the incidence of subsequent infertility averaged 30%, which seems a high price to pay for treatment which has never been evaluated in a randomised controlled trial.

More recently, hysteroscopic metroplasty has been reported, with encouraging results (reviewed by Bennett 1987). The advantages of this technique are that major surgery is avoided, hospital stay may be as short as 24 hours, complications reported to date are few and subsequent pregnancies do not require delivery by Caesarean section. If further studies confirm that fertility is not compromised significantly, this may become the procedure of choice for the septate uterus.

The diagnosis of cervical incompetence is usually based on a history of rapid, painless mid-trimester abortions or pre-term delivery. There is no agreement on the criteria for diagnosis in non-pregnant women. Many uncontrolled studies have reported the benefit of cervical cerclage in terms of the rate of abortion before and after treatment (Crombleholme et al. 1983; Schwartz et al. 1984; McDonald 1987; Edmonds 1988). These and other studies are described in detail in Chapter 12.

Infection. Few data exist at the present time to support the role of infection in the aetiology of recurrent early pregnancy loss and the results of studies claiming benefit from empirical drug regimens require cautious interpretation. For example, several studies suggesting that recurrent miscarriage is associated with *Mycoplasma* infection have claimed an improved pregnancy outcome in women treated with tetracycline (Horne et al. 1974; Quinn et al. 1983; Stray-Pedersen et al. 1978). Controls for the large number of other potential organisms that would be inhibited by such broad spectrum antibiotic therapy have not been included in these studies. Until placebo-controlled treatment studies are conducted in which a variety of genital organisms are cultured, the use of antibiotics for treatment of recurrent pregnancy loss will remain empirical. Maternal infection with CMV may occasionally reactivate or persist despite antibody production, but the low incidence and equivocal interpretation of the serological tests available cannot justify routine screening of patients in the UK. The purpose of preconception of prenatal screening for toxoplasmosis (as practised in France) is to reduce the risk of acute maternal infection, identify the affected mother soon enough to choose appropriate management options and thereby reduce the risk of congenital infection (Daffos et al. 1988).

Endocrine.   There is no reliable method available to diagnose inadequate luteal function in the pregnant patient, hence endocrine evaluation of patients with recurrent miscarriage has usually focused on the luteal phase of the non-fertile menstrual cycle using progesterone estimations and endometrial biopsies. There have been numerous anecdotal reports of the use of human chorionic gona-dotrophin (hCG) and progesterone supplementation and there is some evidence that correction of a deficient luteal phase can improve subsequent pregnancy outcome (Harrison 1985; Balasch et al. 1986; Wentz et al. 1984) but no proof exists to support the efficacy of empirical hormonal therapy in an unselected group of women with repeated miscarriage. Several large controlled studies have failed to show the benefit of hormonal supplementation in the treatment of recurrent abortion (Klopper and Macnaughton 1965; MacDonald et al. 1972; Reijinders et al. 1988).

Our recent understanding that the quality of the luteal phase is dictated in part by endocrine events occurring before ovulation has important implications. Full evaluation of endocrine causes of miscarriage must now include follicular phase endocrine assessment rather than being limited to the measurement of hormones during the luteal phase and early pregnancy. The finding that a raised serum LH level in the mid-follicular phase results in a substantial risk of miscarriage may provide a useful predictive test with which to identify a subgroup of patients who suffer recurrent miscarriage with an endocrine abnormality which may be remediable. Treatment which normalises LH secretion during the first half of the menstrual cycle may result in an increased chance of a successful pregnancy.

There are now several methods available for supression of elevated LH including, using superactive analogues of LHRH followed by human menopausal gonadotrophin (HMG) (Homburg et al. 1990). Preliminary results from our pilot study at St. Mary's Hospital, London, suggest that this regimen results in a high rate of fertility and improved pregnancy outcome in women with recurrent miscarriage and hypersecretion of LH (Watson et al. unpublished data). Furthermore, in some patients with PCO, gonadotrophin therapy alone results in a reduction of endogenous LH secretion (Sagle et al. 1991) and when compared to clomiphene treatment, has been shown to improve the outcome of pregnancy (Johnson and Pearce 1990). The use of ovarian electrodiathermy appears to be beneficial also (Armar et al. 1990) and the recent finding that somatostatin has an inhibitory effect on the secretion of LH and ovarian steroids in PCO (Prelevic et al. 1990), suggests that this may be another therapeutic avenue worth exploring.

There are obvious limitations to single measurements of a hormone usually secreted in a pulsatile fashion. In those recurrent miscarriage patients with normal day-8 serum LH levels and in whom pelvic ultrasonography demonstrates the presence of polycystic ovaries, monitoring daily urinary LH levels may identify more subtle abnormalities of LH secretion in both the follicular and luteal phases in over 40% of cases (Watson et al. 1989), thereby identifying further patients who may benefit from the endocrine treatments outlined above.

Immunological.   In an unselected population of women with recurrent miscar-riage the incidence of antiphospholipid antibodies is about 10% (Tincani et al. 1987; Petri et al. 1987; Lockwood et al. 1986), but if women with recurrent fetal loss associated with placental infarction and maternal thrombotic episodes are investigated a significantly higher yield of positive tests is noted, reaching 100% in some studies (Soulier and Boffa 1980; Firkin et al. 1980; Carreras et al. 1981;

Lubbe et al. 1984). The lupus anticoagulant is an acquired IgM or IgG antiphospholipid antibody and is recognised by its ability to prolong phospholipid-dependent coagulation tests. The tests commonly used for detecting the anticoagulant are the partial thromboplastin time (APPT) and the kaolin clotting time (KCT). The KCT is believed to be the most sensitive screening test, the presence of the lupus anticoagulant being confirmed by the addition of normal plasma. Cross reactivity has been demonstrated between lupus anticoagulant, anticardiolipin and antinuclear antibody. The vast majority of patients with lupus anticoagulant also have positive anticardiolipin tests, but the correlation is not complete (Lockshin et al. 1987).

Although clotting studies (KCT) are the most reliable method of diagnosis, they are time consuming and expensive. The antinuclear antibody test has been proposed but only 60%–80% of patients with lupus anticoagulant have positive tests, and the VDRL test which is easy to perform is positive in only 20%–30% of women (Lubbe and Liggins 1988). The most helpful screening test appears to be the assay for anticardiolipin antibody (ACAb) which can be performed on stored serum (Harris et al. 1987). A positive ACAb test should be followed by full-scale anticoagulant screening.

The first successfully treated pregnancies in women with lupus anticoagulant and recurrent fetal losses, using steroids and low dose aspirin, were reported by Lubbe and colleagues (1984). Other centres have employed similar treatment regimens and success rates of 65%–85% have been reported although the numbers of patients are small (Vermylen et al. 1986; Branch et al. 1985). In order to minimise the number of women subjected to the hazard of high-dose steroid therapy, Lubbe and Liggins (1988) have confirmed the efficacy of low-dose aspirin treatment alone for women with a mild prolongation of the KCT (one and a half times control). If steroids are required to suppress higher KCT values, prednisone and aspirin are started as soon as pregnancy is diagnosed and the prednisone dosage increased if the KCT remains prolonged. The aim of treatment is to achieve a normal KCT value during the gestational period 18–24 weeks, the time recognised as most important for placentation and for fetalisation of maternal spiral arterioles to proceed normally. Dissociation between the antiphospholipid antibodies may be seen during steroid treatment, anticoagulant activity disappearing altogether while cardiolipin titres remain relatively unaltered (Derksen et al. 1986). Other forms of treatment such as azathioprine, high-dose immunoglobulins and subcutaneous heparin in women with a past history of venous thrombosis have also been reported but controlled studies of adequate size are needed to establish whether these potent drug regimens are truly effective.

As clinicians become more aware of patients with an obstetric history suggestive of "anticardiolipin syndrome", an increasing number of women in whom serological screening for antiphospholipid antibody activity is non-informative are emerging. Although it is difficult to justify the use of steroids or heparin in the absence of a serum marker which can be monitored, the data suggesting that low-dose aspirin therapy may be beneficial in preventing pre-term labour, pre-eclampsia, intrauterine growth retardation and miscarriage (McParland et al. 1990; Uzan et al. 1991; Tullpala et al. 1991) has resulted in many patients receiving empirical aspirin treatment. Further controlled studies are urgently needed.

Allo-immune causes, investigation and treatment of recurrent miscarriage are considered elsewhere in this volume. A few caveats for the clinician are mentioned here. Although HLA sharing was one of the original indications for immunological treatment of recurrent miscarriage, most workers have abandoned HLA typing, mixing lymphocyte reaction (MLR) blocking studies and other tests of allo-immune status, since they are costly, only available in a few specialised research centres and of no proven value. For example, the presence of anti-paternal cytotoxic antibody (APCA) in serum provides evidence of maternal immunological recognition of the fetus. That women with recurrent abortion have a significantly lower incidence of this antibody has been used to identify patients for whom immunisation treatment with paternal or donor cells may be beneficial. However, since the development of this antibody is primarily dependent upon the gestational duration of pregnancy (it is a rare finding in pregnancies of less than 28 weeks gestation), it is unlikely to be relevant to the success or failure of an early pregnancy. Furthermore, detectable APCA disappears from the serum in most women, suggesting that APCA is not a useful serum marker with which to identify patients with recurrent miscarriage (Regan et al. 1991).

Based on the hypothesis that successful pregnancy requires positive maternal recognition of the fetus and the production of protective blocking substances, many centres have introduced immunisation treatment regimens for women with recurrent miscarriage, with the aim of inducing this putative response. Trophoblast, paternal and unrelated lymphocytes have all been used as immunogens but, so far, only one randomised controlled trial has demonstrated the benefit of such treatment (Johnson et al. 1988; Mowbray et al. 1985).

Summary and Conclusions

The effective management of women with recurrent episodes of miscarriage has been repeatedly thwarted by the lack of epidemiological data on the incidence and risks of recurrence and the presumption that all cases must have a demonstrable aetiology. Since it is difficult for the patient to accept that three or more consecutive pregnancy losses may be due to chance alone, the search for an abnormal test result often leads to extensive investigations of doubtful practical use and the implementation of treatment regimens on empirical grounds alone.

Some women with recurrent miscarriage do have characteristics distinguishing them from patients who have had sporadic losses. They tend to miscarry chromosomally normal fetuses at later stages in gestation. In approximately one-third of cases a history of subfertility and conception delay will be present, and this confers a poor prognosis for subsequent pregnancy outcome. Details of these contributory factors should be sought routinely when couples with a history of recurrent miscarriage present for investigation, in order to offer them an assessment of future risk and identify avenues for investigation and treatment.

Parental karyotyping of both partners and a search for evidence of auto-immune disease should be performed in all patients. Although the number of positive tests is small in an unselected population of recurrent aborters, the tests will identify a group of patients whose pregnancy prognosis could be improved by appropriate treatment, or whose subsequent pregnancy requires prenatal diagnosis and careful monitoring. The use of HSG to identify anatomical abnormalities of the genital tract need only be performed in selected cases where a high index of clinical suspicion is based on the patients' past obstetric history. Screening for evidence of thyroid dysfunction, diabetes and infection is generally non-contributory.

Ultrasound scanning of the pelvis to document the presence of polycystic ovaries, together with an assessment of early follicular serum LH levels will identify those patients with abnormalities of LH secretion, an endocrine cause which appears to be amenable to treatment. At the present time the value of hormone measurements and endometrial biopsies is uncertain, but preliminary data suggest that these tests will prove useful additions to our investigative checklist for patients with a history of subfertility and recurrent miscarriage.

The clinician must remember that women who have miscarried recurrently from one cause are not protected from a further miscarriage from another cause such as fetal aneuploidy. Most importantly, when assessing the efficacy of any "new" treatment for patients with recurrent miscarriage, it is important to recall that no treatment has been shown to have greater benefit than the tender loving care and psychotherapy offered to patients in a controlled study conducted by the Stray-Pedersens (1984). Since approximately 60% of women with a history of recurrent miscarriage will be successful in their next pregnancy, the importance of randomised controlled trials to assess any new treatment option cannot be overstated.

References

Adamoli A, Bernardi F, Chiaffoni G, Fraccaro M, Giardino D, Romitti L, Simoni G (1986) Reproductive failure and parental chromosome abnormalities. Hum Reprod 1:99–102

Adinolfi M (1986) Recurrent habitual abortion, HLA sharing and deliberate immunisation with partner's cells: a controversial topic. Hum Reprod 1:45–48

Alberman E (1988) The epidemiology of repeated abortion. In: Beard RW, Sharp F (eds). Early pregnancy loss: mechanisms and treatment. RCOG, London, pp 9–17

Armar NA, MacGarrigle HHG, Honour JW, Holownia P, Jacobs HS, Lachelin GCL (1990) Laparoscopic ovarian diathermy in the management of anovulatory infertility in women with polycystic ovaries: endocrine changes and clinical outcome. Fertil Steril 53:45–49

Austin CR (1982) The egg. In: Austin CR, Short RE (eds). Reproduction in mammals. Part 1. Germ cells and fertilisation, 2nd edn. Cambridge University Press, Cambridge, pp 58–73

Baker TG (1982) Oogenesis and ovulation. In: Austin CR, Short RV (eds). Reproduction in mammals. Part 1. Germ cells and fertilisation, 2nd edn. Cambridge University Press, Cambridge, pp 17–45

Balasch J, Creus M, Marquez M, Burzaco I, Vanrell JA (1986) The significance of luteal phase deficiency on fertility: a diagnostic and therapeutic approach. Hum Reprod 1:145–147

Bennett MJ (1987) Congenital abnormalities of the fundus. In: Bennett MJ, Edmonds DK (eds). Spontaneous and recurrent abortion. Blackwell Scientific Publication, Oxford, pp 109–129

Blackwell R, Chang A (1988) Video display terminals and pregnancy. A review. Br J Obstet Gynaecol 95:446–453

Boué J, Boué A (1973) Chromosomal analysis of two consecutive abortuses in each of 43 women. Humangenetik 19:275–280

Boué A, Gallano P (1984) A collaborative study of the segregation of inherited structural arrangements in 1356 prenatal diagnoses. Prenat Diagn 4:45–67

Boué J, Boué A, Lazar P (1975) Retrospective and prospective epidemiological studies of 1500 karyotyped spontaneous human abortions. Teratology 12:11–26

Branch DW, Scott JR, Kochenour NK, Hershgold E (1985) Obstetric complications associated with the lupus anticoagulant. N Engl J Med 313:1322–1326

Bryant HE, Love J (1989) Video and display terminal use and spontaneous abortion. Int J Epidemiol 18:132–133

Buttram VC Jr, Gibbons WE (1979) Müllerian anomalies: a proposed classification (an analysis of 144 cases). Fertil Steril 32:40–46

Byrd JF, Askew DE, McDonough PG (1977) Cytogenetic findings in fifty-five couples with recurrent fetal wastage. Fertil Steril 28:246–250

Campana M, Serra A, Neri G (1986) Role of chromosome aberrations in recurrent abortion: A study of 269 balanced translocations. Am J Med Genet 24:341–356

Carreras LO, Vermylen J, Spitz B, Van Asche A (1981) Lupus anticoagulant and inhibition of prostacyclin formation in patients with repeated abortion, intrauterine growth retardation and intrauterine death. Br J Obstet Gynaecol 88:890–894

Christiansen OB, Riisom K, Lauritsen JG (1989) No increased histocompatibility antigen-sharing in couples with idiopathic habitual abortions. Hum Reprod 4:160–162

Conway GS, Honour JW, Jacobs HS (1989) Heterogeneity of the polycystic ovary syndrome: Clinical, endocrine and ultrasound features in 556 patients. Clin Endocrinol 30:459–470

Cowchock S, Smith JB, Gocial B (1986) Antibodies to phospholipids and nuclear antigens in patients with repeated abortions. Am J Obstet Gynecol 155:1002–1010

Crombleholme WR, Minkoff HL, Delke I, Schwartz RH (1983) Cervical cerclage: an aggressive approach to threatened or recurrent pregnancy wastage. Am J Obstet Gynecol 146:168–174

Daffos F, Forestier F, Capella-Pavlovsky M, Thulliez P, Aufrant C, Valenti D, Cox WL (1988) Prenatal management of 746 pregnancies at risk for congenital toxoplasmosis. N Engl J Med 318:271–275

Derksen RHWM, Biesma D, Bouma B, Gmelig Meyling FH, Kater L (1986) Discordant effects of prednisone on anti-cardiolipin antibodies and the lupus anticoagulant. Arthritis Rheum 29:1295–1296

Derue GJ, Englert HJ, Harris EN et al. (1985) Fetal loss in systemic lupus erythematosus: association with anti-cardiolipin antibodies. J Obstet Gynaecol 5:207–209

Desmonts G, Couvreur J (1974) Congenital toxoplasmosis: a prospective study of 378 pregnancies. N Engl J Med 290:1110–1116

Edmonds DK (1988) Use of cervical cerclage in patients with recurrent first trimester abortion. In: Beard RW, Sharp F (eds). Early pregnancy loss: mechanisms and treatment. RCOG, London, pp 411–417

Firkin BG, Howard MA, Radford SI (1980) Possible relationship between the lupus inhibitor and recurrent abortion in young women. Lancet ii:366

Fitzsimmons J, Wapner RJ, Jackson LG (1983) Repeated pregnancy loss. Am J Med Genet 16:7–13

Fritz MA (1988) Inadequate luteal function and recurrent abortion: Diagnosis and treatment of luteal phase deficiency. Semin Reprod Endocrinol 6:129–143

Gill TJ III (1986) Immunological and genetic factors influencing pregnancy and development. Am J Reprod Immunol Microbiol 10:116–120

Glass RH, Golbus MS (1978) Habitual abortion. Fertil Steril 29:257–265

Harger JH, Archer DF, Marchese SG, Muracca-Clemens M, Garver KL (1983) Etiology of recurrent pregnancy losses and outcome of subsequent pregnancies. Obstet Gynecol 62:574–581

Harlap S, Schiono PH (1980) Alcohol, smoking and incidence of spontaneous abortions in the first and second trimester. Lancet ii:173–176

Harris EN, Gharavi AE, Patel SP, Hughes GRV (1987) Evaluation of the anticardiolipin antibody test: Report of an international workshop held 4 April 1986; Clin Exp Immunol 68:215–222

Harrison RF (1985) Treatment of habitual abortion with human chorionic gonadotrophin; results of open and placebo-controlled trials. Eur J Obstet Gynecol Reprod Biol 20:159–168

Hassold T, Chen N, Funkhouser J et al. (1980) A cytogenetic study of 1000 spontaneous abortions. Ann Hum Genet 44:151–178

Homburg R, Armar NA, Eshel A, Adams J, Jacobs HS (1988) Influence of serum luteinising hormone concentrations on ovulation, conception, and early pregnancy loss in polycystic ovary syndrome. Br Med J 297:1024–1026

Homburg R, Eshel A, Kilborn J, Adams J, Jacobs HS (1990) Combined luteinising hormone releasing hormone analogue and exogenous gonadotrophins for the treatment of infertility associated with polycystic ovaries. Hum Reprod 5:32–35

Horne HW Jr, Kundsin RB, Kosas TS (1974) The role of Mycoplasma infection in human reproductive failure. Fertil Steril 25:380–389

Howles CM, Macnamee MC, Edwards RG, Goswamy R, Steptoe PC (1986) Effect of high tonic luteinising hormone on outcome of in-vitro fertilisation. Lancet ii:521–522

Huisjes HJ (1984) Spontaneous abortion. Churchill Livingstone, Edinburgh

Hunter RHF, Cook B, Baker TG (1976) Dissociation of response to injected gonadotrophin between the graafian follicle and oocyte in pigs. Nature 260:156–158

Jacobs HS, Homburg RR (1990) The endocrinology of conception. In: Clinics in endocrinology and metabolism. 4:195–205

Javert CT (1957) Spontaneous and habitual abortion. McGraw Hill, New York

Jazwinska EC, Kilpatric DC, Smart GE, Liston WA (1987) Feto-maternal HLA compatibility does not have a major influence on human pregnancy except for lymphocytotoxin production. Clin Exp Immunol 68:116–122

Johnson P, Pearce JM (1990) Recurrent spontaneous abortion and polycystic ovary disease: Comparison of two regimes to induce ovulation. Br Med J 300:154–156

Johnson PM, Chia KV, Hart CA, Griffith HB, Francis WJA (1988) Trophoblast membrane infusion for unexplained recurrent miscarriage. Br J Obstet Gynaecol 95:342–347

Kajii T, Ferrier A (1978) Cytogenetics of aborters and abortuses. Am J Obstet Gynecol 131:33–38

Kalter H (1987) Diabetes and spontaneous abortion: a historical review. Am J Obstet Gynecol 156:1243–1253

Klee JG (1979) Undiagnosed Wilson's disease as a cause of unexplained miscarriage. Lancet ii:423

Klopper AI, Macnaughton MC (1965) Hormones in recurrent abortion. J Obstet Gynaecol Br Commonw 72:1022–1028

King A, Loke YW (1990) Human trophoblast and JEG choriocarcinoma cells are sensitive to lysis by IL-2 stimulated decidual NK cells. Cellular Immunology 129:435–438

King A, Wellings V, Gardner I, Loke YW (1989) Immunocytochemical characterisation of the unusual large granular lymphocytes in human endometrium throughout the menstrual cycle. Hum Immunol 24:195–205

King A, Loke YW (1990) Uterine large granular lymphocytes: A possible role in embryonic implantation? Am J Obstet Gynecol 162:308–310

Lauritsen JG (1976) Aetiology of spontaneous abortion. A cytogenetic and epidemiological study of 288 abortuses and their parents. Acta Obstet Gynaecol Scand 53:1–29

Lee RV (1988) The problems of malaria and toxoplasmosis. Clin Perinatol 15:351–363

Lippman-Hand A, Vekemans M (1983) Balanced translocations among couples with two or more spontaneous abortions. Are males and females equally likely to be carriers? Hum Genet 63:252–257

Lockshin MD, Quamar T, Druzin ML, Goei S (1987) Antibody to cardiolipin, lupus anticoagulant and fetal death. J Rheumatol 14:259–262

Lockwood CJ, Reece EA, Romero R, Hobbins JC (1986) Anti-phospholipid antibody and pregnancy wastage. Lancet ii:742–743

Lubbe WF, Butler WS, Palmer SJ, Liggins GC (1984) Lupus anticoagulant in pregnancy. Br J Obstet Gynacol 91:357–363

Lubbe WF, Liggins GC (1985) Lupus anticoagulant and pregnancy. Am J Obstet Gynecol 135:322–327

Lubbe WF, Liggins GC (1988) Role of lupus anticoagulant and autoimmunity in recurrent pregnancy loss. Sem Reprod Endocrinol 6:181–190

Macnaughton MC (1964) The probability of recurrent abortion. J Obstet Gynaecol Br Commonw 71:784

MacDonald RR, Goulden R, Oaker RE (1972) Cervical mucus, vaginal cytology and steroid secretion in recurrent abortion. Obstet Gynaecol 1972; 40:394–402

McDonald IA (1980) Cervical cerclage. Clin Obstet Gynecol 7:461–479

McDonald IA (1987) Cervical incompetence as a cause of spontaneous abortion. In: Bennett MJ, Edmonds DK (eds) Spontaneous and recurrent abortion. Blackwell Scientific Publications, Oxford, pp 168–192

McParland P, Pearce JM, Chamberlain GVP (1990) Doppler ultrasound and aspirin in recognition and prevention of pregnancy-induced hypertension. Lancet 335:1552–1555

Mills JLM, Simpson JLL, Driscoll SG et al. (1988) Incidence of spontaneous abortion among normal women and insulin dependant diabetic women whose pregnancies were identified within 21 days of conception. N Engl J Med 319:1617–1623

Miodovnik M, Mimoumi F, Siddiqi TA, Tsang RC (1988) Periconceptual metabolic status and risk for spontaneous abortion in insulin-dependant diabetic pregnancies. Am J Perinatol 4:368–373

Mowbray JF, Gibbings C, Liddell H, Reginald PW, Underwood JL, Beard RW (1985) Controlled trial of treatment of recurrent spontaneous abortion with paternal cells. Lancet i:941–943

Naylor AF, Warburton D (1979) Sequential analysis of spontaneous abortion. II. Collaborative study data show that gravidity determines a very substantial rise in risk. Fertil Steril 31:282–286

Parazzini F, Acaia B, Ricciardiello O, Fedele L, Liati P, Candiani GB (1988) Short-term reproductive prognosis when no cause can be found for recurrent miscarriage. Br J Obstet Gynaecol 95:654–658

Petri M, Golbus M, Anderson R, Whiting-O'Keefe Q, Corash L, Hellman D (1987) Anti-nuclear antibody, lupus anticoagulant and anti-cardiolipin antibody in women with idiopathic habitual abortion: a controlled prospective study of forty-four women. Arthritis Rheum 30:601–606

Poland BJ, Miller JR, Jones DC, Trimble BK (1977) Reproductive counselling in patients who have had a spontaneous abortion. Am J Obstet Gynecol 127:685–691

Polson DW, Wadsworth J, Adams J, Franks S (1988) Polycystic ovaries—a common finding in normal women. Lancet ii:870–872

Prelevic GM, Wurzburger MI, Balint-Peric L, Nesic JS (1990) Inhibitory effect of sandostatin on secretion of luteinising hormone and ovarian steroids in polycystic ovary syndrome. Lancet 336:900–903

Punnönen R, Heinonen PK, Ashorn R, Kujansuu E, Vilja P, Tuohimaa P (1988) Spontaneous luteinising hormone surge and cleavage of in vitro fertilised embryos. Fertil Steril 49:479–482

Quinn PA, Shewchuk AB, Shuber J et al. (1983) Efficacy of antibiotic therapy in preventing spontaneous pregnancy loss among couples colonised with genital mycoplasmas. Am J Obstet Gynecol 145:239–244

Reijinders F, Thomas CMG, Doesburg WH, Rolland J, Eskes TK (1988) Endocrine effects of 17 alpha hydroxyprogesterone caproate during early pregnancy: a double blind clinical trial. Br J Obstet Gynaecol 95:462–468

Regan L (1988) A prospective study of spontaneous abortion. In: Beard RW, Sharp F (eds). Early pregnancy loss: mechanisms and treatment. RCOG, London, pp 23–27

Regan L (1989) Epidemiology of sporadic and recurrent abortion. MD Thesis. London University

Regan L, Braude PR, Trembath PL (1989) Influence of past reproductive performance on risk of spontaneous abortion. Br Med J 299:541–545

Regan L, Owen EJ, Jacobs HS (1990) Hypersecretion of luteinising hormone, infertility and miscarriage. Lancet 336:1141–1144

Regan L, Braude PR, Hill D (1991) The incidence and time of development of antipaternal lymphocytotoxic antibodies in human pregnancy. Hum Reprod 6:294–298

Reshef E, Lei ZM, Rao ChV, Pridham DD, Chegini N, Luborsky JL (1990) The presence of gonadotrophin receptors in non-pregnant uterus, human placenta, fetal membranes and decidua. J Clin Endocrinol Metab 70:421–430

Risch HA, Weiss NS, Clarke AE, Miller A (1988) Risk factors for spontaneous abortion and its recurrence. Am J Epidemiol 128:420–430

Rock JA, Zacur HA (1983) The clinical management of repeated pregnancy wastage. Fertil Steril 39:123–140

Sachs ES, Jahoda MGJ, Van Hemel JO, Hoogeboom AJM, Sandkuyl LA (1985) Chromosome studies of 500 couples with two or more abortions. Obstet Gynecol 65:375–378

Sagle M, Bishop K, Ridley N et al. (1988) Recurrent early miscarriage and polycystic ovaries. Br Med J 297:1027–1028

Sagle M, Hamilton-Fairley D, Kiddy DS, Franks S (1991) A comparative, randomised study of low dose human menopausal gonadotrophin and follicle stimulating hormone in women with polycystic ovarian syndrome. Fertil Steril 55:1–5

Schwartz S, Palmer CG (1983) Chromosomal findings in 164 couples with repeated spontaneous abortions: with special consideration to prior reproductive history. Hum Genet 63:28–34

Schwartz RP, Chatwani A, Sullivan P (1984) Cervical cerclage: A review of 74 cases. J Reprod Med 29:103–106

Simpson JL (1980) Genes, chromosomes and reproductive failure. Fertil Steril 33:107–116

Simpson JL, Bombard A (1987) Chromosomal abnormalities in spontaneous abortion: Frequency, pathology and genetic counselling. In: Bennett MJ, Edmonds DK (eds). Spontaneous and recurrent abortion. Blackwell Scientific Publications, Oxford, pp 51–76

Simpson JL, Elias S, Martin AO (1981) Parental chromosomal rearrangements associated with repetitive spontaneous abortions. Fertil Steril 36:584–590

Sokol RJ, Miller SI, Reed G (1980) Alcohol abuse during pregnancy: an epidemiologic study. Clin Exp Res 4:135–145

Soulier JP, Boffa MC (1980) Avortéments a répétition, thromboses et anticoagulant circulant anti-thromboplastine. Nouv Presse Med 9:859–864

Stagno S, Pass RF, Dworsky ME, et al. (1982) Congenital cytomegalovirus infection: The relative importance of primary and recurrent maternal infection. N Engl J Med 306:945–949

Stanger JD, Yovich JL (1985) Reduced in-vitro fertilisation of human oocytes from patients with raised basal LH levels during the follicular phase. Br J Obstet Gynaecol 92:385–393

Stenchever MA (1980) Managing habitual abortion. Cont Obstet Gynecol 16:23–24

Stenchever MA, Parks KA, Daines TL, Allen MA, Stenchever MR (1977) Cytogenetics of habitual abortion and other reproductive wastage. Am J Obstet Gynecol 127:143–150

Stoot JEGM (1978) Aangeborn afwijkingen van de uterus en gestoorde voortplanting. PhD Thesis University of Nijmegen, Holland

Stray-Pedersen B, Stray-Pedersen S (1984) Etiologic factors and subsequent reproductive performance in 195 couples with a prior history of habitual abortion. Am J Obstet Gynecol 148:140–146

Stray-Pedersen B, Eng J, Reikvam TM (1978) Uterine T-mycoplasma colonisation in reproductive failure. Am J Obstet Gynecol 130:307–311

Strobino B, Fox HE, Kline J, Stein Z, Susser M, Warburton D (1986) Characteristics of women with recurrent spontaneous abortions and women with favourable reproductive histories. Am J Publ Hlth 76:986–991

Tho PT, Byrd JR, McDonough PG (1979) Etiologies and subsequent reproductive performance of 100 couples with recurrent abortion. Fertil Steril 32:389–395

Thomas ML, Harger JH, Wagener DK, Rabin BS, Gill TJ (1985) HLA sharing and spontaneous abortion in humans. Am J Obstet Gynecol 151:1053–1061

Tibiletti MG, Simoni G, Terzoli GL, Romitti L, Fedele L, Candiani GB (1981) Pericentric inversion of chromosome 9 in couples with repeated spontaneous abortion. Acta Euro Fert 12:245–248

Tincani A, Cattaneo M, Martinelli M et al. (1987) Anti-phospholipid antibodies in recurrent fetal loss: one side of the coin? Clin Exp Rheumatol 4:390–392

Tulpalla M, Viinikka, Ylikorkala O (1991) Thromboxane dominance and prostacyclin deficiency in habitual abortion. Lancet 337:879–881

Uzan S, Beaufils M, Breart G, Bazin B, Capitant C, Paris S (1991) Prevention of fetal growth retardation with low dose aspirin: findings of the EPREDA trial. Lancet 337:1427–1431

Vermylen J, Blockmans D, Spitz B (1986) Thrombosis and immune disorders. Clin Haematol 15:1–20

Verp MS, Simpson JL (1985) Prenatal diagnoses of cytogenetic abnormalities. In: Filkins K, Kaminetsky H (eds). Prenatal diagnosis. Dekker, New York

Warburton D, Fraser FC (1964) Spontaneous abortion risks in man: data from reproductive histories collected in a medical genetics unit. Hum Genet 16:1–25

Waterson AP (1979) Virus infections (other than rubella) during pregnancy. Br Med J 2:564–566

Watson H, Hamilton-Fairley D, Kiddy DS et al. (1989) Abnormalities of follicular phase LH secretion in women with recurrent early miscarriage. Journal Endocrinol suppl, Abstr 25

Watson H, Hamilton-Fairley D, Kiddy DS et al. (1991) The effect of hypersecretion of LH on ovarian steroid hormone secretion in women with recurrent early miscarriage. J Endocrinol 129:suppl, Abstr 205

Watts DH, Eschenbach DA (1988) Reproductive tract infections as a cause of abortion and preterm birth. Semin Reprod Endocrinol 6:203–215

Wentz AC, Herbert CM, Maxson WS, Garner CH (1984) Outcome of progesterone treatment of luteal phase inadequacy. Fertil Steril 41:856–862

Wilcox AJ, Weinberg CR, O'Connor JF (1988) Incidence of early loss of pregnancy. N Engl J Med 319:189–194

8. Septic Abortion

Felicity Ashworth

The term septic abortion describes the occurrence of infection developing in or around the uterus during or after an abortion. The genital tract is particularly susceptible to infection at this time and sepsis is often, but not always, consequent to attempts to cause abortion by untrained persons using non-sterilised instruments.

The incidence of sepsis complicating an incomplete abortion varies between countries and reported series are given in Table 8.1. Munday et al. (1989) report that there were 3050 women discharged from hospitals in the UK with the diagnosis of septic abortion in 1965 compared to only 390 in 1982. Figures from New Zealand (Shepherd and Benny 1984) show a reduction from 6% of all abortions being septic in 1962 to less than 1% in 1979. The incidence of septic abortion has declined in countries where the operation of termination of pregnancy has been legalised and women have more ready access to these services.

Table 8.1. Incidence of incomplete abortion complicated by sepsis

Author	Country	Incidence (%)
Adetoro (1986)	Nigeria	12
Aggarwal and Mati (1980)	Kenya	16
Barnes and Ulfelder (1964)	USA	14
Botes (1973)	South Africa	5.8–34
Munday et al. (1989)	UK	below 1
Shepherd and Benny (1984)	New Zealand	below 1

Relevance of Septic Abortion to Maternal Mortality Statistics

Deaths from abortion, and particularly septic abortion, contribute significantly to a country's maternal mortality. In England and Wales the most dramatic decline in maternal mortality followed the introduction of the Abortion Act in 1967. From 1958 to 1972, abortion was the commonest cause of maternal mortality in England and Wales. There was then a steady decline in deaths from abortion and in the triennium from 1982 to 1984, 8% of all maternal deaths were due to abortion, septic complications accounting for 27% of these deaths (DHSS 1989). Abortion as a cause of maternal death has now been regulated to the sixth commonest cause and in the 1982–1984 report (DHSS 1989) there were no deaths from criminal abortion. Epidemiologists in the USA have described a similar reduction of deaths from abortion after the abortion laws were liberalised (Cates et al. 1978; Grimes et al. 1981) and contraception made more freely available.

By contrast, countries where abortion is not legally available have a high death rate from septic abortion leading to calls for liberalisation of abortion laws (Adetoro 1986; Mathai 1986; Unuigbe et al. 1988). In Nigeria, complications of illegal abortion account for up to 50% of maternal mortality in that country (Adetoro 1986). In the Greater Harare Maternity Unit, Zimbabwe, sepsis accounted for 50% of the deaths from abortion and a total of 8% of the maternal deaths. Abortion ranked joint second with puerperal sepsis and haemorrhage as a cause of maternal death (Ashworth 1990). This figure was an improvement on a previous report from the same unit: post-abortal sepsis accounted for 18% of maternal deaths in 1983 (Crowther 1986). Although the abortion laws had not changed during this period, there had been an expansion of available contraceptive services.

Risk Factors

In spite of the presence of profuse bacterial colonisation in the lower genital tract, infection rarely complicates spontaneous abortion. Kowen et al. (1979) studied 100 women and demonstrated 100% bacterial colonisation of products of conception. Of these patients, 10% showed clinical evidence of infection after curettage, although this is an unusually high rate of infection.

Uterine sepsis results from instrumentation of the uterus to remove retained products of conception or to terminate the pregnancy. The use of unsterilised instruments and the astonishing variety of methods used to induce abortion by illegal abortionists leads to incomplete evacuation of uterine contents and the inevitable introduction of infection. Infection may also arise after a spontaneous incomplete abortion, without surgical evacuation, since the remaining products of conception will act as a nidus of infection.

The intrauterine contraceptive device (IUCD) has been implicated in the aetiology of septic abortion, particularly in the second trimester. Williams et al. (1975) showed a higher incidence of septic abortion in IUCD users but no serious consequences were recorded. Tatum et al. (1976) found 2 cases of septic first-trimester abortion out of a total of 113 abortions occurring in women who had a copper T intrauterine contraceptive device. Templeton (1974) reported 4 fatal cases of septic abortion with a Dalkon shield in situ, an observation which subsequently led to the withdrawal of the Dalkon shield.

Chorionic villus sampling may result in septic abortion. Hogge et al. (1986) have reported this complication in 0.6% of their first 1000 cases using the transcervical route. The abortion may be delayed up to 10 weeks following the procedure (Marini et al. 1988). For this reason, many prefer the transabdominal route for this procedure.

Midtrimester rupture of membranes may lead to ascending infection and colonisation of the uterine cavity followed later by septic abortion. Pre-term rupture of membranes may be idiopathic, or related to the insertion of a cervical suture, or to an amniocentesis or cone biopsy.

The question as to whether human immunodeficiency virus (HIV) infection leads to a higher rate of infection after a spontaneous abortion, or worsens the outcome of a septic abortion, needs to be addressed. There are no published data but clinicians working in areas with a high prevalence of HIV believe that the incidence of severe septic abortion has increased in women who are HIV seropositive. The combination carries a high mortality.

Clinical Features

The following features suggest the possibility of septic abortion: illegally procured abortion; continued bleeding after a spontaneous abortion; fevers; chills and rigors; malaise; nausea; an offensive discharge; and lower abdominal pain.

On examination, there may be:

1. Pyrexia: in order for an abortion to be defined as septic, a temperature of at least 38°C should be recorded on any 2 days or a temperture of 38.3°C and above at any time before or after evacuation (Barnes and Ulfelder 1964). The absence of pyrexia can be an ominous sign of septic shock

2. General features: signs of anaemia and dehydration

3. Cardiovascular system: tachycardia will be present; a pulse rate of more than 110 beats per minute suggests more widespread infection. Hypotension may be due to blood loss or circulating endotoxins

4. Abdominal examination: tenderness with guarding and possibly rebound tenderness in the lower abdomen. Spread of infection will lead to signs of ileus with a distended, generally tender abdomen and absent bowel sounds.

5. Vaginal examination: profuse, offensive vaginal discharge and possibly products of conception or evidence of criminal interference such as sticks, leaves, wire etc. Cervical excitation tenderness will be present. The uterus will be tender, soft and enlarged and there will be tenderness in the fornices. An adnexal mass might be present.

6. Rectal examination: this may detect an abscess in the pouch of Douglas.

Many women with septic abortion are never seriously ill. The best indicator of a serious illness is the presence of chills and fever (Barnes and Ulfelder 1964).

Microbiology

Women presenting with suspected septic abortion should have high vaginal and cervical swabs taken. The main organisms isolated are the non-clostridial anaerobic and micro-aerophilic bacteria; anaerobic streptococci and bacteroides (Rotheram and Schick 1969). The normal vaginal flora can make interpretation of these cultures difficult. Table 8.2 lists the organisms which may be found.

Table 8.2. Pathogenic organisms in septic abortion

Anaerobes	Aerobes
Bacteroides fragilis	*Escherichia coli*
Bacteroides melaninogenicus	*Enterobacter* species
Peptostreptococcus species	*Beta haemolytic streptococci*
Peptococcus species	*Proteus* species
Fusobacterium species	*Klebsiella aerogenes*
Clostridium perfringens	*Pseudomonas aeruginosa*
Clostridium tetani	*Neisseria gonorrhoeae*
	Staphylococcus aureus
	Streptococcus milleri

Of the beta haemolytic streptococci, group A are the most pathogenic and are usually introduced into the vagina by instrumentation since they are not a normal vaginal commensal. Groups B and D are less virulent and are also normal vaginal commensals (Rotheram and Schick 1969).

Clostridium perfringens (welchii) is a gram-positive, anaerobic, spore-forming organism which is often encapsulated. It can be found in up to 29% of cervical cultures in septic abortion (Butler 1945), although only a small percentage of these organisms will be virulent. *Clostridium perfringens* releases many exotoxins, the main ones being an alpha toxin which causes haemolysis, a collagenase, a hyaluronidase, a DNA-ase and a myotoxin. These exotoxins are only produced after 24–48-h incubation in the necrotic host tissue and lead directly to haemolysis, hypotension, jaundice and renal failure. At one time, post-abortal sepsis due to *Clostridium perfringens* was associated with a mortality ranging from 53% to 85% (Decker and Hall 1966). *Clostridium tetani* rarely complicates illegal abortion although it too carries a high mortality (Adadeuoh and Akinla 1970).

Rotheram and Schick (1969) reported positive blood cultures in 60% of patients with septic abortion, anaerobic bacteria predominating. Smith et al. (1970) confirmed *Peptostreptococcus* as the most common organism, found in 41% of positive cultures. Aerobic gram-negative rods are detected in smaller numbers in blood cultures than the anaerobes but they are important since they are the most frequent cause of endotoxic shock (Deane and Russell 1960).

Complications of Septic Abortion

The condition may progress toward shock, with higher fever, tachycardia, tachypnoea, falling blood pressure and diminishing urine output. This is the "septic syndrome" (Balk and Bone 1989) and it is important that it should be identified before full septic shock ensues.

Septicaemia

A systemic response differentiates the septicaemic patient from the bacteraemic one. The dispersion of bacteria into the circulation occurs in approximately 10% of women with septic abortion. Transient bacteraemia is common after uterine curettage, but does not usually lead to septicaemia (Kowen et al. 1979).

The usual organisms found in septicaemia are gram-negatives such as *Escherichia coli*, *Klebsiella*, *Proteus mirabilis* and *Pseudomonas aeruginosa* (Botes 1973). Streptococci and anaerobic organisms are also found.

Endotoxic Shock

Endotoxic shock complicates approximately 0.7% of septic abortions (Botes 1973). The mortality from septic shock is high, ranging from 11% to 82% (Adetoro 1986; Cavanagh et al. 1985; Douglas and Beckman 1966).

The pathophysiology of septic shock involves infection which results in peripheral circulatory failure with inadequate tissue perfusion leading to cellular dysfunction or death. The underlying haemodynamic anomaly is vasoconstriction. Endotoxic shock occurs as a result of the release of a lipopolysaccharide-protein complex from gram-negative bacteria, leading to platelet damage and the activation of the coagulation system. Cytokines, such as tumour necrosis factor and interleukin-1 appear to have an important mediating effect as well as the prostaglandin cascade (Pearlman and Faro 1990). Microemboli are generated which reduce the blood supply to various organs. Pooling of blood in the portal system leads to a relative hypovolaemia with reduced venous return to the heart, resulting in reduced cardiac output to vital organs.

The haemodynamic changes in patients with septic shock commence with "warm" shock when the patient is in a hyperdynamic, vasodilated state and progress to "cold" shock when vasoconstriction occurs with a diminished cardiac output. The clinical manifestations of septic shock are summarised in Table 8.3 (Pearlman and Faro 1990). The organisms which lead to endotoxic shock are the gram-negative bacteria.

Acute Tubular Necrosis

Acute tubular necrosis may result from hypotension and vasoconstriction together with fibrin and immune complex deposition. Clostridia release a nephrotoxic exotoxin, as may certain abortifacient agents such as soap and detergent douches.

Table 8.3. Common clinical manifestations of septic shock

Organ system	Clinical findings	Mechanism
Cardiovascular hypotension	Systolic BP <60 mmHg	Vasodilation Decreased circulating volume due to increased vascular permeability
Cardiac dysfunction	Increase in cardiac index (early) Decrease in CI (late) Decrease in ejection fraction	Myocardial depressant factor Decreased myocardial blood flow
Pulmonary ARDS	Bilateral diffuse infiltrates on CNR Hypoxemia Normal PACWP (<18 mmHg)	Increased vascular permeability Direct endothelial damage
Renal oliguria	Less than 30 ml/h	Hypotension and renal vasoconstriction
ATN		Prolonged cortical hypoxia secondary to decreased renal blood flow
Interstitial nephritis		Immune mechanism
Haematologic DIC	Elevated FDP, PT, PTT Decreased platelets, and fibrinogen Spontaneous bleeding (uncommon)	Endotoxin activation of Hageman factor
Leukocytosis	>20 000 cells/mm³	Demargination Neutrophil releasing substance
Neurologic mental status changes	Somnolence, coma, combative (uncommon, usually due to hypoxia)	Decreased cerebral blood flow Hypoxia
Fever	Temperature >38°C	Direct endotoxin/TNF effect on hypothalamus

From Pearlman M, Faro S (1990) Clinical Obstetrics and Gynecology 33:482–492. Reproduced with permission.

Management of Septic Abortion

Prevention

The incidence of septic abortion has dramatically declined in countries where abortion laws have been liberalised. If access to legal termination of pregnancy were universally available, there would be a significant improvement in maternal mortality from septic abortion.

Uterine evacuation should be performed following incomplete abortion in order to prevent subsequent infection of retained products of conception. This may be a problem in those countries in which women have limited access to health services. Antibiotics should be given to a woman with an incomplete abortion if there are signs of infection at initial presentation.

Infection may follow elective termination of pregnancy. Women should be screened pre-operatively and treated with a full course of antibiotics if infection is detected (Mills 1984). Some units use a single prophylactic dose of antibiotics peri-operatively, doxycycline 500 mg orally, but this may be insufficient to treat established infection.

When pregnancy occurs with an IUCD in situ, the coil should be removed during the first trimester in order to reduce the risk of septic abortion (Foreman et al. 1981).

Prophylactic antibiotics do not reduce the risk of intrauterine infection in midtrimester rupture of membranes (Keirse et al. 1989). However, they do reduce the problems of postpartum infection in the mother although it is not yet clear whether giving antibiotics at the time of delivery would be as efficacious.

Antibiotic Therapy

Once the diagnosis of septic abortion is made, antibiotics should be given immediately, after vaginal and cervical swabs and blood cultures have been taken.

The recommended combination is amoxycillin (500 mg every 8 h) and metronidazole (400 mg every 8 h) or a cephalosporin (500 mg every 8 h), and metronidazole. If the patient's condition is more serious, a combination of gentamicin (80 mg every 8 h), amoxycillin (500 mg every 8 h) and metronidazole (500 mg every 8 h) given intravenously should cover most organisms whilst awaiting results of bateriological cultures. If the expense or availability of drugs is a problem, a combination of chloramphenicol (500 mg every 6 h) and penicillin (5 MU every 6 h) is also effective (Chow et al. 1977). If clostridial infection is suspected, high-dose intravenous penicillin or ampicillin should be given.

Curettage

Once the patient's condition has been stabilised and antibiotics given intra-venously, the uterus must be evacuated within 6 h (Cavanagh et al. 1985). There is no advantage to be gained in waiting for the antibiotics to take effect since this will only delay removal of the source of infection.

Uterine evacuation must be performed by an experienced operator, preferably using suction curettage, since there is a risk of uterine perforation. An oxytocin agent should also be given to reduce the uterine bleeding.

Surgery

If the patient's condition does not improve within 6–12 h of initial treatment, laparotomy and hysterectomy should be considered. The indications for laparotomy are as follows (Botes 1973; Richards et al. 1985):

1. Pelvic peritonitis or septicaemic shock not responding to medical treatment
2. Uterine size more than 16 weeks
3. Uterine perforation
4. Uncontrollable uterine haemorrhage

5. Abortion induced with chemical agents e.g. soaps and detergents
6. Superimposed clostridial infection

Medical stabilisation and resuscitation and correction of anaemia and fluid and electrolyte balance is very important prior to laparotomy. The anaesthetic should be performed by an experienced anaesthetist.

The laparotomy should be performed through a midline incision to give full access. Purulent fluid may be found between loops of bowel in the abdominal cavity, as well as in the peritoneal spaces, particularly the subphrenic. Loops of bowel should be separated and inspected for evidence of perforation; careful handling is essential since they are extremely friable. Purulent exudate should be removed from the abdominal cavity. The peritoneal cavity should be lavaged thoroughly with warm saline. At the end of the procedure, large-bore Portex drains should be inserted in all four quadrants of the abdomen.

Hysterectomy is necessary if the uterus is larger than 16 weeks; shows evidence of perforation or necrosis or is actively bleeding (Richards et al. 1985). If the ovaries appear normal, they may be preserved (De Jonge and Venter 1988). However, if they are involved in tubo-ovarian masses, one or both should be removed. This is mutilating surgery since the patients are often young and primigravid, but early hysterectomy does improve survival (Richards et al. 1985).

The merits of early hysterectomy in clostridial infections are disputed. Decker and Hall (1966) recommend immediate hysterectomy if there are general signs of sepsis, uterine tenderness and clostridial organisms are identified from a cervical swab. In their series, mortality was reduced to 9% compared to previous reported rates of up to 70%. However, O'Neill and Schwartz (1970) managed their 7 cases conservatively without fatalities. They recommend curettage, antibiotics and a readiness to perform hysterectomy if the woman's condition does not improve.

If diffuse peritonitis is found at laparotomy, further management should be considered as well as debridement and drainage. Continuous peritoneal lavage may be instituted by inserting three large Portex drains through separate incisions, one to each sub-phrenic space and one to the pouch of Douglas. Rivlin and Hunt (1986) have described a method of irrigating the abdominal cavity with 2 l of warm peritoneal dialysis solution every 3 h. Each litre of solution contains 15 mg gentamicin and 4 mEq potassium chloride. Each tube was used in turn to irrigate, leaving the other two tubes to drain. The tubes were removed when the lavage fluid became clear, usually after 2 to 3 days. These authors reported a mortality of 27% in women with septic abortion. However, an important aspect of their improved survival figures was the addition of an anti-anaerobic antimicrobial to the systemic treatment.

Another method of management is to leave the abdominal wound open after the first laparotomy in order to allow infected peritoneal fluid to drain. The wound can be covered with gauze (Korepanov 1989) or a polypropylene mesh (Richardson and Polk 1981). However, Maetani and Tobe (1981) have shown that open drainage will not always drain residual collections and repeat laparotomy was necessary in 30% of their patients.

Repeat laparotomy is indicated if there are signs of continuing intra-abdominal sepsis. A policy of planned repeat laparotomy is carried out in some units (Schein et al. 1988): laparotomy is repeated every 2 to 3 days, irrespective of the patient's clinical condition, until a clean abdominal cavity is found. Between laparotomies, the open abdominal wound is covered with a Marlex mesh over the bowel and a plastic adhesive drape over the skin defect. Schein et al. (1988) reported a 32% mortality rate using this technique in general surgical patients, an average of 2.5 reoperations being required. A Marlex mesh with a zip sewn to the fascia of the wound allows easy access for abdominal exploration and debridement 1 to 3 times per day (Walsh et al. 1988).

All women should be nursed on an intensive care unit with close supervision of ventilation, fluid balance, antibiotic therapy and total parenteral nutrition. Unfortunately, countries in which the problem of septic abortion is common often do not have these facilities.

Management of Septic Shock

The patient must be treated in an intensive care unit with a multidisciplinary team approach. On admission, a large bore intravenous cannula is inserted and blood drawn for the investigations outlined in Table 8.4. Various bacteriological and radiological investigations are instituted. Monitoring of haemodynamic changes and urine output is essential. An indwelling urinary catheter is inserted. If the patient remains hypotensive after initial resuscitation, a central venous pressure line should be inserted and, if necessary, a Swan Ganz cannula to the pulmonary artery to measure pulmonary capillary wedge pressure (PCWP). The main steps of treatment are as follows: maintain oxygenation, support the circulation and control infection.

Table 8.4. Investigations in suspected septic shock

Full blood count
Clotting studies: prothrombin time, partial thromboplastin time, fibrin degradation products
Cross match blood
Urea and electrolytes
Glucose
Liver function tests
Arterial blood gases
Chest X-ray
Bacteriological specimens
Midstream specimen of urine
High vaginal swab
Endocervical swab
Swab products of conception
Blood cultures

Oxygenation

Respiratory failure is usually related to the onset of adult respiratory distress syndrome (ARDS). ARDS occurs in approximately 10%–40% of septic patients (Balk and Bone 1989). It is characterised by hypoxaemia with pulmonary oedema detectable on chest X-ray in the absence of fluid overload or cardiac failure.

Ventilation should be commenced when there is evidence of respiratory failure with a pO_2 of <50 mmHg and a pCO_2 of >50 mmHg in room air with a decreasing pH (Lee et al. 1989). Early ventilation may also allow blood flow to be directed away from the respiratory muscles to improve circulation to the brain and other vital organs. Positive end-expiratory ventilation is usually necessary in patients with ARDS.

There has been much debate as to the value of high-dose corticosteroids in patients with septic shock. In a recent review, Nicholson (1989) concluded that high-dose glucocorticoid treatment in the early septic state neither improves outcome nor prevents or reverses ARDS. There remains uncertainty as to whether steroids might reduce mortality in patients with gram-negative septicaemia (Veterans Administration 1987) and further studies are awaited.

Circulatory Support

Resuscitation must be initiated rapidly by fast infusion of 1–2 l of normal saline or similar crystalloid. Colloid solutions should also be used when there is significant hypotension. While monitoring the PCWP with a Swan Ganz catheter, a monitored fluid challenge of 500 ml normal saline over 10 min can be given. If the PCWP rises by more than 7 mmHg the next bolus is withheld. If it does not increase by at least 3 mmHg, then a further bolus of fluid is given. This is known as the "7–3" rule (Pearlman and Faro 1990) and may be sufficient to achieve the required PCWP of 12–16 mmHg.

Following abortion, a large quantity of blood may be lost which should be replaced within the fluid requirements. Anaemia may also be secondary to haemolysis caused by the septicaemia. Disseminated intravascular congestion (DIC) must be treated in consultation with the haematology department. This will involve giving fresh frozen plasma and possibly other clotting factors and platelets.

If fluid and blood fail to restore cardiovascular function, inotropic drugs are necessary. Dopamine, which has dose-dependent actions, is the first choice. At the lowest rate (0.5–3.0 $\mu g/kg/min$), it should increase urine output and cause naturesis (Boyd et al. 1989). At a higher dose (5–10 $\mu g/kg/min$), it has a β-adrenergic effect with a positive inotropic action on the heart; at a dose of more than 15 $\mu g/kg/min$ it has an α-adrenergic effect causing general vasoconstriction. The usual starting dose is 2–5 $\mu g/kg/min$.

The systemic blood pressure may still remain low, due either to depressed left ventricular function or to persistent vasodilatation. If the myocardium is depressed, further inotropic drugs such as dobutamine, isoprenaline or amrinone may be used. Phenylephrine or noradrenaline are given as vasoconstrictors to treat periperhal vasodilatation. The above scheme is depicted in Fig. 8.1 in the form of an algorithm obtained from Lee et al. (1988).

Infection Control

Antibiotic therapy must be initiated immediately using a combination with broad spectrum activity. These can then be adjusted once bacteriological results are available. An intravenous combination of high-dose ampicillin (2 mg every 6 h),

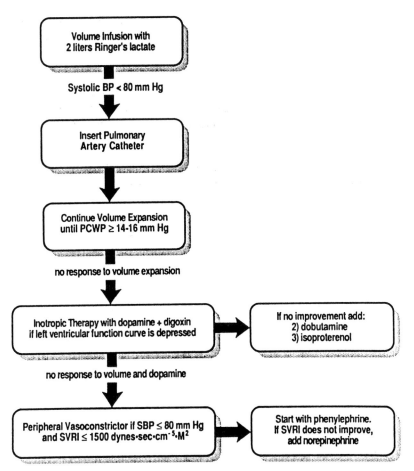

Fig. 8.1. Haemodynamic algorithm for obstetric septic shock. BP, blood pressure; PCWP, pulmonary catheter wedge pressure; SBP, systolic blood pressure; SVRI, systemic vascular resistance index. Reproduced with permission from Lee W, Clark SL, Cotton DB et al. (1988) American Journal of Obstetrics and Gynecology 159:410–416

gentamicin (2 mg/kg loading then 1.5 mg/kg every 8 h) and metronidazole (500 mg every 8 h) is effective against the usual organisms causing septic abortion. Ampicillin is omitted if the patient is allergic to penicillin. In countries with limited access to antibiotics, the combination of benzyl penicillin, chloramphenicol and metronidazole is usually effective. When gentamicin is used, peak and trough blood levels must be routinely monitored to avoid nephrotoxic effects.

Surgical removal of retained products of conception must be expedited and further surgery may be necessary, as already discussed.

If pyrexia continues in spite of the above treatment, septic pelvic vein thrombosis should be considered and full heparin anticoagulation commenced. Some authors consider that heparin should be used routinely in the management of septic abortion since platelet aggregation is one of the underlying pathological mechanisms (Margulis et al. 1971; Botes 1973). The dose is 5000 units i.v.

followed by an infusion of 500–700 units/h, closely monitored by clotting times. More recent reviews on the management of septic shock do not advocate heparin (Pearlman and Faro 1990), though it might be useful in the very early hypercoagulable phase of DIC, if this were recognised in time (Beller 1985).

There are exciting developments in the use of monoclonal antibodies directed at the lipid A domain of endotoxins. Ziegler et al. (1991) have reported a multicentre study of the use of HA–1A (a monoclonal antibody that binds to lipid A) in septic patients. There was a statistically significant reduction in mortality in those patients with gram-negative septicaemic shock treated with the antibody compared to a placebo.

The technology of monoclonal antibodies leads to the possibility of antibodies directed against other pathogenic factors in bacterial shock such as the cytokines, tumour necrosis factor and interleukin 1 (Wolff 1991).

Conclusion

Septic abortion can present with various degrees of severity, but the medical staff must be prepared for the rapid decline in the patient's condition and must not hesitate to perform a laparotomy if she does not respond to supportive therapy, antibiotics and uterine curettage. The obvious way to reduce the incidence of septic abortion and associated mortality is to liberalise abortion laws worldwide.

References

Adadeuoh BK, Akinla O (1970) Postabortal and postpartum tetanus. J Obstet Gynaec Brit Comm 77:1019–1023
Adetoro OO (1986) Septic induced abortion at Ilorin, Nigeria: an increasing gynaecological problem in the developing countries. Asia Oceania J Obstet Gynaecol 12:201–205
Aggarwal VP, Mati JK (1980) Review of abortions at Kenyatta National Hospital, Nairobi. East Afr Med J 57:138–143
Ashworth MF (1990) Harare hospital maternal mortality report for 1987 and a comparison with previous reports. Cent Afr J Med 36:209–212
Balk RA, Bone RC (1989) The septic syndrome: definition and clinical implications. Crit Care Clin 5:1–8
Barnes AB, Ulfelder H (1964) Septic abortion. JAMA 189:919–923
Beller FK (1985) Sepsis and coagulation. Clin Obstet Gynecol 28:46–52
Botes M (1973) Septic abortion and septic shock. S Afr Med J 47:432–435
Boyd JL, Stanford GG, Chernow B (1989) The pharmacotherapy of septic shock. Crit Care Clin 5:133–150
Butler HM (1945) Bacteriological studies of clostridium welchii infections in man. Surg Gynecol Obstet 81:475–486
Cates W, Rochat RW, Grimes DA, Tyler CW (1978) Legalized abortion: effect on national trends of maternal and abortion-related mortality (1940 through 1976). Am J Obstet Gynecol 132:211–214
Cavanagh D, Rao SP, Roberts WS (1985) Septic shock in the gynaecologic patient. Clin Obstet Gynecol 28:355–364
Chow AW, Marshall JR, Guze LB (1977) A double blind comparison of clindamycin with penicillin plus chloramphenicol in treatment of septic abortion. J Infect Dis 135:S35–39

Crowther C (1986) The prevention of maternal deaths: a continuing challenge. Cent Afr J Med 32:11–14

Deane RM, Russell KP (1960) Enterobacillary septicaemia and bacterial shock in septic abortion. Am J Obstet Gynecol 79:528–541

Decker WH, Hall W (1966) Treatment of abortions infected with *Clostridium welchii*. Am J Obstet Gynecol 95:394–399

De Jonge ETM, Venter PF (1988) Hysterectomy for septic abortion – is bilateral salpingo-oophorectomy necessary? S Afr Med J 74:291–292

Department of Health and Social Security (1989) Report on Confidential Enquiries into Maternal Deaths in England and Wales 1982–1984. Her Majesty's Stationery Office, London

Douglas GW, Beckman EM (1966) Clinical management of septic abortion complicated by hypotension. Am J Obstet Gynecol 96:633–644

Foreman H, Stadel BV, Schlesselman S (1981) Intrauterine device usage and fetal loss. Obstet Gynecol 58:669–677

Grimes DA, Cates W, Selik RM (1981) Fatal septic abortion in the United States, 1975–1977. Obstet Gynecol 57:739–744

Hogge WA, Schonberg SA, Golbus MS (1986) Chorionic villus sampling: experience of the first 1000 cases. Am J Obstet Gynecol 154:1249–1252

Keirse MJNC, Ohlsson A, Treffers PE, Kanhai HH (1989) Prelabour rupture of the membranes preterm. In: Chalmers I, Enkin M, Keirse MJNC (eds) Effective care in pregnancy and childbirth, Oxford University Press, Oxford, pp 663–693

Kowen DE, Hanslo DH, Botha PL, Davey DA (1979) Incidence of aerobic and anaerobic infection in patients with incomplete abortion. S Afr Med J 55:129–132

Korepanov VI (1989) Open abdomen technique in the treatment of peritonitis. Br J Surg 76:471

Lee W, Clark SL, Cotton DB et al. (1988) Septic shock during pregnancy. Am J Obstet Gynecol 159:410–416

Lee RM, Balk RA, Bone RC (1989) Ventilatory support in the management of septic patients. Crit Care Clin 5:157–175

Maetani S, Tobe T (1981) Open peritoneal drainage as an effective treatment of advanced peritonitis. Surgery 90:804–809

Margulis RR, Dustin RW, Lovell JR, Robb H, Jabs C (1971) Heparin for septic abortion and the prevention of endotoxin shock. Obstet Gynecol 37:474–483

Marini A, Suma V, Baccichetti C, Lenzini E (1988) A case of septic miscarriage, a probable complication of chorion villus sampling. Prenat Diagn 8:399–400

Mathai S (1986) Abortion and its associated problems – editorial. East Afr Med J 63:769–770

Mills AM (1984) An assessment of pre-operative microbial screening on the prevention of post-abortion pelvic inflammatory disease. Br J Obstet Gynaecol 91:182–186

Munday D, Francome C, Savage W (1989) Twenty one years of legal abortion. Br Med J 298:1231–1234

Nicholson DP (1989) Review of corticosteroid treatment in sepsis and septic shock: pro or con. Crit Care Clin 5:151–155

O'Neill RT, Schwarz RH (1970) Clostridial organisms in septic abortion. Obstet Gynecol 35:458–461

Pearlman M, Faro S (1990) Obstetric septic shock: a pathophysiologic basis for management. Clin Obstet Gynecol 33:482–492

Richards A, Lachman E, Pitsoe SB, Moodley J (1985) The incidence of major abdominal surgery after septic abortion – an indicator of complications due to illegal abortion. S Afr Med J 68:799–800

Richardson JD, Polk HC (1981) Newer adjunctive treatments for peritonitis. Surgery 90:917–918

Rivlin ME, Hunt JA (1986) Surgical management of diffuse peritonitis complicating obstetric/gynecologic infections. Obstet Gynecol 67:652–655

Rotheram EB, Schick SF (1969) Nonclostridial anaerobic bacteria in septic abortion. Am J Med 46:80–89

Schein M, Saadia R, Freinkel Z, Decker GAG (1988) Aggressive treatment of severe diffuse peritonitis: a prospective study. Br J Surg 75:173–176

Shepherd JM, Benny PS (1984) Septic abortion in Wellington 1960–1979. NZ Med J 97:322–324

Smith JW, Southern PM, Lehmann JD (1970) Bacteraemia in septic abortion: complications and treatment. Obstet Gynecol 35:704–708

Tatum HJ, Schmidt FH, Jain AK (1976) Management and outcome of pregnancies associated with the copper T intrauterine contraceptive device. Am J Obstet Gynecol 126:869–879

Templeton JS (1974) Septic abortion and the Dalkon shield. Br Med J ii:612

Unuigbe JA, Oronsaye AU, Orhue AAE (1988) Abortion related morbidity and mortality in Benin City, Nigeria: 1973–1985. Int J Gynaecol Obstet 26:435–439

Veterans Administration Systemic Sepsis Cooperative Study Group (1987) Effect of high-dose glucocorticoid therapy on mortality in patients with clinical signs of sepsis. N Engl J Med 317:659–665

Walsh GL, Chiasson P, Hedderich G, Wexler MJ, Meakins JL (1988) The open abdomen. The Marlex mesh and zipper technique: a method of managing intraperitoneal infection. Surg Clin North Am 68:25–40

Williams P, Johnson B, Vessey M (1975) Septic abortion in women using intrauterine devices. Br Med J iv:263–264

Wolff SM (1991) Monoclonal antibodies and the treatment of gram negative bacteremia and shock – editorial. N Engl J Med 324:486–488

Ziegler EJ, Fisher CJ, Sprung CL et al. (1991) Treatment of gram-negative bacteremia and septic shock with HA–1A human monoclonal antibody against endotoxin. N Engl J Med 324:429–436

9. Miscarriage Following Assisted Conception

A. H. Balen and J. L. Yovich

Miscarriage occurs in between 10% and 30% of all spontaneous pregnancies (Shoham et al. 1991). Infertility is also common, affecting about 30% of couples (Hull et al. 1985). The causes of infertility are multiple and diverse, yet some, for example endometriosis and the polycystic ovary syndrome, may also affect successful implantation and pregnancy outcome. With the development of the techniques of assisted conception it is now possible either to overcome or to circumvent the majority of problems presented by the subfertile couple. One of the main questions to have arisen from the various therapies available is: Do they increase the rate of miscarriage or fetal malformations? And if they are found to do so, is this secondary to the treatment or a reflection of the underlying fertility disorder?

We shall address these questions by examining both the influence on miscarriage of the drugs that are used in ovulation induction and the effect of the different techniques that are employed in assisted conception. We shall also include data from the first 1000 pregnancies in the in-vitro fertilisation (IVF) programme at the Hallam Medical Centre.

Miscarriage in the Infertile Couple

Couples attending the infertility clinic tend to be older than the average couple attending an antenatal clinic. They may have tried for a pregnancy for several years before seeking medical advice, and may then have attended both their general practitioner and gynaecologist for investigation and possibly simple treatments, prior to being referred for assisted conception. Women may also choose to delay starting a family, for example whilst establishing a career. Such a delay leads to a greater incidence of ovulatory dysfunction, endometriosis and the possibility of developing gynaecological pathology necessitating surgery, such as ovarian cysts, fibroids and tubal damage. In our clinic the mean age of the women attending is 33 years (range 22–44).

In addition to the problem of becoming pregnant, the older woman has a high chance of miscarriage. In a recent series of 2730 sonographically confirmed pregnancies the overall first trimester spontaneous abortion rate was 14.6% (Brambati 1990). The incidence of abortion in those women under 35 was 6.4%, rising to 14.7% in women between 35 and 40, and to 23.1% in women over 40. The frequency of chromosomal abnormalities in this series was 82.7% and was greatest in the first 6–8 weeks (86.5%). There are extensive data that confirm a rising risk of chromosomal anomalies with maternal age (Penrose 1933; Trimble and Baird 1978; Hook et al. 1979; Hassold et al. 1980), and this accounts, in a large part, for the increasing miscarriage rate. If a pregnancy continues there appears to be no association between birth defects of unknown aetiology and advancing maternal age (Baird et al. 1991). These data were compiled from 26859 children with birth defects from 576 815 consecutive live births, in whom chromosomal abnormalities and defects of known aetiology (e.g., maternal illness (infection, diabetes, alcohol), teratogenic drugs etc.) had been excluded.

There has been disagreement concerning male factors in spontaneous abortion. Chromosomally abnormal spermatazoa that achieve fertilisation may result in a chromsomally abnormal abortus. Polyploidy should be excluded during IVF procedures as embryos are screened at the pronuclear stage. The uncertainty remains with respect to the influence of abnormal semen parameters severe enough to affect fertility. Some authors have described an adverse effect on pregnancy outcome (Furuhjelm et al. 1962; Joel 1966), whereas more recent reports have found no correlation between abortion and sperm count or motility (Steinberger et al. 1982; Lev-Gur et al. 1990). The use of donor sperm does not appear to have an adverse effect on miscarriage rate (Smith et al. 1981; Lev-Gur et al. 1990).

Apart from the considerations of parental age, the couple with secondary infertility often presents with a poor obstetric history, and with pregnancy losses prior to treatment in 70%–80% (Goldfarb et al 1968; Weir and Hendricks 1969; Hack et al. 1972).

Pregnancy Diagnosis

A major difference between spontaneous and assisted conception is the intensity of early pregnancy monitoring. Pregnancy can be diagnosed as early as 24 h after conception, with the measurement of early pregnancy factor. It is, however, human chorionic gonadotrophin (hCG) that is usually assayed. hCG can be measured in maternal serum and urine from between 8 and 11 days post-ovulation. It is, therefore, possible to determine the success of an assisted conception cycle in the late luteal phase, and so women may know whether they are pregnant before the expected commencement of menses. The usual practice after assisted conception treatements is to wait until day 16 following the day of ovulation or egg collection procedure.

With the advent of sensitive assays for hCG it has been possible to obtain a better idea of the incidence of pregnancy failure in both natural and assisted conceptions. In 1967, Hertig suggested that in natural cycles 85% of oocytes fertilise, 70% of these implant, yet only 58% of these survive until the end of the second week and 16% of them are abnormal and abort shortly after this time. In a series of women trying to conceive, an elevated urinary hCG was found in 59.6% of 198 ovulatory cycles (Edmonds et al. 1982), yet 62% of conceptuses were lost by 12 weeks and most of the losses (92%) were subclinical. The overall fecundability was therefore 22%, which is similar to that expected for a normal population.

It should be remembered that hCG is usually given in most assisted conception regimens in order to mimic the mid-cycle luteinising hormone (LH) surge. This is required in order to initiate oocyte maturation prior to a timed oocyte collection procedure. The exogenous hCG should have been cleared from the circulation by 9–10 days after ovulation or oocyte retrieval (Jones et al. 1985), so hCG at a concentration of greater than 10 IU/l on luteal days 11–13 indicates a pregnancy (and one can be certain of the hCG had been less than 5 IU/l on days 9–10). Many regimens also include hCG for luteal support, administered in one or multiple doses either alone or in combination with a progestogen. In these cases pregnancy can only be diagnosed by a rising titre of hCG, which is usually measured 14–16 days after oocyte retrieval.

A preclinical, or biochemical, abortion occurs with a measurable hCG, usually less than 50 IU/l, which remains elevated for a few days only and results in a delay of menses of no more than 14 days (Jones et al. 1985). A clinical abortion occurs after the hCG has continued to rise to a time when an intrauterine gestation sac can be seen sonographically, either with or without a fetal pole or heart beat.

The Influence on Miscarriage of the Drugs used in Assisted Conception

Ovulatory failure accounts for 21% of cases of infertility (Hull et al. 1985). Over the last 30 years drug regimens of increasing complexity have evolved to induce ovulation. The drugs prescribed to anovulatory women are also used to induce multifollicular growth in women who ovulate normally. These women benefit from superovulation as the production of several oocytes increases the success of assisted conception therapies. The most commonly used preparations are the anti-oestrogens (e.g., clomiphene citrate), the gonadtrophins and gonadotrophin-releasing-hormone agonists. Information about the sequelae of the use of fertility drugs therefore chiefly refers to these three groups.

Anti-oestrogens

The most widely prescribed anti-oestrogen is clomiphene citrate (CC). Its use in ovulation induction was first reported in 1961 (Greenblatt et al. 1961) at a time when human pituitary, and menopausal urinary, gonadotrophins were also beginning to be extracted and standardised. Because of worries about ovarian cyst formation and the difficulties in monitoring the response to the drug, the use of clomiphene was restricted to anovulatory women with a "moderately intact pituitary-ovarian axis" (Karow and Payne 1968).

In an early report of pregnancy outcome in a small number of women, Greenblatt found the incidence of spontaneous abortion to be 22% (Greenblatt et al. 1962). It was to be a few years before the results of larger series were published. Karow and Payne (1968) reported on a heterogeneous group of 410 infertile women, in whom a pregnancy rate of 39.8% was achieved. The spontaneous abortion rate was 19% and similar to that seen in infertility patients prior to the advent of the drug (Karow and Payne 1968). The incidence of twins was 8.6%, contributing to a premature delivery rate of 12%. There was no confirmation of an earlier theory that conception in the first treatment cycle resulted in an increased chance of miscarriage or multiple pregnancy. Also in 1968, a series of 2196 CC-induced pregnancies were reported (MacGregor et al. 1968), in which miscarriage rate was 17.6%, multiple pregnancy rate 10.2% and the incidence of congenital anomalies 2.5%. In a smaller series (160 pregnancies) a lower miscarriage rate of 10.8% was attributed to the use of various combined oestrogen-progestin preparations which were prescribed from the sixth to the twenty-second week of pregnancy (Goldfarb et al. 1968).

Although CC was found to achieve ovulation in about 90% of infertile women and pregnancy in 50%, the multiple pregnancy rate was sometimes as high as 50% (Gemzell 1967). In general the miscarriage rate has been found to be between 20% and 27%, the rate of multiple pregnancy 10%–15% and the incidence of congenital abnormalities about 2%–3% (Bishop 1970; Garcia et al. 1977; Adashi et al. 1979; Kurachi et al. 1983).

One series reported an overall miscarriage rate of 9.3%, yet a rate of 28.1% if conception occurred during the first cycle of treatment and as high as 70.0% if conception resulted after 7 cycles (Toshinobu et al. 1979). It is thought that prolonged usage of CC may have a deleterious effect on the endometrium, causing atrophy and implantation failure (Wall et al. 1964). The relatively high miscarriage rate during the first cycle of treatment that was seen in this study was postulated as being secondary to the release of "over ripe" oocytes after a prolonged period of anovulation (Toshinobu et al. 1979).

Interpreting data from the early use of CC is made difficult by the lack of uniformity in presenting details of maternal age and the cause of infertility. The monitoring of an individual's response to the drug was limited to urinary oestrogens or vaginal cytology, and often monitoring was omitted (Bishop 1970). Pregnancy diagnosis was not as advanced as we have described above and so it is difficult to compare miscarriage data between the different series.

Congenital Abnormalities with Clomiphene Citrate

The incidence of congenital abnormalities and physical development of infants born to mothers who had received CC has not been found to be different to the general population (Bishop 1970; Hack et al. 1972; Garcia et al. 1977; Adashi et al. 1979; Kurachi et al. 1983), yet concern was expressed by the finding of an increased frequency of chromosomal abnormalities after induced ovulation (Boué and Boué 1973), an effect that appeared to persist during the subsequent, non-stimulated cycle.

Following the report of two cases of neural tube defects following CC therapy

(Dyson and Kohler 1973), other isolated cases of congenital abnormalities appeared in the literature (Sandler 1973; Berman 1975; Singh 1978; Czeizel 1989). Others have felt that factors related to infertility itself may be to blame, rather than induction of ovulation (James 1974; Field and Kerr 1974; Ahlgren et al. 1976) and that babies born after ovulation induction are no more at risk of being malformed than if they were conceived spontaneously (Harlap 1976).

Whereas there continue to be reports that suggest a more than coincidental association between ovulation induction specifically using CC, and neural tube defects (Cornel et al. 1989), other reports are reassuring and suggest no evidence for this (Mills et al. 1990). Shoham recently reviewed 3751 births after CC therapy and found an overall incidence of major and minor malformations of 32.5 per 1000 births (Shoham et al. 1991), this figure being within the range found among the normal population (Harlap 1976).

Hypersecretion of Luteinising Hormone

It has been postulated that CC may either reduce the chance of conception in some women, and similarly increase the risk of miscarriage, by inducing an abnormal hormonal environment for the developing oocyte. CC causes an exaggerated early follicular phase release of both gonadotrophins and the resultant luteinising hormone (LH) is thought to have a deleterious effect (Shoham et al. 1990).

In recent years there has been increasing evidence that hypersecretion of luteinising hormone (LH) is deleterious both to fertility and pregnancy outcome (Stanger and Yovich 1985; Abdulwahid et al. 1985; Howles et al. 1986; Homburg et al. 1988). Treatment has therefore been tailored to try to correct the gonadotrophin abnormality.

LH has several functions in the control of the developing follicle: in the early follicular phase low levels of LH induce a change in function of the theca interstitial cells from progesterone to androgen production (Erickson et al. 1985). Follicle stimulating hormone (FSH) then promotes the conversion of androgen to oestradiol by the granulosa cells. Of equal importance is the role of LH in the suppression of the oocyte maturation inhibitor (OMI). The precise nature of OMI is uncertain; it is known that cyclic adenosine monophosphate (cAMP) activates OMI or is itself OMI (Downs 1990). The action of OMI is to maintain the meiotic arrest of the oocyte at the diplotene stage of prophase 1. By reducing cAMP in the oocyte, LH enables the reactivation of meiosis and hence the attainment of oocyte maturity prior to ovulation (Dekel et al. 1990). Inappropriate release of LH may profoundly affect this process such that the released egg is either unable to be fertilised (Homburg et al. 1988) or, if fertilised, miscarries (Regan et al. 1990).

Recently there has been debate about the predictive value of an elevated follicular phase LH for either conception or pregnancy outcome. It was first demonstrated in 1985 that oocytes obtained from women undergoing IVF who had a serum LH value greater than one standard deviation above the mean on the day of human chorionic gonadotrophin (hCG) administration had a significantly reduced rate of fertilisation and cleavage (Stanger and Yovich 1985). This relationship has subsequently been confirmed with urinary LH measurements in the Bourn Hall IVF programme (Howles et al. 1986) and in the ovulation induction clinic at the Middlesex Hospital (Homburg et al. 1988). It has also been shown that not only are ovulation and fertilisation affected by high tonic LH levels but also miscarriage is more likely (Homburg et al. 1988).

The only syndrome to result in a tonic elevation of LH is the polycystic ovary syndrome (PCOS), and it is in women with this condition that CC may induce an exaggerated follicular phase LH rise (Shoham et al. 1990).

A study of women attending a clinic for those who had suffered recurrent miscarriage demonstrated that 82% had PCO (Sagle et al. 1988) and women attending this clinic were also found to have abnormalities in follicular phase LH secretion (Watson et al. 1989). A recent study of 193 women planning to become pregnant showed that mid-follicular phase LH levels of greater than 10 IU/l were associated with both a significant drop in conception rate (67%) and a major increase in miscarriage rate (65%), compared with those women with normal LH levels (88% and 12% respectively) (Regan et al. 1990).

There has been some disagreement on the effect of an elevated LH with one group suggesting no deleterious effect in IVF cycles (Thomas et al. 1989). In this study it was considered that only cycles that result in a pregnancy should be used to provide the normal range of LH concentrations and that by taking LH levels above the 75th centile no adverse effect on fertilisation or cleavage was detected. An effect on miscarriage was not addressed.

While the precise mechanism resulting in hypersecretion of LH in the PCOS is unclear (Conway et al. 1989) we are currently exploring a possible deficiency of a follicular peptide (different from inhibin, and termed "gonadotrophin surge attenuating factor") that has been found by others to suppress pituitary LH release (Fowler et al. 1989; Knight et al. 1990). Irrespective of the aetiology of LH hypersecretion, the therapeutic approach to ovulation induction in women with PCOS should be aimed at preventing inappropriate gonodotrophin levels.

To this end, recent work at the Middlesex Hospital has explored the use of oral Tamoxifen as an alternative regimen to CC, as this antiandrogen has been found to induce ovulation without increasing serum LH concentrations (MacDougall, unpublished data).

Ovulation Induction with Gonadotrophins

Women who do not respond to oral CC therapy may succeed in having ovulation induced with gonadotrophin therapy. The preparations available are either human menopausal gonadotrophin (hMG), which contains 75 IU of both LH and FSH, or "purified" FSH (which contains 75 IU of FSH and less than 1 IU of LH). It was thought that the use of the latter would benefit women with the PCOS by minimising circulating LH levels (Jones et al. 1985). However, these women are usually very senstive to both forms of treatment and the use of "purified" FSH confers no advantage (Homburg et al. 1990). Preparations of recombinant FSH are currently being evaluated and may have a role in future therapies. Whatever the preparation, the main problems with exogenous gonadotrophin therapy are multiple pregnancy and miscarriage (Wang and Gemzell 1980).

Pulsatile administration of luteinising hormone releasing hormone (LHRH) (Mason et al. 1984; Homburg et al. 1989) or FSH (Polson et al. 1987) results is a more physiological response. Another advantage of pulsatile infusion regimens is the low multiple pregnancy rate (Shoham et al. 1990). The use of gonadotrophin releasing hormone analogues (GnRHa) to suppress endogenous gonadotrophins is of uncertain benefit in ovulation induction regimens (Homburg et al. 1990), although there may be a reduction of the miscarriage rate via the suppression of excess LH (Johnson and Pearce 1990).

As for the actual reported miscarriage rate after gonadotrophin-induced ovulation, this varies between 11.3% and 27.5% (Shoham et al. 1991), with an average of 18.8% in a total of 1340 pregnancies, from 6 separate series (Spadoni et al. 1974; Caspi et al. 1976; Schwartz et al. 1980; Kurachi et al. 1983; Lunenfeld et al. 1986; Brown 1986). Lunenfeld also reports an analysis of the abortion rates in both the first and subsequent treatment cycles and the first and subsequent pregnancies (Lunenfeld et al. 1981). In this study it was found that whereas the abortion rate was 28.8% in a first pregnancy, it was only 12.8% in a second pregnancy. This figure is similar to the 13% of women who aborted after a spontaneous conception that followed a successful gonadotrophin-induced pregnancy. There was no difference in the abortion rates of patients who became pregnant after the first or subsequent treatment cycles. This goes against a commonly proposed theory that women who are anovulatory release eggs of "poor quality" in their first ovulation induction cycle (Boué and Boué 1973).

Other groups have also found a higher miscarriage rate in the first gonadotrophin-induced pregnancy. One series demonstrated a reduction in miscarriage rate from 28.5% in first hMG pregnancies to 11.9% in those conceiving for a second time (Ben-Rafael et al. 1983); another series found these figures to be 33% and 9.8% respectively (Miyake et al. 1988). In contrast to these studies a more recent paper reported an overall spontaneous abortion rate in first treatment cycles of 24.2%, yet a 48% abortion rate in women whose first hMG pregnancy ended in a spontaneous abortion; this compared to an incidence of abortion of 6.7% if the first hMG-induced pregnancy was normal (Corsan and Kemmann 1990). This large study looked at 4113 treatment cycles in 996 women, of whom 350 achieved a total of 424 pregnancies. There were no differences in terms of age, weight, duration of infertility, parity or peak oestradiol levels. These data are in keeping with the knowledge that the risk of miscarriage following a natural conception is directly related to a woman's past obstetric history (Poland et al. 1977; Regan et al. 1989).

Various factors have been proposed in the aetiology of spontaneous abortion following gonadotrophin therapy, including an increased incidence of chromosomal abnormalities (Boué and Boué 1973), increased maternal age and obesity (Bohrer and Kemmann 1987), abnormal hormone patterns (Lam et al. 1989) and luteal phase deficiency (Olson et al. 1983). The ovarian hyperstimulation syndrome (OHSS) has also been implicated. This condition may occur when superovulation results in the development of 15 or more follicles and concomitant serum oestradiol levels of greater than 10000 pmmol/l. There may then follow a range of endocrine, haematological and metabolic disturbances. Several groups have reported a higher than expected miscarriage rate when the OHSS has occurred (Hack et al. 1970; Caspi et al. 1976; Lunenfeld et al. 1981; Ben-Rafael et al. 1983). We have not found this to be the case at the Hallam Medical Centre, where the incidence of miscarriage in moderate to severely hyperstimulated women was 14.3% in a recent series (MacDougall et al. 1992).

Congenital Abnormalities after Gonadotrophin Treatment

An analysis of 7 studies that addressed the outcome of gonadotrophin-induced pregnancies concluded that this treatment results in the same incidence of congenital malformations expected for the general population (Shoham et al., 1991). These studies included a total of 1160 newborn infants, in whom the overall incidence of malformations was 54.3 per 1000 (21.6/1000 major and 32.7/1000 minor malformations) (Hack et al. 1970; Spadoni et al. 1974; Harlap 1976; Caspi et al. 1976; Kurachi et al. 1983; Lunenfeld et al. 1986).

Miscarriage after IVF and Related Procedures

Clomiphene or gonadotrophins used for induction of ovulation for either "natural" conception or insemination procedures are aimed to stimulate the development of one, two or at the most three ovulatory follicles. In in-vitro fertilisation (IVF) and other related methods of assisted conception, the usual aim is to achieve superovulation and multifollicular development, with at least 4 oocytes and often many more. However, the usual number of oocytes obtained is between 8 and 15 at the Hallam Medical Centre, with a mean number of 10 oocytes; occasionally 30 or more oocytes are collected. Both CC and the gonadotrophins are used, either singly or in combination, but in recent years there has been a move towards pituitary desensitisation with a gonadotrophin releasing hormone agonist (Porter et al. 1984). The reversible hypogonadotrophic hypogonadism produced permits unimpeded control over follicular development (Fleming et al. 1985) leading to improved pregnancy rates in IVF programmes (Rutherford et al. 1988; Frydman et al. 1988).

The suppression of endogenous LH by GnRH agonists is of particular relevance and advantage to the woman with the PCOS (Jacobs et al. 1987; Fleming and Coutts 1988). Thus many oocyte-containing follicles may develop in the sensitive polycystic ovary free from the adverse environment of high tonic LH levels. These oocytes appear to fertilise better than those from cycles without pituitary desensitisation (Fleming et al. 1988; Abdalla et al. 1990) suggesting that it is indeed the abnormal hormonal milieu, rather than the polycystic ovary itself, that is the problem for women with the PCOS.

Since the birth in 1978 of Louise Brown, the first baby born following in-vitro fertilisation and embryo transfer – in an unstimulated, "natural" cycle – many groups worldwide have reported their experience with IVF and related procedures. It is now possible to determine the rate of miscarriage from the publication of series with large numbers of pregnancies, both from individual clinics and collated national registers (Table 9.1).

It is important to note the criteria that are used both to diagnose pregnancy and to determine the gestational age at miscarriage, as these influence the interpretation of data from different series (Steer et al. 1989). Some groups record "biochemical" pregnancies and miscarriage separately, whilst others classify both together under the heading "miscarriage". The mean age of patients and the methods used to stimulate follicular growth are not always recorded. Up to 1989

Table 9.1. Analysis of multicentre studies on pregnancy outcome following various ovarian stimulation regimes for IVF–ET

Series	Time span	No. of cycles	Regimen	Pregnancies	Live births	Biochemical	Miscellaneous (%)
Trounson and Wood 1984	1979–82	874	CC/hMG	80	55	–	24 (30)
Seppala 1985	1978–84	10028	CC/hMG	1084	600+	–	324 (29.9)
Australian IVF Collab. 1985	1979–83	–	–	244	135	18%	50 (27)
Frydman et al. 1986	1981–84	1280	CC/hMG	142	100	15.5%	27 (19)
Andrews et al. 1986	1981–84	–	hMG/FSH	155	115	18%	23 (15)
Yovich and Matson 1988	1981–86	–	CC/hMG CC/FSH	205	139	9.7%	30 (14.6)
Cohen et al. 1988	1979–85	–	CC/hMG	2329	1456+	–	577 (24.8)
Sharma et al. 1988	1984–86	2232	CC/hMG	306	265	13.3%	26 (8.6%)
NPSU 1988	1979–87	–	CC/hMG	3247	1993	15%	1090 (33.6)
Corson et al. 1989	–	870	CC/hMG	242	187	–	39 (16.1)
Med Res Int 1989	1987	14647	–	1909	1858	–	472 (25%)
Total				9943	6903+	–	2682 (27%)

+ indicates ongoing pregnancies at time of publication

the most popular stimulation regimens were clomiphene citrate with either hCG or purified FSH, and there were also a small number of treatments performed in natural cycles.

The first large series was the World Collaborative Report compiled in 1984 by Seppala from the results of 200 groups worldwide. There was a miscarriage rate of 29.9% in the 1084 pregnancies reported and the 1.5% incidence of congenital anomalies was considered to be similar to that after natural conception. The Australian IVF Collaborative Group reported the results from 8 centres recording a miscarriage rate of 21% and a biochemical pregnancy rate of 18% (Australian IVF Collaborative Group 1985). When the "biochemical" pregnancies were excluded the spontaneous abortion rate was 27%, and this was greatest in older women, as expected after spontaneous conception. It was suggested that some causes of infertility may be associated with a high risk of spontaneous abortion and even premature delivery. The overall live-birth rate was 55% of all diagnosed pregnancies. Again the 1.1% incidence of major congenital abnormalities was equivalent to the Australian national average of 1.5%–2.0%.

Frydman et al. (1986) found that 34.5% of pregnancies conceived in their unit ended either as a biochemical pregnancy or a miscarriage, although with the exclusion of the former group the overall miscarriage rate of 22.5% is not very different from those reported for both fertile and infertile populations (Boué and Boué 1977; Weir and Hendricks 1969). Other authors concur with this finding and stress both the older age of treated women and the greater intensity of pregnancy monitoring, which leads to the detection of biochemical pregnancies and early spontaneous abortions (Andrews et al. 1986; Yovich et al. 1988; Corson et al. 1989).

Early ultrasonography has also demonstrated the spontaneous absorption of a gestation sac in 11 of 42 twin pregnancies and in 5 of 13 sets of triplets (in which two were reduced to singleton pregnancies) (Corson et al. 1989). In another study, 140 pregnancies were scanned weekly from the fifth to the thirteenth week of conception (Tan et al. 1989). In the patients with one sac seen initially, 27% of the sacs disappeared; when there were two sacs, 25% disappeared; and with three sacs, 47% disappeared. The percentage of women who ended up with a viable pregnancy was 72%, 94% and 100% respectively for those initially with 1, 2 and 3 sacs.

The collaborative study by Cohen et al. (1988) looked at 2342 clinically detected pregnancies from 55 centres. With the exclusion of biochemical pregnancies, the miscarriage rate was 24.8% and was greatest in older women. The incidence of malformation was also higher in women of 34.7 years and older; this was 3.4% compared to an incidence of 2.7% in those under 32.9 years. The incidence of congenital malformations was also found to be higher in multiple births (3.6%) compared to singletons (2.5%). This is an interesting observation as the chance of a multiple pregnancy (Cohen et al. 1988) after IVF and its associated procedures is 19% (because of the usual transfer of 2 or more eggs/embryos). The incidence of multiple pregnancy after natural conception is about 1%.

Two other large collaborative studies report the results of conceptions by both IVF and gamete intrafallopian transfer (GIFT) (National Perinatal Statistics Unit (NPSU) 1988; Medical Research International (MRInt) 1989). In 96 clinics in the United States in 1987 the miscarriage rate after IVF was 25% and after GIFT 24% (MRInt 1989). There was similarly little difference between the two procedures in Australia (22.9% for IVF and 24.7% for GIFT) (NPSU 1988). Again the incidence of miscarriage rose markedly with maternal age, being 14% in women under the age of 25 years and 40% in those over 40. This has been a consistent finding and many centres do not treat women over the age of 40 because of the reduced chance of achieving a pregnancy and the increased risk of miscarriage. This issue was addressed by Romeu et al. (1987) who actually found a surprisingly good response to ovulation induction and in-vitro fertilisation in older women, and also found that the abortion rate is only slightly higher than in the younger age group, at 60% overall (33.3% biochemical pregnancies and 26.6% clinical abortions). The incidence of chromosomal abnormalities is increased in this group of patients and so careful counselling and prenatal diagnosis is suggested.

The first 1000 pregnancies at the Hallam Medical Centre occurred as a result of treatment from 1984 to Feburary 1989. 680 pregnancies resulted in the birth of 901 live children (147 twins, 34 triplets and 2 sets of quadruplets). There were 52 ectopic pregnancies – an incidence of 5.2%, which is similar to the mean of 4.7% from other large series (Table 9.2). There were 13 cases of heterotopic pregnancy; in 7 of these there was a viable intrauterine pregnancy and the pregnancy progressed uneventfully after the ectopic pregnancy had been removed.

There were 80 biochemical pregnancies (8%) and 188 miscarriages (18.8%) resulting in an early pregnancy loss rate of 26.8%, excluding ectopic pregnancies. It is interesting that there is no difference between the mean age of the women

Table 9.2. Analysis of multicentre studies on the incidence of ectopic pregnancy and fetal congenital abnormality following treatment by IVF–ET

	Ectopic (%)	Congenital anomalies (%)
Trounson and Wood 1984	1.25	1.25
Seppala 1985	1.8	1.5
Australian IVF Collab. 1985	5	1.1
Frydman et al. 1986	2.1	2.6
Andrews et al. 1986	1.6	
Yovich and Matson 1988	7.8	
Cohen et al. 1988	5.2	3
Corson et al. 1989	5.8	
Med Res Int 1989	7	1.4
MRC 1990		2.9
Total	4.7	2

who miscarried (32.8 years (range 22–41)) and those who had successful pregnancies (32.1 years (range 22–44)). The primary diagnosis of sub-fertility was also the same in the two groups (Table 9.3) and this is similar to the experience of other centres. The mean gestation at the time of miscarriage was 9.75 weeks.

Luteal support was given in the form of 2 injections of hCG 2000 U, the first on the day of embryo transfer and the second three days later. We have since changed to the regimen of 5 daily intramuscular injections of Gestone 50 mg (Paines and Byrne UK) followed by hCG 1000 U on days 4, 7, 10 and 13 after oocyte recovery (Yovich et al 1991).

A variety of regimens are used in different centres for supporting the luteal phase of assisted conception cycles. Published reports of randomised controlled trials assessing the use of progesterone (P) (Leeton et al. 1985; Yovich et al. 1985; Trounson et al. 1986) or hCG (Yovich et al. 1984; Mahadevan et al. 1985; Buvat et al. 1990) fail to show significant improvements in pregnancy rates, although

Table 9.3. Analysis of multicentre studies of diagnostic categories of couples undergoing IVF-ET

	Tubal damage (%)	Endometriosis (%)	Male factor (%)	Immunological (%)	Unknown (%)	Other (%)
Trounson and Wood 1984	52	8	20		20	
Seppala 1985	78	8.7			13.1	
Frydman et al. 1986	90		12	3.2	2.5	
Cohen et al. 1988	67.9		3.5		11.9	16.7
Sharma et al. 1988	44.5	12.3	5.4	3.6	27.2	6.9
Corson et al. 1989	42	31	8	4	10	9
MRC 1990	65	6	8		11	8
Mean	62.8	13.2	9.5	3.6	12.2	10.2

there is usually a trend implying benefit. All of these studies have suffered by being too small and comprising heterogeneous populations of patients.

The study of Yovich et al. (1991), compared four groups: group 1 received no luteal support; group 2, hCG 1000 U given by intramuscular injection on days 4, 7, 10 and 13 of the luteal phase (the day of oocyte recovery being day 0); group 3, 50 mg progesterone in oil, given by intramuscular injection on days 0, 1, 2, 3 and 4; and group 4 being a combination of groups 2 and 3. 280 couples were randomised into the four groups during GIFT treatment cycles, although only 207 completed the treatment. Those in group 4 achieved the best pregnancy rate of 41.2%, compared to 27.5% in group 1, 34.6% in group 2 and 32.0% in group 3. These differences were not significant. However, the birth rates were significantly better in those women receiving luteal support (29.4% group 4, 26.0% group 3, 25.5% group 2) compared to those who received none (11.8%). Thus luteal support appears to reduce the miscarriage rate and improve the ongoing pregnancy rate.

Summary

In conclusion, we have found that the incidence of early pregnancy loss in our IVF practice differs little from that of other clinics. However, in contrast to the experience of others, and that expected for the general population, there was no difference in age between those women who miscarried and those who carried a pregnancy to term. When one accounts for the intensity of early pregnancy monitoring after assisted conception procedures, and hence the relatively frequent diagnosis of "biochemical" pregnancy, the overall spontaneous miscarriage rate is similar to that expected for the general population. Indeed it has been pointed out by Shoham et al. (1991) that as a mean age of under 30 is usually quoted for patients in studies of miscarriage after spontaneous conception, the abortion rate is treated, subfertile women might be "even lower than that of the so called normal population when adjusted for age". It is also encouraging to note that the drugs used in assisted conception regimens do not appear to adversely affect the incidence of congenital abnormalities.

References

Abdalla HI, Ahuja KK, Leonard T, Morris NN, Honour JW, Jacobs HS (1990) Comparative trial of luteinising hormone releasing hormone analogue/HMG and clomiphene citrate/HMG in an assisted conception programme. Fertil Steril 53:473–478

Abdulwahid NA, Adams J, Van der Spuy ZM, Jacobs HS (1985) Gonadotrophin control of follicular development. Clin Endocrinol 23:613–626

Adashi EY, Rock JA, Sapp KC, Martin EJ, Wentz AC, Jones GS (1979) Gestational outcome of clomiphene-related conceptions. Fertil Steril 31:620–626

Ahlgren M, Kallen B, Rannevik G (1976) Outcome of pregnancy after clomiphene therapy. Acta Obstet Gynecol Scand 55:371–375

Andrews MC, Muasher SJ, Levy D, Jones HW, Garcia JE, Rosenwaks Z, Jones GS, Acosta AA

(1986) An analysis of the obstetric outcome of 125 consecutive pregnancies conceived in vitro and resulting in 100 deliveries. Am J Obstet Gynecol 154:848–854

Australian IVF Collaborative Group (1985) High incidence of preterm births and early losses in pregnancy after IVF. Br Med J 291:1160–1163

Baird PA, Sadovnick AD, Yee IML (1991) Maternal age and birth defects: a population study. Lancet 337:527–530

Ben-Rafael Z, Dor J, Mashiach S, Blankstein J, Lunenfeld B, Serr DM (1983) Abortion rate in pregnancies following ovulation induced by human menopausal gonadotropin/human chorionic gonadotropin. Fertil Steril 39:157

Berman P (1975) Congenital abnormalities associated with maternal clomiphene ingestion. Lancet i:878

Bishop PMF (1970) Clomiphene. Br Med Bull 26:22–25

Bohrer M, Kemmann E (1987) Risk factors for spontaneous abortion in menotropin-treated women. Fertil Steril 48:571

Boué JG, Boué A (1973) Increased frequency of chromosomal anomalies in abortions after induced ovulation. Lancet i:679

Boué A, Boué J (1977) Le role des anomalies chromosomiques dans les echecs de la reproduction. J Gynecol Obstet Biol Reprod 6:5–21

Brambati B (1990) Fate of human pregnancies. In: Edwards RG (ed): Establishing a successful human pregnancy, Serono Symposia, vol. 66. Raven Press, NY, pp 269–281

Brown GB (1986) Gonadotropins. In: Insler V, Lunenfeld B (eds) Infertility: male and female. Churchill Livingstone, New York, pp 359–373

Buvat J, Marcolin G, Guittard C, Herbaut JC, Louvet AL, Dehaone JL (1990) Luteal support after LHRH agonist for IVF: superiority of human chorioinic gonadotropin over oral progesterone. Fertil Steril 53:490–494

Caspi E, Ronen J, Schreyer P, Goldberg MD (1976) The outcome of pregnancy after gonadotropin therapy. Br J Obstet Gynaecol 83:967–971

Cohen J, Mayaux MJ, Guihard-Moscato ML (1988) Pregnancy outcomes after in vitro fertilization: A collaborative study on 2342 pregnancies. Ann NY Acad Sci 541:1–6

Conway GS, Honour JW, Jacobs HS (1989) Heterogeneity of the polycystic ovary syndrome: clinical, endocrine and ultrasound features in 556 patients. Clin Endocrinol 30:459–470

Cornel MC, Kate LPT, Dukes MN, de Jong VD, Berg LTW, Meyboom RHB, Garbis H, Peters PW (1989) Ovulation induction and neural tube defects. Lancet i:1386

Corsan GH, Kemmann E (1990) Risk of a second consecutive first-trimester spontaneous abortion in women who conceive with menotropins. Fertil Steril 53:817–821

Corson SL, Dickey RP, Gocial B, Batzer FR, Eisenberg E, Huppert L, Maislin G (1989) Outcome in 242 in vitro fertilization-embryo replacement or gamete intrafallopian transfer-induced pregnancies. Fertil Steril 51:644–650

Czeizel A (1989) Ovulation induction and neural tube defects. Lancet i:167

Dekel N, Galiani D, Aberdam E (1990) Regulation of rat oocyte maturation: involvement of protein kinases. In: Bavister BD, Cummins J, Roldan ERS (eds) Fertilisation in mammals. Serono Symposia, Norwell, USA, pp 17–24

Downs SM (1990) Maintenance of meiotic arrest in mammalian oocytes. In: Bavister BD, Cummins & Roldan ERS (eds) Fertilisation in mammals. pp 5–16. Serono Symposia, Norwell, USA

Dyson JL, Kohler HG (1973) Anencephaly and ovulation stimulation. Lancet i:1256–1257

Edmonds DK, Lindsay KS, Miller JF, Williamson E, Wood PJ (1982) Early embryonic mortality in women. Fertil Steril 38:447–453

Erickson GF, Magoffin DA, Dyer CA, Hofeditz C (1985) The ovarian androgen producing cells: a review of structure/function relationships. Endo Rev 6:371–399

Field B, Kerr C (1974) Ovulation stimulation and defects of neural-tube closure. Lancet ii:1511

Fleming R, Haxton MJ, Hamilton MPR, McCune GS, Black WP, Macnaughton MC, Coutts JRT (1985) Successful treatment of infertile women with oligomenorrhoea using a combination of a luteinising hormone releasing hormone agonist and exogenous gonadotrophin. Br J Obstet Gynaecol 92:369–374

Fleming R, Jamieson ME, Hamilton MPR, Black WP, Macnaughton MC, Coutts JRT (1988) The use of gonadotrophin releasing hormone analogues in combination with exogenous gonadotropins in infertile women. Acta Endocrinol, suppl 288, 119:77–84

Fleming R, Coutts JRT (1988) luteinising hormone releasing hormone analogues for ovulation induction, with particular reference to polycystic ovary syndrome. In: Healy D (ed) Anti-Hormones in Clinical Gynaecology, Bailliere's Clin Obstet Gynaecol 2:677–688

Fowler PA, Messinis IE, Templeton AA (1989) Gonadotrophin surge-attenuating factor activity in human follicular fluid is different from inhibin. J Repro Fert, Abs series 4 no. 17

Frydman R, Belaisch-Allart JC, Fries N, Hazout A, Glissant A, Testart J (1986) An obstetric assessment of the first 100 births from the in vitro fertilization program at Clamont, France. Am J Obstet Gynecol 154:550–555

Frydman R, Fries N, Testart J et al. (1988) Luteinising hormone releasing hormone agonists in in-vitro fertilisation: different methods of utilization and comparison with previous ovulation stimulation treatments. Hum Reprod 3:559–561

Furuhjelm M, Jonson B, Lagergren CC (1962) The quality of human semen in spontaneous abortion. Int J Fertil 7:17–21

Garcia J, Jones GS, Wentz AC (1977) The use of clomiphene citrate. Fertil Steril 28:707–717

Gemzell CA (1967) Clomiphene induction of ovulation. In: Westlin B, Wiqvist N (eds). Fertility and sterility. Excerpta Medica Foundation, Amsterdam, p 43

Goldfarb AF, Morales A, Rakoff AE, Protos P (1968) Critical review of 160 clomiphene related pregnancies. Obstet Gynecol 31:342–345

Greenblatt RB, Barfield WE, Jungck EC, Ray AW (1961) Induction of ovulation with MRL–41. JAMA 178:101

Greenblatt RB, Roy S, Mahesh VB, Barfield W, Jungck EC (1962) Induction of ovulation. Am J Obstet Gynecol 84:900–907

Hack M, Brish M, Serr DM, Insler V, Lunenfeld B (1970) Outcome of pregnancy after induced ovulation. Follow-up of pregnancies and children born after gonadotropin therapy. JAMA 211:791–976

Hack M, Brish M, Serr DM, Insler V, Salomy M, Lunenfeld B (1972) Outcome of pregnancy after induced ovulation. JAMA 220:1329–1333

Harlap S (1976) Ovulation induction and congenital malformations. Lancet ii:961

Hassold T, Jacobs P, Kline J, Stein Z, Warburton D (1980) Effect of maternal age on autosomal trisomies. Ann Hum Genet 44:29–36

Hertig AT (1967) The overall problem in man. In Benirschke K (ed) Comparative aspects of reproductive failure. Springer-Verlag, NY, pp 11–41

Homburg R, Armar NA, Eshel A, Adams J, Jacobs HS (1988) Influence of serum luteinising hormone concentrations on ovulation, conception and early pregnancy loss in polycystic ovary syndrome. Br Med J 297:1024–1026

Homburg R, Eshel A, Armar NA, Tucker M, Mason PW, Adams J, Kilborn J, Sutherland IA, Jacobs HS (1989) One hundred pregnancies after treatment with pulsatile luteinising hormone hormone to induce ovulation. Br Med J 298:809–812

Homburg R, Eshel A, Kilborn J, Adams J, Jacobs HS (1990) Combined luteinising hormone releasing hormone analogue and exogenous gonadotrophins for the treatment of infertility associated with polycystic ovaries. Hum Repro 5:32–35

Hook EB, Woodbury DF, Albright SG (1979) Rates of trisomy 18 in livebirths, stillbirths and at amniocentesis. Birth defects: original article series. New York: A. R. Liss, 15(5c):81–89

Howles CM, Macnamee MC, Edwards RG, Goswamy R, Steptoe PC (1986) Effect of high tonic levels of luteinising hormone on outcome of in-vitro fertilisation. Lancet i:521–522

Hull MGR (1990) Indications for assisted conception. In: Edwards RG (ed) Assisted Human Conception. Br Med Bull 46:580–595

Hull MGR, Glazener CMA, Kelly NJ et al. (1985) Population study of causes, treatment and outcome of infertility. Br Med J 291:1693–1697

Jacobs HS, Porter R, Eshel A, Craft I (1987) Profertility uses of luteinising hormone releasing hormone agonist analogues. In: Vickery BH, Nestor JJ (eds) LHRH and its Analogs. MTP Press Ltd, Lancaster, pp 303–322

James WH (1974) Anencephaly, ovulation stimulation and subfertility. Lancet ii:1353

Joel CA (1966) New etiologic aspects of habitual abortion and infertility with special reference to the male factor. Fertil Steril 17:374–379

Johnson P, Pearch JM (1990) Recurrent spontaneous abortion and polycystic ovarian disease: comparison of two regimens to induce ovulation. Br Med J 301:154–156

Jones GS, Acosta AA, Garcia JE, Bernadus RE, Rosenwaks Z (1985) The effect of follicle stimulating hormone without additional luteinising hormone on follicular stimulation and oocyte development in normal ovulatory women. Fertil Steril 43:696–702

Karow WG, Payne SA (1968) Pregnancy after clomiphene citrate treatment. Fertil Steril 19:351–362

Knight PG, Lacey M, Peter JLT, Whitehead SA (1990) Demonstration of a non-steroidal factor in human follicular fluid that attenuates the self-priming action of gonadotrophin-releasing hormone on pituitary gonadotropes. Biol Repro 42:613–618

Kurachi K, Aono T, Minagawa J, Miyake A (1983) Congenital malformations of newborn infants after clomiphene-induced ovulation. Fertil Steril 40:187–189

Lam S-Y, Baker HWG, Evans JH, Pepperell RJ (1989) Factors affecting fetal loss in induction of ovulation with gonadotrophins: increased abortion rates related to hormonal patterns in conceptual cycles. Am J Obstet Gynecol 160:621–629

Leeton J, Trounson A, Jessup D (1985) Support of the luteal phase in in vitro fertilization programs: result of a controlled trial with intramuscular Proluton. J In Vitro Fert Embryo Transfer 2: 166–171

Lev-Gur M, Rodriguez LJ, Smith KD, Steinberger E (1990) Risk factors for pregnancy loss apparent at conception in infertile couples. Int J Fert 35:51–57

Lunenfeld B, Serr DM, Mashiach S et al. (1981) Therapy with gonadotropins: Where are we today? Analysis of 2890 menotropin treatment cycles in 914 patients. In: Insler V, Bettendorf G (eds) Advances in diagnosis and treatment of infertility. Elsevier Inc, Amsterdam, pp 27–31

Lunenfeld B, Blankstein J, Kotev-Emet S, Kokia E, Geier A (1986) Drugs used in ovulation induction: safety of patients and offspring. Hum Reprod 1:435–439

MacDougall J, Tan SL, Jacobs HS (1992) Ovarian Hyperstimulation Syndrome after in-vitro fertilisation. Fertil Steril (in press).

MacGregor AH, Johnson JE, Bunde CA (1968) Further clinical experience with clomiphene citrate. Fertil Steril 19:616–622

Mahadevan MM, Leader A, Taylor PJ (1985) Effects of low dose human chorionic gonadotrophin on corpus luteum function after embryo transfer. J In Vitro Fert Embryo Transfer 2:190–194

Mason P, Adams J, Morris DV, Tucker M, Price J, Voulgaris Z, Van der Spuy ZM, Sutherland I, Chambers GR, White S, Wheeler MJ, Jacobs HS (1984) Induction of ovulation with pulsatile luteinising hormone releasing hormone. Br Med J 288:181–185

Medical Research International (1989) In vitro fertilization/embryo transfer in the United States: 1987 results from the National IVF-ET Registry. Fertil Steril 51:13–15

Mills JL, Simpson JL, Rhoads GG et al. (1990) Risk of neural tube defects in relation to maternal fertility and fertility drug use. Lancet 336:103–104

Miyake A, Kurachi H, Wakimoto H, Hirota K, Terakawa N, Aono T, Tanizawa O (1988) Second pregnancy with spontaneous ovulation following clomiphene- or gonadotropin-induced pregnancy. Eur J Obstet Gynecol Reprod Biol 27:1–5

National Perinatal Statistics Unit (NPSU) and the Fertility Society of Australia and New Zealand (1988) IVF and GIFT Pregnancies Australia and New Zealand, 1987. NPSU, 1988

Olson JL, Rebar RW, Schreiber JR, Vaitukaitis JL (1983) Shortened luteal phase after ovulation induction with human menopausal gonadotropin and human chorionic gonadotropin. Fertil Steril 39:284–289

Penrose LS (1933) The relative effects of maternal and paternal age in mongolism. J Genet 27:219–224

Poland BJ, Miller JR, Jones DC, Trimble BK (1977) Reproductive counselling in patients who have had a spontaneous abortion. Am J Obstet Gynecol 127:685–691

Polson DW, Mason HD, Saldahna MB, Franks S (1987) Ovulation of a single dominant follicle during treatment with low-dose pulsatile follicle stimulating hormone in women with polycystic ovary syndrome. Clin Endocrinol 26:205–212

Porter RN, Smith W, Craft IL, Abdulwahid NA, Jacobs HS (1984) Induction of ovulation for in-vitro fertilisation using buserelin and gonadotrophins. Lancet ii:1284–1285

Regan L, Braude PR, Trembath PL (1989) Influence of past reproductive performance on risk of spontaneous abortion. Br Med J 299:541–545

Regan L, Owen EJ, Jacobs HS (1990) Hypersecretion of luteinising hormone, infertility and miscarriage. Lancet ii:1141–1144

Romeu A, Muasher SJ, Acosta AA, Veeck LL, Diaz J, Jones GS, Jones HW, Rosenwaks Z (1987) Results of in vitro fertilization attempts in women 40 years of age and older: the Norfolk experience. Fertil Steril 47:130–136

Rutherford AJ, Subak-Sharpe RJ, Dawson MJ, Margara RA, Franks S, Winston RML (1988) Improvement of in-vitro fertilisation after treatment with buserelin, an agonist of luteinising hormone releasing hormone. Br Med J 296:1765–1768

Sagle M, Bishop K, Alexander FM, Michel M, Bonney RC, Beard RW, Franks S (1988) Recurrent early miscarriage and polycystic ovaries. Br Med J 297:1027–1028

Sandler B (1973) Anencephaly and ovulation stimulation. Lancet ii:379

Schwartz M, Jewelewicz R, Dyrenfurth I, Tropper P, Vande Wile RL (1980) The use of human menopausal and chorionic gonadotropins for ovulation induction. Am J Obstet Gynecol 138:801–806

Seppala M (1985) The World Collaborative Report on in vitro fertilization and embryo replacement: current state of the art in January 1984. Ann N Y Acad Sci 442:558–563

Sharma V, Riddle A, Mason BA, Pampiglione J, Campbell S (1988) An analysis of factors influencing the establishment of a clinical pregnancy in an ultrasound-based ambulatory in-vitro fertilisation program. Fertil Steril 49:468–478

Shoham Z, Borenstein R, Lunenfeld B, Pariente C (1990) Hormonal profiles following clomiphene citrate therapy in conception and nonconception cycles. Clin Endocrinol 33:271–278

Shoham Z, Zosmer A, Insler V (1991) Early miscarriage and fetal malformations after induction of ovulation (by clomiphene citrate and/or human menotropins), in vitro fertilization, and gamete intrafallopian transfer. Fertil Steril 55:1–11

Singh M (1978) Possible relationship between clomiphene and neural tube defects. J Ped 93:152

Smith KD, Rodriguez-Rigau LJ, Steinberger E (1981) The influence of ovulatory dysfunction and timing of insemination on the success of AID with fresh or cryopreserved semen. Fertil Steril 36:496–499

Spadoni LR, Cox DW, Smith DC (1974) Use of human menopausal gonadotropin for the induction of ovulation. Am J Obstet Gynecol 120:988–992

Stanger JD, Yovich JL (1985) Reduced in-vitro fertilisation of human oocyte from patients with raised basal luteinising hormone levels during the follicular phase. Br J Obstet Gynaecol 92:385–393

Steer C, Campbell S, Davies M, Mason B, Collins W (1989) Spontaneous abortion rates after natural and assisted conception. BMJ 299: 1317–1318

Steinberger E, Rodriguez-Rigau LJ, Smith KD (1982) Interaction of the two partners in the couple. In Menchini Fabris GF, Pasini W, Martini L (eds) Therapy in Andrology. Int Cong Ser 596: 21–29

Tan SL, Riddle A, Sharma V, Mason B, Campbell S (1989) The relation between the number of gestation sacs seen after IVF-ET and outcome of pregnancy. Proceedings of the XIIth Asian and Oceanic Congress of Obstetrics and Gynaecology

Thomas A, Okamoto S, O'Shea F, Maclachlan V, Besanko M, Healy D (1989) Do raised serum luteinising hormone levels during stimulation for in-vitro fertilisation predict outcome? Br J Obstet Gynaecol 96:1328–1332

Toshinobu T, Seiichiro F, Noriaki S, Kihyoe I (1979) Correlation between dosage or duration of clomid therapy and abortion rate. Int J Fert 24:193–197

Trimble BK, Baird PA (1978) Maternal age and Down syndrome. Age specific incidence rates by single year maternal age intervals. Am J Med Genet 1:1–5

Trounson A, Wood C (1984) In vitro fertilisation results, 1972–1982, at Monash University, Queen Victoria, and Epworth Medical Centres. J IVF-ET 1:42–47

Trounson A, Howlett D, Rogers P, Hoppen HO (1986) The effect of progesterone supplementation around the time of oocyte recovery in patients superovulated for in vitro fertilization. Fertil Steril 45:532–537

Wall JA, Franklin RR, Kaufman RH (1964) Reversal of benign and malignant endometrial changes with clomiphene. Am J Obstet Gynecol 88:1–7

Wang CF, Gemzell C (1980) The use of human gonadotrophins for the induction of ovulation in women with polycystic ovary syndrome. Clin Endocrinol 12: 479–486

Watson H, Hamilton-Fairly D, Kiddy D, Bray C, Armstrong P, Beard R, Bonrey R, Franks S (1989) Abnormalities of follicular phase luteinising hormone secretion in women with recurrent early miscarriage. J Endocrinol 123 suppl, Abstract 25

Weir WC, Hendricks CH (1969) The reproductive capacity of an infertile population. Fertil Steril 20:289–298

Yovich JL, Stanger JD, Yovich JM, Tuvik A (1984) Assessment and hormonal treatment of the luteal phase of IVF cycles. Aus N Z J Obstet Gynaecol 24:125

Yovich JL, McColm SC, Yovich JM, Matson PL (1985) Early luteal serum progesterone concentrations are higher in conception cycles. Fertil steril 44:185–191

Yovich JL, Matson PL (1988) Early pregnancy wastage after gamete manipulation. Br J Obstet Gynaecol 95:1120–1127

Yovich JL, Edirisinghe WR, Cummins JM (1991) Evaluation of luteal support therapy in a randomized controlled study within a gamete intrafallopian transfer program. Fertil Steril 55:131–139

10. Abortion Following Invasive Diagnostic Procedures in the First Trimester

M. D. Griffith-Jones and R. J. Lilford

Introduction

Prenatal diagnostic tests can be divided into those involving measurement of chemicals in maternal blood, those in which the fetus is imaged, and invasive tests are used to remove tissues of fetal origin. The latter may be further divided into those carried out beyond 14 weeks gestational age, before 14 weeks but after implantation, and those in the pre-implantation period. The first group (beyond 14 weeks) includes fetal blood sampling, fetal tissue biopsy, mid-pregnancy amniocentesis and transabdominal chorion biopsy. Pre-implantation diagnosis includes embryo biopsy and polar body analysis. This chapter, however, is concerned with those tests that may be performed in the first trimester with early amniocentesis, transabdominal chorion villus biopsy or sampling (CVS) and transcervical CVS being considered. Less frequently used methods such as aspiration of chorionic villi, amniotic or blastocyst fluid through the vaginal fornices and cytological sampling of the lower uterine pole are not considered in this chapter.

Safety

Evaluating Safety of Invasive Prenatal Diagnostic Tests

The technique which is safest in general is not always the method which is safest in a particular practitioner's hands. Nevertheless established centres will wish to monitor pregnancy outcomes and audit these against reported results and doctors planning early pregnancy diagnostic services will wish to compare the safety of various procedures. Comparisons may be drawn from different centres doing different tests, or from particular centres offering alternative procedures (i.e., direct comparative studies). Non-randomised studies of both types are subject to numerous potential biases (some examples are given in Table 10.1) and practitioners should also be aware of these when comparing their results with those reported in the literature or published by other centres.

Table 10.1. Sources of bias of particular relevance in non-randomised studies of the miscarriage risks of prenatal diagnostic procedures

Factor	Mechanism of Bias
Maternal age	Miscarriage rate rises with age and younger age distribution in one group could bias results away from the other
Removal of aneuploid fetuses from follow-up	Many fetal losses have aneuploidy losses and these are removed from follow-up by testing, thereby biasing results in favour of a diagnostic test vs background risk. This factor may counterbalance the above maternal age effect, but to an unspecified degree
Gestational age at testing	Ultrasonically intact pregnancies may be lost at any time. First trimester procedures may be carried out at slightly different mean gestational ages, e.g., transabdominal CVS is usually done slightly later than the transcervical method
Operator	Bias results against test where operators are on earlier part of the learning-curve. Tests may have differently shaped learning curves
Unequal follow-up	If good news travels better than bad, results biased against test with better follow-up and vice versa

The principal maternal risk of prenatal tests is septicaemia. The principal fetal risks are of miscarriage and of a degree of pulmonary hypoplasia with amniocentesis (Tabor et al. 1986). However, as with drug effects in pregnancy, any rare complications cannot be distinguished with confidence from the natural incidence of these outcomes (Orrell and Lilford 1990). For example, if transabdominal CVS was associated with, say, a one-in-300 risk of massive placental abruption or if amniocentesis caused brain damage, through pre-term birth, in one baby in 400, then we would never know about these risks. On the other hand, certain poor outcomes will occur in sporadic clusters from time to time and isolated reports from specific centres linking CVS and, say, a rare congenital abnormality are difficult to interpret.

Transabdominal versus Transcervical CVS

A good overview of the results of different types of CVS are presented in Professor Laird Jackson's Newsletters from the Division of Medical Genetics, Jefferson Medical College, Philadelphia. The May 1990 report presents a non-randomised study in the State of Victoria giving fetal loss rates of 5.9% and 2.4% for transcervical and transabdominal CVS respectively, though operator experience and gestational age at sampling may have differed between techniques, thereby biasing the comparison. Amalgamating all data in the Newsletter, the transabdominal technique is associated with a consistently lower fetal loss rate. In March 1987 the total register had 25 000 patients. Transabdominal sampling was then very new and results may have been biased away from this technique. Nevertheless, this method was associated with a total loss rate of 2.1%, in contrast to over 4% for all transcervical methods. However, the most experienced centres had fetal loss rates close to 2%. The tentative conclusion of these studies is that, with skill and experience, transcervical CVS can be as safe as transabdominal CVS but the learning curves are different.

One of the concerns with transcervical CVS is the fear of maternal septicaemia and septic abortion. While it cannot be claimed that these complications never occur after transabdominal procedures, they would appear to occur much more commonly following transcervical aspiration; this accords with our knowledge of the bacteriology of the cervix, together with the experience in countries where abortion is illegal. Finikiotis and Gower (1990), on direct comparison of the two techniques, found two septic abortions in 84 transcervical CVS compared to no such cases amongst 126 transabdominal procedures.

Non-randomised studies are subject to selection bias, especially that which would arise if transabdominal sampling was done at a greater mean gestational age. A large randomised comparison of the two techniques was carried out by Brambati and colleagues and reported in two parts (Brambati et al. 1988, 1990). They found that the transabdominal method was easier to learn. Samples suitable for analysis were produced more frequently with transabdominal CVS while uterine infection was more common after the transcervical method. However, total fetal loss rates were very similar with both techniques; 3.2% transabdominal (29/850) versus 3.9% transcervical (53/1350). Nevertheless, this group has come to prefer the transabdominal method, having originally been pioneers of transcervical sampling. R. J. Wapner and colleagues have also undertaken a randomised trial as part of the, as yet unpublished, NIH trial, and compare abortion rates among pregnancies which were not terminated following the transabdominal and transcervical methods. They report 15 miscarriages among 659 pregnancies with transabdominal CVS (2.4%) versus 11 miscarriages among 698 unterminated pregnancies following transcervical CVS (1.6%). The difference is not significant. These authors also report two cases of clinical infection among 1636 transcervical procedures and none among 964 transabdominal procedures. Bovicelli et al. (1986) in a small randomised study (120 patients) report identical miscarriage risks with each method.

CVS versus Midtrimester Amniocentesis

Abortion rates for pregnancies destined to continue following both transabdominal and transcervical CVS in centres with the greatest experience are of the order of 2% (Brambati et al. 1990). Background total abortion rates at various stages of pregnancy have been documented (Gustavii et al. 1984; Hobbins 1984) but these are of little relevance to the risk of miscarriage where the fetus is seen to be intact on ultrasound. A number of studies have now addressed the probability of fetal loss in pregnancies which are shown by ultrasound to be intact and viable at around 10 weeks gestation (Wilson et al.1984). Exclusion of patients with missed abortions shows that the background abortion rate for viable pregnancies at ten weeks gestation is about two per cent (Liu et al. 1987). This could be an overestimate for women of unselected maternal age, as patients having ultrasound in the first trimester may be a selected group with a high risk of miscarriage because of previous or threatened miscarriage. Furthermore, simple subtraction of background abortion risk from the total abortion rate following the procedure may not give an accurate measurement of the procedure-related risks. Patients requiring CVS are often older and may have a higher background risk of abortion than unselected populations. For example Gilmore and McHay (1985) estimate a 4% background fetal loss rate before 28 weeks for women aged 35–39 years of age. On the other hand, the higher rate of fetal loss in older mothers could be due to a higher incidence of chromosomally abnormal conceptions. Direct comparison of miscarriage risks following CVS and amnio-centesis may also be confounded by gestational age at testing since the possibility of fetal loss in the interval between these procedures would bias results in favour of the later test. Despite this a prospective trial found no increased risk of abortion with CVS (Crane et al. 1988). The issue can only be resolved by randomised trials using amniocentesis patients as controls. Of the two large series that have employed such an approach, the Canadian trial has suggested an excess fetal loss of at least 1% with transcervical CVS although losses were remarkably high in both groups and the relatively small sample size (2600) of this trial makes measurement imprecise. The larger European trial, however, found a much greater difference with 4.6% fewer patients assigned to the CVS group having a successful outcome to their pregnancy (MRC Working Party European Trial of Chorionic Villus Sampling 1991). Nonetheless, experienced centres claim total fetal loss rates of under 2% with CVS. The background loss rate of euploid fetuses of similar-aged mothers may be 1%. Therefore, the procedure-related loss rate is likely to be little higher than the 0.3%–1% rate associated with amniocentesis (Tabor et al. 1986; NICHHD 1976).

Abortions after invasive tests follow two patterns. A proportion occur within the first week of chorion villus sampling and manifest with bleeding followed by abortion. A second, and equally common form of abortion occurs between 1 and 5 weeks after the procedure. In many cases the fetus grows initially but this is followed by severe oligohydramnios, loss of the fetal heart and then abortion. The first pattern can be ascribed to mechanical disruption of the placenta and this is seldom seen in units with considerable experience. The second pattern of abortion, however, is presumed to be due to chronic infection (Maxwell and Lilford 1985), with an organism such as *Listeria, Chlamydia* or *Mycoplasma* since these are commonly found in the pregnant cervix (Scialli et al. 1985). A number of factors are thought to increase the risk of abortion following *transcervical* chorion biopsy. These include the need for repeated aspiration, a gestational age of greater than 11 weeks and immediate bleeding or sac puncture. In addition, ultrasonic demonstration of a subchorial haematoma after the procedure may be associated with a higher chance of subsequent abortion (Maxwell and Lilford 1985). Unfortunately, it is not possible to predict which pregnancies are at greatest risk of spontaneous abortion; gestational-age related human chorionic gonadotrophin or gestation sac volume measurements correlate very poorly with pregnancy outcome (Jouppila et al. 1984).

Risks of CVS/amniocentesis other than miscarriage must also be considered such as the risk of pulmonary hypoplasia with amniocentesis. Firth et al. (1991) in Oxford have described a cluster of cases of limb anomalies associated with CVS. All cases were associated with biopsy before 9 weeks and it is possible that this complication is specific to CVS carried out at the very early stages of gestation. We do not know whether to attribute these abnormalities to random clustering or to the invasive procedure, but the rarity of the anomaly favours the latter hypothesis.

Early Amniocentesis

Transabdominal amniocentesis before 14 weeks of gestation is a somewhat deceptive technique since, unlike mid-trimester amniocentesis, the membranes are easily indented and the needle tip may appear to lie within the amniotic cavity when it has not, in reality, penetrated the amnion. Obtaining an adequate volume of amniotic fluid for analysis may not be, therefore, as elementary as it would seem. The safety of early amniocentesis (amniocentesis at less than 15 weeks) is less well explored than for mid-trimester amniocentesis (available data is summarised in Table 10.2) and no randomised trials are available for review. However, individual series are available with Nevin et al. (1990) reporting an abortion risk of 1.4% and Miller et al. (1987) reporting early amniocentesis as being safer than transcervical chorionic sampling, but they do not give fetal loss rate of either. Garrison et al. (1988) do not give their overall miscarriage risks while Elejalde and de Elejalde (1988) claimed no miscarriages in some 300 cases. Arnovitz et al. (1988) quote a miscarriage rate of 1% and Godmilow et al. (1988) of 3%. These results are preliminary but suggest that early amniocentesis is as safe as, or safer than CVS. To ensure that miscarriage rates are kept as low as possible a number of measures are recommended to decrease the chance of miscarriage (although none of these have achieved universal acceptance). These measures include:

1. A small needle should be used, and in practice this usually involves gauge 23 or 22
2. As little fluid as possible should be removed

Table 10.2. Reported rates of miscarriage following early amniocentesis from major studies

Study	Gestational ages	No. of patients	Incidence of miscarrage
Hanson et al. (1987)	11–14 weeks	541	3.6% within 4 weeks
Arnovitz et al. (1988)	12.5–14.5 weeks	142	0.97% within 4 weeks
Elejalde and de Elejalde (1988)	9–16 weeks	310	0% at time of press
Godmilow et al. (1988)	12–14 weeks	600	3.1%
Stripparo et al. (1990)	11–15 weeks	505	3.2% (2% within 2 weeks)
Nevin et al. (1990)	9–14 weeks	222	1.4%
Hanson et al. (1990)	10–14 weeks	517	1.9% before 28 weeks
Penso et al. (1990)	11–14 weeks	407	2.3% within 4 weeks

3. The placenta should be avoided and if the procedure is guided by ultrasound in real time, then it is almost always possible to thread the needle into the amniotic cavity, while avoiding both the placenta and the fetus. The fetal surface of the placenta contains a large number of thin walled veins, which do not have the retractile properties of the main umbilical vein and fatal haemorrhage following puncture of these chorial vessels has been documented
4. Full aseptic technique should be followed since both acute and chronic infections are possible following amniocentesis.

Early amniocentesis may be more likely than later sampling to lead to pulmonary hypoplasia. Animal experiments show that this occurs to a greater degree when amniotic fluid is removed very early in pregnancy (Hislop et al. 1984). Nevin et al. (1990) showed no increase in this complication. However, small series of cases cannot detect even large proportional increases in relatively rare events. It is, therefore, essential that perinatal follow-up should be carried out whenever early amniocentesis is performed. Meanwhile it is possible that this technique will largely supplant CVS for chromosome diagnosis, especially in low-risk women. It is at least as safe as transabdominal sampling and the problem of mosaicism will almost certainly be less. Although the karyotype will be available somewhat later than with CVS, it will be available by 14 weeks. Most practitioners are prepared to perform transcervical termination up to this stage of pregnancy. This prediction is preliminary since only 10% of published early amniocentesis cases have been carried out before 12 weeks gestational age (Table 10.3). Chorionic sampling will remain the test of first choice for patients with single gene defects and those with a high cytogenetic risk, such as translocation carriers.

Table 10.3. Documented gestational age of early amniocentesis

Gestation (weeks)	Stripparo et al. (1990)	Nevin et al. (1990)	Hanson et al. (1990)	Penso et al. (1990)	Rebello et al. (1991)	Total
9	0	1 (0.4%)	0	0	0	1 (0.06%)
10	0	2 (0.9%)	2 (0.4%)	0	0	4 (0.2%)
11	13 (2.6%)	2 (0.9%)	9 (1.7%)	9 (2.2%)	5 (4.4%)	38 (2.1%)
12	42 (8.3%)	26 (11.7%)	46 (8.7%)	179 (44%)	23 (20.2%)	316 (17.8%)
13	158 (31.2%)	61 (27.4%)	215 (40.8%)	177 (43.5%)	49 (43.0%)	660 (37.2%)
14	182 (36%)	130 (58.7%)	255 (48.4%)	42 (10.3%)	37 (32.4%)	646 (36.4%)
15	110 (21.7%)	0	0	0	0	110 (6.2%)
Total	505	222	527	407	114	1775

Accuracy

The risk of miscarriage with diagnostic techniques must be viewed, not in isolation, but in context of test accuracy and genetic risk.

Single Gene Defects

Enzyme assays and gene probe diagnosis may be inaccurate, because of the problems inherent in a laboratory technique (e.g., meiotic cross-over between marker and genetic locus in the case of DNA linkage studies) or because of sampling errors. The latter can result from maternal cell overgrowth of cultured tissue or, in the case of direct analysis of CVS samples, from inadvertent sampling of the placental remnant of a resorbing second sac. Chorionic sampling would seem to have the advantage over amniocentesis for diagnosis of single gene defects, since time is of the essence in these cases, and this technique usually provides sufficient tissue for direct analysis without culture. Transcervical CVS has been consistently shown to produce larger samples than those obtained by transabdominal methods (Brambati et al. 1988; Bovicelli et al. 1986; Mackenzie et al. 1988), but we and others seldom fail to obtain adequate samples for enzyme of DNA diagnosis. The availability of the polymerase chain reaction (PCR) has decreased the demand for large samples for the purposes of gene probe diagnosis.

Chromosomal Abnormalities

The situation is far more complex for cytogenetic diagnosis. Firstly, in these cases, the fetus is usually at much lower genetic risk and, therefore, the relative importance of early diagnosis is not as great as in cases of higher risk (Lilford 1990). Secondly, diagnostic inaccuracy, inherent in sampling technique, is greater than in the case of single gene defects. This is the result of cytogenetic disparity between different cell lines within the placenta and between placenta and fetus. Chorionic sampling seldom provides a complete false-negative or false-positive diagnosis provided that short (e.g., overnight) and long-term cultures are used. However, cytogenetic disparity resulting from post-zygotic mitotic errors (mosaicism), between long- and short-term culture, or within either of these methods, is a formidable problem, occurring in 0.5%–4% of cases. The anxiety caused to parents and the expense to the Heath Service are extremely important factors and probably constitute the single strongest argument against CVS as the standard method for cytogenetic diagnosis, especially in women of relatively low genetic risk.

Transabdominal CVS has not been shown to be any more accurate than transcervical methods, but laboratories report that the samples are much "cleaner" in the case of the former and one could hypothesise that maternal contamination will be less of a probelm. However, it is not difficult to dissect decidual fragments away from chorionic villi when contaminating material is present. This is necessary, not only as a prelude to long-term culture, but also before short-term cultures (direct preparations) as maternal metaphases can be found in decidua in the first trimester (Blakemore et al. 1985).

It would appear that ambiguous karyotype results are less common after first trimester amniocentesis than after CVS (carried out by any route). However, a note of caution must be sounded. Since the proportion of chorion-derived cells in amniotic fluid is higher in earlier gestation, it is likely that chromosome mosaicism or perhaps even false-negative results will be more common in cells from amniotic fluid sampled at an earlier gestational age than in conventional amniotic samples. However, trophoblast, the predominant tissue in short-term

CVS cultures and that having the greatest potential cytogenetic disparity with the fetus, is not represented in long-term amniotic fluid cell cultures. It is, therefore, almost certain that the rate of mosaicism will be lower in early amniocentesis than in chorion samples. Initial experience would seem to bear this out (MacLachlan et al. 1989; Godmilow et al. 1988; Arnovitz et al. 1988; Miller et al. 1987; Hanson et al. 1987, Stripparo et al. 1990; Hanson et al. 1990). The advantage that amniotic fluid may be analysed for alphafetoprotein and acetylcholinesterase is not as great as might at first be suspected, since false-positive results may be more common at earlier gestations (Burton and Pettenati 1988).

Multiple pregnancy always presents a special challenge in prenatal diagnosis. Amniocentesis is feasible because ultrasonic identification of the septum separating all dizygotic and many monozygotic fetuses allows liquor to be drawn from each sac independently (Rodeck and Ivan 1981). Selective fetocide can then be carried out if one twin is found to be affected. Separate sampling from the relatively amorphous placental mass by CVS is more difficult to ensure. Again, the transabdominal method is advantageous as it affords precise localisation of the needle tip. Confirmation of the separate origin of each sample is virtually assured if they are of opposite sexes, if the results are different or if different chromosomal banding patterns are observed. If these differences do not exist, identification must rely on HLA antigens which have been demonstrated on cultured mesenchymal cells (Niazi et al. 1979) or on genetic finger-printing. We have found the latter very useful and use this routinely when cytogenetic and other laboratory results are the same. Following diagnosis it may be more difficult to ensure selective termination of the appropriate fetus, although this has been accomplished in the first trimester for a haemophiliac fetus (Mulcahy et al. 1984). We obtain a tissue sample at the time of fetocide for retrospective confirmation that the correct fetus has been selected and this is particularly important if fetuses are of the same sex since ultrasound of the fetus itself cannot help in this case.

Cost Considerations

Chorionic villus sampling is more expensive than amniocentesis for the diagnosis of cytogenetic disorders. The clinical costs of early techniques (amniocentesis or CVS) are greater because the operator (usually highly trained and therefore expensive) is required for larger periods of time (Lilford et al. 1991). Similarly the laboratory costs of CVS are more than double those of amniocentesis because:

1. Both direct (or short-term cultures) and long-term preparations are necessary
2. Ancilliary investigations (to elucidate ambiguous results) are required more often

For most cytogenetic indications, where genetic risk is low, these costs outweigh the financial advantages of early versus late termination of pregnancy. Foregoing long-term culture for cost reasons would increase the risk of a false-negative result for both aneuploidy (a mosaic cell line may be missed in trophoblast or a trisomic chromosome might have been lost in the progenitors of this tissue) and chromosome re-arrangements (banding is less clear in short-term preparations). Foregoing the short-term culture increases the risk of maternal cell overgrowth and removes an attractive feature of CVS versus early amniocentesis – namely a reassuring result within 24 h of sampling.

Transcervical and transabdominal techniques have no significant advantages in relative cost except those contingent upon any difference in rates of fetal loss. However, transabdominal sampling may be more acceptable and certainly less embarrassing to patients. Monni et al. (1988) asked 72 Italian women with experience of both techniques to give their preference for sampling method and all but one (who had a long history of needle phobia) voted for the transabdominal route, on the grounds of privacy and comfort.

If the probable greater safety of transabdominal CVS (especially regarding infection and miscarriage risk in the early phases of the learning curve) is added to the other advantages of the transabdominal technique, then this emerges as the best technique for general use. Furthermore, it can be carried out later in pregnancy and staff can therefore learn one technique for application over a wide range of gestational ages.

References

Arnovitz KS, Priest JH, Elsas LJ, Strumlauf E (1988) Amniocentesis prior to 14.5 weeks gestation: experience in 142 cases (Abstract). Am J Hum Genet 43 (Suppl 3): A225

Blakemore KJ, Samuelson J, Breg WR, Mahoney MJ (1985) Maternal metaphases on direct chromosome preparation of first trimester decidua. Hum Genet 69:380

Bovicelli L, Rizzo N, Montacuti V, Morandi R (1986) Transabdominal versus transcervical routes for chorionic villus sampling. Lancet ii:290

Brambati B, Oldrini A, Lanzani A, Terzian E, Tognoni G (1988) Transabdominal versus transcervical chorionic villus sampling: A randomized trial. Hum Reprod 3:811–813

Brambati B, Lanzani A, Tului L (1990) Transabdominal and transcervical chorionic villus sampling: efficiency and risk evaluation of 2,411 cases. Am J Med Genet 35:160–164

Burton BK, Pettenati MJ (1988) False positive acetylcholinesterase with early amniocentesis (Abstract) Am J Hum Genet 43 (Suppl 3): A903

Crane JP, Beaver HA, Cheung SW (1988) First trimester chorionic villus sampling versus mid-trimester genetic amniocentesis. Preliminary results of a controlled prospective trial. Prenat Diagn 8:355–661

Canadian Collaborative CVS – Amniocentesis Clinical Trial Group. Multicentre randomised clinical trial of chorion villus sampling and amniocentesis (1989). Lancet i:1–6

Elejalde BR, de Elejalde MM (1988) Early genetic amniocentesis, safety, complications, time to obtain results and contradictions (Abstract). Am J Hum Genet 43 (Suppl 3): A232

Finikiotis G, Gower L (1990) Chrion villus sampling – transcervical or transabdominal? Aust NZ J Obstet Gynaecol 3:63–65

Firth HV, Boyd PA, Chamberlain P, Mackenzie IZ, Lindenbaum RH, Huson SM (1991) Severe limb abnormalities after chorion villus sampling at 56–66 days gestation. Lancet 337:762–763

Garrison CP, Berry PK, Mitter NS, Snoey DM, Johnston JS (1988) Early amniocentesis and rapid prenatal diagnosis. Am J Hum Genet 43 (Suppl 3):A234

Gilmore DH, McHay MB (1985) Spontaneous fetal loss rate in early pregnancy. Lancet i:107

Godmilow L, Weiner S, Dunn LK (1988) Early genetic amniocentesis: experience with 600 consecutive procedures and comparison with chorionic villi sampling (Abstract). Am J Hum Genet 43 (Suppl 3): A234

Gustavii B, Chester MA, Edvall H, et al. (1984) First-trimester diagnosis on chorionic villi obtained by direct vision technique. Hum Genet 65:373–376

Hanson FW, Zorn EM, Tennant FR, Marianos S, Samuals S (1987) Amniocentesis before 15 weeks gestation: outcome, risks and technical problems. Am J Obstet Gynecol 156:1524–1531

Hanson FW, Happ RL, Tennant FR, Hune S, Peterson AG (1990). Ultrasonography-guided early amniocentesis in singleton pregnancies. Am J Obstet Gynecol 162:1376–1383

Hobbins JC (1984) Consequences of chorionic biopsy. New Engl J Med 310:1121

Hislop A, Howard S, Fairweather DVI (1984) Morphometric studies on the structural development of the lung in Macaca fascicularis during fetal and postnatal life. J Anat 138:95–112

Jackson Newsletter (Chorion Villus Sampling), Jefferson Medical College, Philadelphia, March 1987

Jackson Newsletter (Early Prenatal Diagnosis), Jefferson Medical College, Philadelphia. May 1990

Jouppila P, Huhtaniemi I, Herva R, Piiroinen O (1984) Correlation of human chorionic gonadotrophin secretion in early pregnancy failure with site of gestational sac and placental histology. Obstet Gynecol 63:537–542

Lilford RJ (1990) Does the tradeoff between the gestational age and miscarriage risk of a prenatal diagnostic test vary according to genetic risk? Lancet 336:1303–1305

Lilford RJ, Irving H, Gupta JK, O'Donovan P, Linton G (1991) Transabdominal chorion villus biopsy versus amniocentesis for diagnosis of aneupolidy: safety is not enough. In Chapman M, Grudzinskas JG, Chard T (eds) The embryo; normal and abnormal growth. Springer-Verlag, London, pp 91–100

Liu DT, Jeavons B, Preston C, Pearson D (1987) A prospective study of spontaneous miscarriage in ultrasonically normal pregnancies and relevance to chorionic villus sampling. Prenatal Diagnosis 7:223–227

Mackenzie WE, Holmes DS, Newton JR (1988) Study comparing transcervical with transabdominal sampling (CVS). Br J Obstet Gynaecol 95:75–78

MacLachlan NA, Rooney DE, Coleman D, Rodeck CH (1989) Prenatal diagnosis: early amniocentesis or chorionic villus sampling. Contemporary Reviews in Obstetrics and Gynaecology 1:173–180

Maxwell DJ, Lilford RJ (1985) An interesting ultrasonic observation following chorionic villus sampling. J Clin Ultrasound 13:343–344

Miller WA, Davies RM, Thayer BA, Peakman D, Harding K, Henry G (1987) Success, safety and accuracy of early amniocentesis. Am J Hum Genet 41(Suppl):A281

Monni G, Olla G, Cao A (1988) Patient's choice between transcervical and transabdominal chorionic villus sampling. Lancet i:1057

Medical Research Council European Trial of Chorion Villus Sampling (1991) Lancet, ii:1491–1499

Mulcahy MT, Roberman B, Reid SE (1984) Chorion biopsy, cytogenetic diagnosis and selective termination in a twin pregnancy at risk of haemophilia. Lancet ii:866–867

National Institute of Child Health and Human Development (1976) Mid-trimester amniocentesis for prenatal diagnosis. Safety and accuracy. J Am Med Assoc 236:1471–1476

Nevin J, Nevin NC, Dornan JC, Sim D, Armstrong JC (1990) Early amniocentesis: experience of 222 consecutive patients, 1987–1988. Prenatal Diagnosis 10:79–83

Niazi M, Coleman DV, Mowbray JF, and Blunt S (1979) Tissue typing amniotic fluid cells: potential use for detection of contaminating maternal cells. J Med Genet 16:21–23

Orrell RW, Lilford RJ (1990) Chorionic villus sampling and rare side-effects. Will a randomised controlled trial detect them? Int J Gynecol Obstet 32:29–34

Penso CA, Sandstrom MM, Garber MF, Ladoulis M, Stryker JM, Bernacerraf BB (1990) Early amniocentesis: Report of 407 cases with neonatal follow-up. Obstet Gynaecol 76:1032–1036

Rebello MT, Gray CTH, Rooney DE et al. (1991) Cytogenetic studies of amniotic fluid taken before the 15th week of pregnancy for earlier prenatal diagnosis: A report of 114 consecutive cases. Prenatal Diagnosis 11:35–40

Rodeck CH, Ivan D (1981) Sampling pure fetal blood in twin pregnancies by fetoscopy using a single uterine puncture. Prenatal Diagnosis 7:43–49

Scialli AR, Neugebauer DL, Fabros S (1985) Microbiology of the endocervix in patients undergoing chorionic villi sampling. In: Fraccaro M, Simoni G, Brambati B (eds) First trimester fetal diagnosis. Springer-Verlag, London, pp 69–73

Stripparo L, Bruscaglia M, Longatti L et al. (1990) Genetic amniocentesis: 505 cases performed before the sixteenth week of gestation. Prenatal Diagnosis 10:359–364

Tabor A, Masden M, O'Bell EB et al. (1986) Randomised controlled trial of genetic amniocentesis in 4,606 low risk women. Lancet i:1287–1292

Wilson RD, Kendrick V, Wittman BK, McGillivray BC (1984) Risk of spontaneous abortion in ultrasonically normal pregnancies. Lancet ii:290

11. Diagnosis and Management of Ectopic Pregnancy

Isabel Stabile

Introduction

A pregnancy in which gestational trophoblast implants at a site other than the uterine endometrium is defined as ectopic. The terms extrauterine and ectopic pregnancy are often used interchangably, although this is not strictly accurate, since cervical and interstitial pregnancy are ectopic nidations, albeit located within the uterus. These subgroups of ectopic pregnancy are exceedingly rare, however, and hence will only command a brief description in the discussion on the use of ultrasound. This chapter will address the incidence and causes of ectopic pregnancy, as well as its management with particular reference to the use of diagnostic tests in this life-threatening condition.

Incidence of Ectopic Pregnancy

Those industrialised countries that collect and publish national figures on the incidence of ectopic pregnancy record a consistent increase in recent years. In the USA, for instance, the Center for Disease Control has reported a fourfold increase in incidence between 1970 and 1983 (CDC 1986). It is not certain whether this increase applies to the same extent in other western countries. The only figures routinely collected in the UK concern the mortality from ectopic pregnancy, a figure which has remained constant since 1972 and accounts for 11.5% of direct maternal deaths in the triennium 1985–1987 (DHSS 1990).

Ectopic pregnancy occurs in approximately 8 to 10 per 1000 maternities in the UK. Calculating the rate of ectopic pregnancy is a contentious point because, firstly, it may be difficult to accurately diagnose an early ectopic pregnancy (even at laparotomy, unless all blood and tissue are thoroughly examined), and, secondly, rates are variously reported as the percentage of the total number of births, the number of live births or even total number of pregnancies. Consistency in reporting is clearly the answer, and since the number of live births is the least inaccurate of the denominators available, it should probably be used to document the ectopic pregnancy rate.

Comparison of incidence rates across geographical regions is hampered by the fact that different population groups may have quite distinct risk factors. For example, race and socio-economic status are inextricably linked and together with widespread sexually transmitted pelvic inflammatory disease (PID), may be responsible for the unusually high rates of ectopic pregnancy reported in poor countries. Local variation in contraceptive use, the availability of assisted conception techniques and, perhaps most importantly, improved methods of diagnosis and consistent reporting have been responsible for the documented rise in the incidence of ectopic pregnancy. Within the same geographical region, there may also be quite dramatic differences. A recent report of a threefold increased risk of dying from ectopic pregnancy amongst black as compared with white women and among young as compared with old women (Atrash et al. 1987) probably reflects the poor quality of health care available to the economically disadvantaged population of the United States. It is unknown whether the same appalling statistics apply in Britain and other European countries.

One subgroup of ectopic pregnancy which deserves particular attention is heterotopic gestation, the combination of intrauterine and extrauterine pregnancy. Although the incidence in spontaneous conceptions is approximately 1:4000 to 1:7000, there is accumulating evidence that it is significantly higher following in vitro fertilisation (IVF), the reported rate ranging from 1% to 3% of all clinical pregnancies (Rizk et al. 1991). Theories abound as to why heterotopic pregnancies occur more frequently after IVF (Lower and Tyack 1990). Although the diagnosis is being made earlier in most cases by recourse to transvaginal sonography (TVS), heterotopic pregnancy remains a difficult diagnostic and management problem. Delay in diagnosis is commonly due to the symptoms being attributed to complications of intrauterine pregnancy. Moreover, hCG levels are often in the normal range. Therefore, early diagnosis is based on maintaining a high index of suspicion, particularly following gamete manipulation. This should be combined with the least invasive therapeutic regime available to ensure continuing viability of the much-longed-for intrauterine pregnancy.

Aetiology of Ectopic Pregnancy

The increasing incidence of ectopic pregnancy has focused interest on its complex causes which are difficult to untangle from each other. This subject has been addressed exhaustively in a recent review (Stabile and Grudzinskas 1990), and we shall summarise only the main findings here.

Factors which interfere with the unique functioning of the Fallopian tube in transporting spermatozoa and ova in opposite directions confer an additional risk of ectopic implantation; the challenge lies in elucidating the mechanisms involved in interrupting the passage of the fertilised ovum from the Fallopian tube (where fertilisation occurs) to the uterus some 5 days later. Pulkkinen and Jaakkola (1989) have recently demonstrated the relationship between serum progesterone levels and tubal electrical activity in non-pregnant pre-menopausal women with normal tubes. Progesterone levels less than 20 nmol/l were associated with primarily ovarian directed electrical activity of the fimbrial end of the tube, the reverse being the case when progesterone levels exceeded 20 nmol/l, thus helping to propel the ovum in the direction of the uterus. Whether these phenomena are related to the higher incidence of ectopic pregnancy in patients with late ovulation and short luteal phase (Iffy 1963) awaits further investigation.

By contrast to these postulated mechanisms, the anatomical changes caused by pelvic infection, tubal surgery and a previous ectopic pregnancy are a major cause of ectopic gestation. Whether this is purely a mechanical obstruction, or whether the inflamed and possibly infected tube provides a better implantation site for the blastocyst is unknown. The importance of tubal factors in the aetiology of ectopic pregnancy is highlighted by the observation that the incidence rises when pregnancy occurs in vitro (Riddle et al. 1987). Whether accidental injection of the embryo into the tubes occurs during embryo transfer, or whether the embryo migrates back out of the uterine cavity into the Fallopian tube remains to be elucidated. The volume of transfer medium as well as the quality and number of embryos transferred are also considered important in the aetiology of ectopic and specifically heterotopic pregnancy. These hypotheses are currently the subject of intensive experimental work in an attempt to discover those functional aspects of the Fallopian tube which are important in the aetiology of ectopic pregnancy.

Although instinctively obvious, the contribution of PID to the aetiology of ectopic pregnancy remains controversial. From the epidemiological point of view, correlations between time trends and the geographical distribution of hospital admissions for salpingitis and those for ectopic pregnancy are not convincing (Beral 1975). However, Westrom (1975) has reported a sevenfold increase in the ectopic pregnancy rate in women with laparoscopically verified salpingitis, a finding which lends credence to the view that the dramatic increase in PID will be reflected in an "epidemic" of ectopic pregnancy in the future.

Systematic studies of protein synthesis and secretion by tubal mucosa have revealed the presence of at least two proteins which may be unique to the Fallopian tube (Verhage et al. 1988; Buhi et al. 1989). This subject has been reviewed extensively elsewhere (Maguiness et al. 1992). It is likely that these substances will provide further insight into the tubal microenvironment both in normal and abnormal states.

Clinical Features of Ectopic Pregnancy

It is well recognised that the history and clinical signs of ectopic pregnancy overlap those of other gynaecological conditions, such as threatened or incomplete abortion and PID. The likelihood of reaching a diagnosis based on clinical features alone is only 50% (Tuomivaara etal. 1986). Thus symptoms and signs cannot be relied upon to make or exclude the diagnosis of ectopic gestation.

The clinical presentation of women with ectopic pregnancy can largely be divided into three distinct groups (Table 11.1). The first step in clinical practice is to identify which clinical group the patient falls in, and act accordingly. In the first "emergency" group there is clear evidence of haemoperitoneum with clinical shock, falling blood pressure and rising pulse rate. Ectopic pregnancy should be high on the differential diagnosis list in this emergency situation, with little room for delay in instituting appropriate management. Apart from a rapid bedside hCG measurement to confirm pregnancy, if available, the emergency situation dictates rapid transfer to the operating theatre for diagnostic laparoscopy or laparotomy. The second "at risk" group consists of women at risk of developing ectopic pregnancy for a variety of reasons, such as a past history of ectopic gestation, previous tubal surgery and subfertile women undergoing assisted conception. This group of women, albeit small, has a high risk of developing ectopic, including heterotopic, pregnancy. The detection rate of ectopic pregnancy is typically high in this group since intensive surveillance is generally offered. The third and most common situation is that of subacute presentation with typically vague symptoms of amenorrhoea, abdominal pain and sometimes irregular vaginal bleeding. The remainder of this chapter will focus on this third group, in whom the prospect for early treatment is dependent on maintaining a high index of suspicion and the deployment of a few additional diagnostic tests, the choice of which is dictated by local availability and cost.

Table 11.1. Clinical presentation of ectopic pregnancy

Group	Name	Choice of investigations
1	Acute/emergency	Laparatomy or laparoscopy
2	At risk	Intensive surveillance with serial TVS and hCGs
3	Subacute	TVS and/or hCG

Diagnostic Tests

It is generally accepted that the morbidity and mortality associated with ectopic pregnancy are directly related to the length of time elapsing between the onset of symptoms and appropriate treatment. It is only in the last two decades that culdocentesis, dilatation and curettage and laparoscopy have been replaced as first-line investigative tools by the largely non-invasive biochemical and sonographic modalities which give virtually instantaneous results. The controversy today concerns which of these latter two techniques should be used first if both are available, and whether there is any advantage in using them in combination. In addition, the introduction of TVS has revolutionised the quality of imaging available, thus calling for a re-evaluation of the role of ultrasound in the diagnosis of ectopic pregnancy. A number of promising new biochemical tests have been the subject of clinical research, although their widespread introduction into practice is as yet premature. These aspects will be addressed in the sections that follow.

Biochemical Tests

This section is dominated by recent improvements in the technology available for measuring human chorionic gonadotrophin (hCG) in various body fluids. Early and fast detection of low levels of hCG is related to the sensitivity of the test used, which in turn is a reflection of the sample fluid tested and the assay characteristics. For example, ectopic pregnancy occasionally presents with hCG levels less than 10 IU/l which would be missed altogether by employing hCG assays with a detection limit above this (Poulsen et al. 1987). Until recently the only hCG tests available to clinicians were laboratory-based radioimmunoassays, the use of which led to unavoidable delays in instituting appropriate management. These tests have largely been replaced by rapid bedside techniques capable of qualitatively and in some cases quantitatively detecting low levels of beta-hCG. Simple dipstick tests for the measurement of beta-hCG in urine based on enzyme-labelled monoclonal antibodies or immunofluorometric assays are recent additions to the clinical armamentarium. The high sensitivity (generally greater than 95%), combined with the speed of the new generation assays (typically less than 1 h), have contributed greatly to the management of the clinically stable woman suspected of harbouring an ectopic pregnancy.

The last decade has seen the introduction of serial quantitative beta-hCG estimations to distinguish accurately between normal and abnormal pregnancies (the discriminatory hCG zone: Table 11.2). The threshold level of hCG above which a normal intrauterine gestational sac can be seen ultrasonically is clearly dependent on the resolution of the equipment used. However, failed pregnancies (both ectopics and spontaneous abortions) typically produce lower hCG levels which increase at a lower rate compared with normal pregnancy. This gives TVS a distinct advantage over transabdominal sonography (TAS) in that it can identify the site of nidation at a lower level of hCG (Table 11.2). The use of TVS allows a gestational sac to be consistently identified as early as 33–34 days following the missed period, thus allowing accurate interpretation of the hCG result.

Table 11.2. Published discriminatory hCG levels for the identification by transabdominal (TAS) and transvaginal (TVS) ultrasound of an intrauterine gestational sac. The level of the First International Reference Preparation (IRP) of human chorionic gonadotrophin (hCG) is approximately twice that of the second International Standard (IS)

Authors	hCG (First IRP)	Ultrasound	hCG (2nd IS)
Kadar et al. 1981	6500	TAS	
Nyberg et al. 1985	3600	TAS	
Romero et al. 1985		TAS	3250
Nyberg et al. 1987	1800	TAS	
Cacciatore et al. 1988	1800	TAS	
Fossum et al. 1988	1398	TVS	914
Goldstein et al. 1988		TVS	1025
Nyberg et al. 1988		TVS	1000
Bernaschek et al. 1988		TVS	300
Bree et al. 1989	1000	TVS	
Cacciatore et al. 1990	935	TVS	

A Swedish group have recently introduced the concept of the hCG score, obtained by plotting the initial hCG value against the rate of change in hCG levels (Lindblom et al. 1989). This test appears to have a useful role in distinguishing normal from pathological pregnancy (but not ectopic pregnancy from spontaneous abortion) in that group of patients with hCG levels between 100 and 4000 IU/l (First IRP), in whom clinical examination and TVS fail to give a clear diagnosis.

A word of caution in the interpretation of this new generation of tests is in order. These assays are capable of detecting levels of beta-hCG as low as 1 IU/l. Such incredibly low hCG levels are found a few days after oocyte retrieval in successful IVF pregnancy. This is equivalent to before the missed period in spontaneous conceptions. The clinician is thus faced with the problem of locating the site of nidation in a woman who is biochemically pregnant. If the doubling time of hCG is 1.8 days (Hamori et al. 1989), then 14 days would have to elapse from biochemical detection of implantation (commonly accepted as a beta-hCG level of greater than 10 IU/l) to visualisation of a gestational sac by TVS. Using the abdominal route this interval is even longer (Table 11.2). This problem is discussed in greater detail below.

Among the patients undergoing IVF (our Group 2 patients), the incidence of ectopic pregnancy is reportedly about 5 times higher than in the normal population. In spite of the fact that most patients receive hCG, it is generally agreed that serial hCG determinations can be used to predict early pregnancy failure (i.e, spontaneous abortion and ectopic pregnancy), but not to distinguish between the two (Liu et al. 1986). These authors also demonstrated that patients receiving 10 000 IU hCG (day 0) had a serum hCG level of 200–700 IU on day 1, falling to less than 5 IU by days 8 to 12. In pregnant patients hCG rose rapidly thereafter with an average doubling time of 33 hours. Further detail of the role of biochemical tests in the diagnosis of ectopic pregnancy following assisted conception procedures will be found in Chapter 9.

Other trophoblasic proteins such as Schwangerschafts protein 1 (SP1) and pregnancy-associated plasma protein A (PAPP-A) have been subjected to intensive scrutiny as possible ancillary diagnostic tests in suspected ectopic pregnancy. SP1 is a glycoprotein with a molecular weight of 90 kD. Although it appears in the maternal circulation shortly after implantation, and hence is a useful marker of pregnancy, quantitative estimations have not been proven to be of greater value than hCG in distinguishing between intrauterine and extrauterine pregnancy (Braunstein and Asch 1983). In spite of encouraging early results published by several groups in Denmark, Sydney and London, PAPP-A has failed to live up to its promise as a clinically useful marker of ectopic pregnancy. The main reason for this disappointing conclusion is the observation that PAPP-A appears relatively late in the maternal circulation (after 5 to 6 weeks of gestation). Nevertheless, the results of these clinical studies support the hypothesis that PAPP-A synthesis by the trophoblast is severely and selectively compromised in ectopic gestation. Immunohistochemical techniques have confirmed the low levels of PAPP-A in tubal trophoblastic tissue (Tornehave et al. 1986). In spite of normal hCG production, trophoblast explants from ectopic gestation synthesise minimal amounts of PAPP-A in vitro (Stabile 1988). This observation supports the hypothesis that factors related to the site of implantation may be important in regulating synthesis of this protein, but the promise that PAPP-A may be the much-sought-after biochemical marker of ectopic pregnancy has not been fulfilled.

Several new candidates for the biochemical marker of ectopic pregnancy have recently emerged. Among them are the two major proteins synthesised by the human endometrium: progesterone-dependent endometrial protein (PEP, also known as placental protein 14, PP14) and insulin-like growth-factor-binding protein (IGF-bp, also known as placental protein 12, PP12). PP14 appears to derive mainly from the glandular endometrium, while IGF-bp is produced principally by stromal cells of the gestational endometrium. Maternal circulating PP14 levels bear a striking resemblance to the pattern of hCG secretion in early pregnancy. It was logical, therefore, to subject PP14 to the same scrutiny that other trophoblastic proteins received a decade ago. Preliminary results by Westergaard and his colleagues (1988) suggest that patients with ectopic pregnancy have generally levels depressed of PP14 and that in combination with progesterone estimations, they may provide a useful biochemical test for ectopic pregnancy. A recent report from Scandinavia has described depressed levels of serum PP14 in ectopic pregnancy prior to the development of symptoms (Pedersen et al. 1991).

By contrast, IGF-bp measurements have proven to be of little clinical value, as there is considerable overlap in levels between failed intrauterine pregnancy and ectopic pregnancy (Stabile et al. 1989c). Although these results are disappointing from the clinical perspective, the observation of normal IGF-bp levels in all but one of the 33 patients with ectopic pregnancy examined (Stabile et al. 1990) provides support for the hypothesis that decidual synthesis of IGF-bp does not depend upon anatomical contact between decidua and trophoblast.

It is now well established that the ovaries are a source of extrarenal renin. Meunier et al. (1991) have evaluated the diagnostic value of hCG, progesterone and the enzymes prorenin and active renin produced by the trophoblast and corpus luteum, either alone or in combination for the diagnosis of ectopic pregnancy. In this study, the combination of low hCG (less than 15 000 IU/l) and low active renin (less than 30 pg/ml) provided the best discriminatory value for ectopic pregnancy with a predictive value positive of 75% and a predictive value negative of 97%. These encouraging early results await confirmation in prospective studies of women clinically suspected of harbouring an ectopic pregnancy.

Alphafetoprotein (AFP), an alpha-1-globulin of fetal origin has recently undergone re-evaluation of its diagnostic role in early pregnancy failure (Stabile et al. 1989a). Generally normal or elevated levels were observed in women with live ectopic pregnancy (Stabile et al. 1989b). However the clinical value of these observations is limited because only 15%–20% of ectopic pregnancies fall into this category, whether assessed by TVS (Nyberg et al. 1991) or pathological examination (DiMarchi et al. 1989). Therefore, it is unlikely that the measurement of AFP will provide additional information of clinical value when ectopic pregnancy is suspected.

It has been assumed that, at least in the very early stages, the fetoplacental unit and corpus luteum of the ectopic gestation are functioning normally. Lower and colleagues (1992) have contested this view, having demonstrated depressed serum progesterone levels in asymptomatic women with ectopic pregnancy 14–21 days after spontaneous conception despite normal hCG levels. Early studies demonstrating depressed progesterone levels in patients with ectopic pregnancy have been confirmed using more sensitive and rapid (within 2–4 h) progesterone determinations, both alone (Yeko et al. 1987) and in combination with hCG (Hubinont et al. 1987; Hahlin et al. 1991). Whether ectopic implantation causes the shut-down of progesterone synthesis by the corpus luteum or whether low levels of progesterone actually lead to ectopic implantation is as yet uncertain, although the electrophysiological studies of Pulkkinen and Jaakkola (1989), described above, suggest the latter may be the case. In the patient suspected of harbouring an ectopic pregnancy on clinical grounds, a progesterone level below 20 ng/ml suggests early pregnancy failure, whatever the gestational age (Sauer et al. 1989). Using receiver operating characteristic curves, Hahlin et al. (1990) demonstrated that, at a progesterone cut-off level of 9.4 ng/ml, the specificity for abnormal pregnancy was in excess of 95%. However the problem lies in distinguishing failed intrauterine pregnancy (spontaneous abortion) from ectopic pregnancy. Gelder et al. (1991) have recently reviewed the published studies that have addressed this point and concluded that no single progesterone value reliably predicts the presence or absence of ectopic pregnancy. In conclusion, provided good quality ultrasound is available, serum progesterone measurements are a useful adjunct in distinguishing normal from failed pregnancy, although their value in the diagnosis of ectopic pregnancy remains unproven.

These biochemical studies suggest that ectopic pregnancy is not a homogeneous disease. Apart from differences in clinical presentation (Groups 1 to 3 described above), there is the question of whether the ectopic pregnancy is viable or not as well as the gestational age at presentation. Moreover, the diagnostic value of any biochemical test may be lower the earlier in pregnancy it is used. These factors combine to make the diagnosis more difficult as the test which can confidently be applied in one situation proves less useful in another. Furthermore, the ability of biochemical tests to predict viability or to screen asymptomatic women for either ectopic pregnancy or abortion cannot be extrapolated to the symptomatic population in which the exclusion of ectopic pregnancy is a genuine problem. Ideally, one should selectively utilise the available biochemical tests depending on the clinical situation. For example, in the acute situation (Group 1) in which the tube has ruptured, both luteal and trophoblastic function as reflected in progesterone, hCG or even PAPP-A secretion are generally normal. Depressed protein and steroid secretion in ectopic pregnancy is a reflection of necrosis of chorionic tissue and luteal insufficiency and is associated with failure of the pregnancy. These women generally present with subacute symptoms, i.e., our Group 3 patients.

The interpretation of quantitative biochemical tests depends on the gestational age at presentation. Since recurrent vaginal bleeding is a common symptom, occurring sometimes days or even weeks before pain supervenes, it is often impossible to have reliable menstrual data upon which to calculate gestational age. Herein lies the major limitation of most biochemical tests except progesterone, which can be used to distinguish normal from abnormal pregnancy irrespective of gestational age (Sauer et al. 1989).

In conclusion, the sensitive assays now available to detect hCG in both urine and blood allow it to retain its primary role in diagnosing pregnancy. Progesterone estimations are probably most useful in distinguishing between viable intrauterine pregnancy and pathological pregnancy, whether intra- or extrauterine. Distinguishing between ectopic pregnancy and spontaneous abortion is probably best achieved by diagnostic ultrasound.

Sonographic Tests

Published investigations in this rapidly changing field fall into three main categories:

1. Descriptive studies of the sonographic features of ectopic pregnancy, whether studied by the vaginal or abdominal route
2. Comparisons between transvaginal and transabdominal ultrasound
3. Studies of the combination of ultrasound and biochemical tests

Each of these will be described in turn, so as to allow an informed decision concerning the role of ultrasound and biochemical tests in the diagnosis of ectopic pregnancy.

Descriptive Studies

The reader is referred to our recent review of the sonographic features of ectopic pregnancy as determined using the abdominal route (Stabile and Grudzinskas 1990). In essence, apart from live ectopic gestation, the sonographic diagnosis of ectopic pregnancy is based on demonstrating an enlarged but empty uterus with or without an adnexal mass and/or fluid in the Pouch of Douglas. More frequently, ultrasound is used to exclude ectopic pregnancy when an intrauterine pregnancy is visualised (remembering that heterotopic pregnancy occurs, albeit rarely).

Over the last few years attention has turned to the novel technique of TVS which undoubtedly has the advantage of improved resolution and patient acceptance. What are the sonographic features of tubal pregnancy as seen through the vaginal transducer? The answer to this question is threefold. Firstly, a live embyro within a gestational sac in the adnexa remains the gold standard for the sonographic diagnosis of ectopic pregnancy. This typically appears as an intact well-defined tubal ring (euphemistically described as the bagel sign by our transAtlantic colleagues) in which the yolk sac and/or the embryonic pole with or without cardiac action are seen within a completely sonolucent sac (Fig. 11.1). Prior to 6 weeks gestation the echogenic contour of the sac is typically less than 5 mm in diameter. These features are identical with those seen via the abdominal route in this situation. In our prospective study of high resolution abdominal sector scanning, a live embryo was seen in 12% of the patients with ectopic pregnancy, but only after 7 weeks amenorrhoea (Stabile et al. 1988). The major advantage of TVS is reportedly the gestational age at which this diagnosis can confidently be made. However there are some pathological data to suggest that many ectopic pregnancies are in fact anembryonic (Emmrich and Kopping 1981). If this is the case then one would not expect TVS to diagnose more intact viable ectopic pregnancies than have hitherto been demonstrated.

The second picture of tubal pregnancy as seen with TVS is a poorly defined tubal ring, with or without contained echogenic structures. Typically the Pouch of Douglas also contains fluid and/or blood. These features are consistent with a tubal pregnancy which is aborting.

Thirdly, tubal pregnancy can present with varying amounts of fluid in the Pouch of Douglas, representing a ruptured tubal pregnancy (Fig. 11.2). In one study, echogenic fluid alone was seen in 15% of patients with ectopic pregnancy

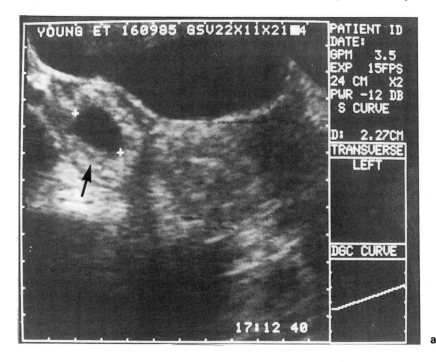

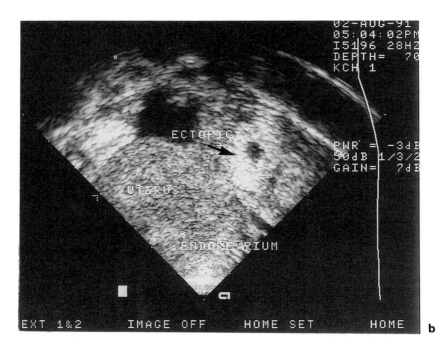

Fig. 11.1. Ectopic pregnancy as seen by **a** TAS and **b** TVS, showing an intact tubal ring.

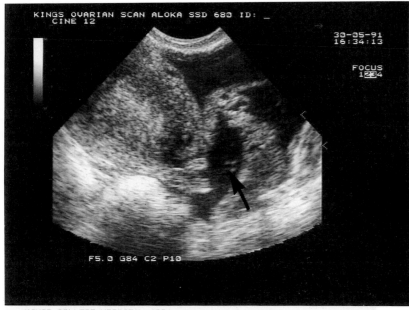

KINGS COLLEGE HOSPITAL 1991

Fig. 11.2. Ruptured tubal pregnancy as seen with TVS, showing extensive blood clot in the pelvis.

(Nyberg et al. 1991). The diagnostic tubal ring is often not visualised, but when it is, it is often blurred and unrecognisable within the blood clot. The one consistent feature noted in these studies is the improved image quality generated by the transvaginal approach. This is a composite sonographic description which includes resolution, contrast and anatomical delineation.

Patients with ruptured tubal pregnancy (Group 1) are often haemodynamically compromised, requiring urgent resuscitation and access to emergency surgery. Abdominal ultrasound is not a practical test in this situation, partly because of delays incurred in filling the bladder and partly because of poor image quality especially in the obese patient. These disadvantages do not apply to the vaginal route since it only takes a few seconds to recognise the bizarre unmistakable appearance of blood clot in the pelvis (Fig. 11.2). Patients with subacute ectopic pregnancy presenting with non-specific symptoms and signs (Group 3) typically have the second group of sonographic features, although a viable ectopic pregnancy in the adnexae is noted in approximately 20% of cases.

Arguments persist as to whether or not a pseudogestational sac is seen using TVS. In the experience of some (Timor-Tritsch et al. 1988), a pseudogestational sac is not present in the uterus at the time the early tubal gestation is detected. Others admit that it may be difficult, even with TVS, to evaluate a very early intrauterine sac (less than 4 mm in diameter). They rightly point out that eccentric placement within the endometrial cavity is a hallmark of intrauterine nidation. In the absence of this, especially if the uterine texture is homogeneous (Fig. 11.3), a pseudogestational sac should be suspected (Cacciatore et al. 1989; Hill et al. 1990).

A number of recent studies have addressed the predictive value of specific sonographic features in the diagnosis of ectopic pregnancy (Stabile et al. 1988;

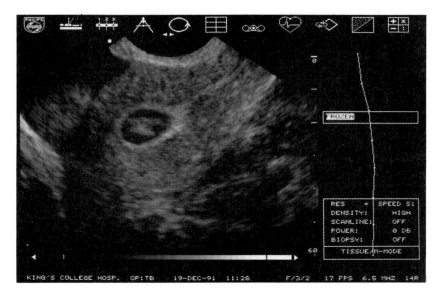

Fig. 11.3. Early ectopic pregnancy (4 and a half weeks) as seen with TVS, showing a pseudo-gestational sac within the uterus.

deCrespigny 1988; Nyberg et al. 1991). These studies included consecutive women with clinically suspected ectopic pregnancy, although the study by Nyberg et al. (1991) incorporated a positive serum pregnancy test as an entry requirement. The last two studies both used transducers of identical frequency, making comparison of the ultrasound results more reliable. Whereas the positive predictive value for ultrasonic parameters such as adnexal abnormalities (Fig. 11.4) with or without pelvic fluid examined in each study was comparably good (63%–100%), in 7 of 36 (19%) women with ectopic pregnancy studied by deCrespigny (1988) there were no abnormalities on TVS. Although Nyberg and colleagues do not state how often this occurred, careful reading of their results reveals that in 13 of 68 (19%) patients there were no extrauterine abnormalities such as an embryo, sac, adnexal mass or pelvic fluid. Therefore, although a positive pregnancy test was essential for entry into Nyberg's study, it did not apparently improve the diagnostic value of TVS for ectopic pregnancy. This point is addressed in greater detail later in this chapter.

Some of the common pitfalls of TVS, especially when used by inexperienced operators, are usefully described here. The intact well-defined tubal ring may occasionally be confused by the tiro for the corpus luteum of pregnancy, a Graafian follicle, loops of small bowel or other tubal pathology such as a hydrosalpinx imaged in cross section. These mistakes are most often made when static films are interpreted and can, therefore, be eliminated by real time TVS. Typically the corpus luteum and Graafian follicle can be identified by defining the ovary itself, a matter that practice will perfect. Peristalsis of the small bowel, when identified, helps to avoid this particular mistake. The remaining errors can be minimised by meticulous examination using multiple reproducible sections. Finally, unless the myometrium of the uterus is always identified (which can be surprisingly difficult on occasions), the beginner may miss the tubal gestation altogether.

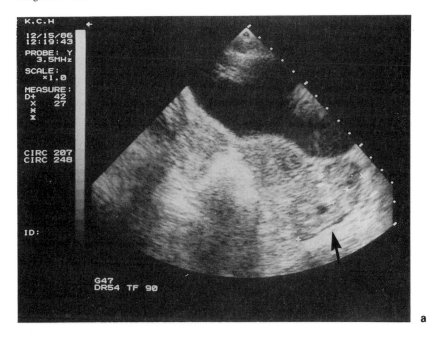

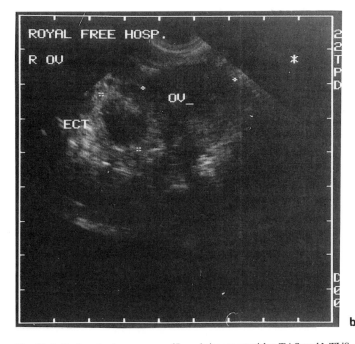

Fig. 11.4. Early ectopic pregnancy (5 weeks) as seen with **a** TAS and **b** TVS, showing an adnexal mass seen separate from the ovary (see arrow).

Are there any limitations to the use of TVS in the differential diagnosis of ectopic pregnancy? Apart from the 19% false-negative rate noted above (a figure which would be expected to fall as experience with TVS increases), the study of Goldstein et al. (1988) identified a particular problem. They studied an unselected group of 235 potentially normal early pregnancies presenting to an abortion clinic. Among them were 10 women with hCG levels between 394 and 6000 IU/l, in whom TVS failed to demonstrate an intrauterine sac. Two of these women had an ectopic pregnancy, although in one the diagnosis was sonographically obvious due to an extrauterine sac. Three missed abortions (early embryonic demise), two complete abortions and three normal intrauterine pregnancies completed the group. All three normal pregnancies missed by TVS were associated with either a fibroid uterus or a co-existing intrauterine device, which presumably masked the intrauterine sac. The authors emphasised that when the uterus appears empty at an hCG level above the accepted discriminatory zone for TVS (Table 11.2), then ultrasound cannot distinguish between the various types of pregnancy failure.

In summary, TVS remains an operator-dependent diagnostic modality, the training for which should be no less rigorous than for the abdominal approach. The technique can be relied upon to provide virtually instantaneous answers to some, but not all, difficult clinical problems. It has the advantage of simplicity of use, patient acceptability and improved resolution, which in experienced hands leads to the earier diagnosis of ectopic pregnancy in the majority of cases. Although uncommon, the possibility of a non-tubal (cornual, interstitial or cervical) ectopic pregnancy should be considered, when none of the classical sonographic features are identified. In addition, when abdominal pregnancy is suspected, abdominal scanning is preferable unless the gestational sac implants in the pelvis. However non-tubal pregnancies are exceedingly rare in clinical practice. The lesser known disadvantages of TVS include a small field of view and limited mobility of the transducer which may lead to the abnormality being incompletely visualised or missed altogether, particularly by the inexperienced.

Comparison between Transabdominal and Transvaginal Ultrasound

TVS is now extensively used in clinical practice. Its superiority in the diagnosis of viable early pregnancy as well as its unique advantages in assisted reproduction are well documented. Image quality is said to influence the diagnostic capability of ultrasound although it is unclear whether this also applies in the situation where detection of the embryonic heart action is not critical. The majority of studies purporting to evaluate the usefulness of TVS in gynaecological disease (as compared to obstetric problems) have been either retrospective (Lande et al. 1988) or not designed to compare the two techniques (Lande et al. 1988; Coleman et al. 1988). Most studies have failed to correlate the sonographic findings with surgical outcome in the whole study group (Leibman et al. 1988; Mendelson et al. 1988; Coleman et al. 1988; Lande et al. 1988). Andolf and Jorgensen (1990) have avoided these common pitfalls in their prospective comparison of TVS and TAS in the diagnosis of gynaecological disease. Eighty five patients underwent TAS and then TVS 24 h before elective surgery for a variety of gynaecological diseases.

In spite of better image quality, the diagnostic value of TVS was not signicantly better than that of TAS, particularly in the evaluation of large ovarian cysts and sizeable fibroids.

The ultrasound literature is now littered with studies claiming to have comparatively evaluated both ultrasound modalities in the diagnosis of early pregnancy failure. Table 11.3 lists the study design, results and false-negative rates reported for TAS and TVS in those comparative studies that have addressed the diagnosis of ectopic pregnancy. Not only are there significant differences in the criteria for entry into these studies, most of them were in fact retrospective analyses and, in some cases, examinations were performed by multiple operators, sometimes submitting hard copy images for later interpretation. In evaluating the false-negative rates of TAS and TVS it should be made clear that since no clinical, surgical or pathological follow-up was available in some of the studies listed in Table 11.3, it is impossible to determine whether the observations were present but missed, or absent altogether. Review of this table reveals another important point. If the aim of a study is to evaluate the clinical benefit of a diagnostic test (TVS, in this case), then it is important that the patient group studied represents a true diagnostic problem, rather than being a simple exercise in data collection. The latter is clearly true of a number of studies listed in Table 11.3. The issue is whether TVS, when utilised prospectively in the investigation of amenorrhea, abdominal pain and bleeding in women of reproductive age, is better than TAS in the diagnosis of ectopic pregnancy. Bearing in mind the limitations described above, the consensus view is that not only is ectopic pregnancy more frequently identified using TVS, but normal intrauterine pregnancy is diagnosed at an earlier stage too. Whether earlier diagnosis of ectopic pregnancy leads to improved management is another matter which has not, as yet, been addressed by studies of this kind.

Another advantage of TVS highlighted by the majority of studies in Table 11.3 is the early diagnosis of normal intrauterine pregnancy (IUP), which is often missed by TAS. This means that surgery for the investigation of an adnexal mass may be avoided in patients with a haemorrhagic corpus luteum cyst. Such complex adnexal masses were seen in 7% of patients with normal IUP in one study (Nyberg et al. 1991), emphasising the need for careful evaluation of adnexal cysts. However, in certain situations e.g., marked PID with distortion of pelvic anatomy or when large adnexal cysts extend above the bladder into the lower abdomen, TVS may be at a disadvantage. It would be expected, though, that with increasing experience these disadvantages can largely be overcome.

In conclusion, what are the diagnostic advantages of TVS over TAS? First, ectopic pregnancy is more frequently identified and second, normal intrauterine pregnancy is identified at an earlier stage. As demonstrated by the data in Table 11.3, there is no question that improved resolution confers upon TVS the advantage of accurate diagnosis with low false-positive and false-negative rates, at least in the hands of experts in tertiary centres (most likely to publish their results). It remains to be seen whether this is also true of the majority of ultrasound departments within general hospitals, especially if reports are based on retrospective review of hard copy images. Moreover, in certain circumstances the diagnosis of ectopic pregnancy is difficult even for TVS and it is here that the combination with biochemical tests may be of value.

Table 11.3. Comparative studies of TAS and TVS in the diagnosis of ectopic pregnancy

	Entry criteria	Equipment
Nyberg et al. 1987	84 women with pos hCG in whom TAS failed to show viable embryo.	GE 3000 and 3600, ATL VM4, Philips 1550 3.5/5.0/7.5 MHz: TAS then TVS. Observer number and bias not stated.
Vilaro et al. 1987	21 women with suspected pelvic mass or vaginal bleeding unrelated to IUP.	Acuson GE 3000, Philips 1550, Aloka 280 SL, Technicare MCC, ATL 600, 3.5/5 MHz; TAS then TVS by different observer. Review of previously recorded images by two radiologists independently.
Nyberg et al. 1991	232 consecutive women with pos preg test, suspicion of EP and failure to demonstrate viable intra- or extrauterine preg with TAS.	Acuson 128; Philips 1500/3000; ATL Um4; GE 5 MhZ.
Rempen 1988	404 women between 4–13 weeks. Pos preg test 361.	Combison 320; 5 MHz.
Jain et al. 1988	Pos preg test: 15 bleeding ± pain; 47 tubal surgery/IVF/symptoms/ signs of EP; 28 asymptomatic.	GE 3600 3.5/5 6.5 MHz. At least two radiologists interpreted sonograms. Not blinded to TAS results.
Tessler et al. 1989	147 unselected consecutive women referred for US. 35 excluded for a variety of reasons.	ATL and Acuson 3.5/5 MHz. Four radiologists; TAS then TVS blinded. Real-time interpretation.
Coleman et al. 1988	215 women with suspected abnormality on pelvic examination.	GE 3600 3.5/5 MHz. Six radiologists not blinded. TAS then TVS.
Pennell et al. 1987	38 pregnant women with vaginal bleeding/cramps or previous tubal surgery in which TAS was equivocal.	Philips 3.5/5 MHz. Two radiologists not blinded. Review of previously recorded images.
Mendelson et al. 1988	200 women with suspected pelvic masses, PID, fibroids, pain or bleeding.	Philips, Diasonics, GE Acuson, 3.5/5 MHz. Retrospective review of previously recorded images by two radiologists.
Dashefsky et al. 1988	53 women at risk for EP with pos urine/serum preg test.	Acuson; 3.5/5 MHz. TAS then TVS; radiologists not blinded to results.
Lande et al. 1988	67 women with suspected adnexal mass. TVS performed when TAS gave equivocal results. 14 women had pos preg test.	Diasonics ATL 3.5/5 MHz. Bruel & Kjaer 7 MHz. Two radiologists independently reviewed previously recorded images.
Cacciatore et al. 1989	100 women with suspected EP and hCG >10 IU/l.	Aloka 3/3.5 MHz. Kretz Technik GE Aloka 5 MHz. Independent review of hard copy images.
Funk and Fendel 1988 (English abstract only)	44 women with suspected EP.	Not stated, 'vaginal probe'.
Degenhardt 1988 (English abstract only)	70 women with suspected EP after pelvic examination.	Not stated, 'transvaginal scanning'.
Shapiro et al. 1988	25 women with pain, bleeding and pos preg test or rising hCG titres.	GE 3000, 3.5/5 MHz, TAS then TVS different ultrasonographer.
Leibman et al. 1988	67 women for evaluation of palpable pelvic masses.	Philips 5 MHz. TAS then TVS. Retrospective review of images by two radiologists unaware of clinical surgical or F/U US findings.

Table 11.3. (*Continued*)

Outcome	Results/Conclusion	False-negative TAS	TVS
Clinical sonographic and surgical F/U. EP 25, IUP 32, non-viable IUP 27.	TVS better 60%, same 32%, worse 8%, 1 false pos by each technique.	Ectopic sac 10. Non-viable ectopic fetus 2. Adnexal mass 3.	Two missed EP.
Clinical follow-up only.	New information 62%; same 33%; worse 5%.	One ectopic sac missed.	One mass posterior to uterus poorly defined.
Review of surgical and clinical records; 68 EP; 83 IUP; 55 non-viable IUP.	TVS echogenic fluid: sens 56%; spec 96%; PVP 93%; PVN 72% for EP.	Not estimated.	4/25 patients without fluid at TVS had EP.
Unclear what parameters were used.	Sens of TVS 86%; spec 99.7%; PVP 95%; PVN 99.2% for EP.	Not estimated.	3 EP classified as IUP by TVS.
Clinical surgical and/or pathologic confirmation.	Mean sac diameter >10 mm: embryo always seen; fetal pole >4 mm: FH always seen; GSD >1.7 cm without fetus/yolk sac: anembryonic pregnancy.	Missed ectopic embryonic pole: 3.	Missed fluid in POD 3; missed adnexal ring 4.
Determined by clinical F/U in 44; surgical confirmation in 16; no F/U in 48.	Equal 36.1%. TVS superior 60.2%; TAS superior 3.7%.	Four uterine masses missed on TAS.	Three normal ovaries missed: clinical outcome unaffected.
Clinical and/or surgery in all but 5 patients. No pathological confirmation of diagnosis.	TVS: new information 60%; better visualisation 22%; no difference 16%; worse images 2%.	FH action missed in 2 viable pregnancies at 6.5 weeks.	None.
Clinical FU: 23 IUP; 18 incomplete abortions; 2 missed abortions; 6 EP.	All IUP diagnosed correctly by TVS. FH always seen in fetal pole >14 mm. No difference between TAS/TVS for 8 incomplete abortions.	Tubal ring not seen in 4/6 EP.	Pseudo-gestational sac not seen in 2/6 EP. Tubal ring not seen in 3/6 EP.
Unclear what parameters were used.	TVS image quality better in up to 87%. Equivalent diagnostic information in 60–84%.	Not stated.	Not stated.
Clinical and pathologic correlation with sonographic data.	TVS live ectopic 17%; TAS live ectopic 6%; adnexal mass diagnosis identical for both. PVP for EP of absent mass or free fluid: TVS 29%; TAS 16%.	8 normal IUP, 4 abnormal IUP missed. Yolk sac missed in 6 patients.	One adnexal mass missed.
Surgical findings 34; clinical outcome 5; US F/U 13; other techniques 11.	12/14 TVS diagnostically more useful for EP; 2/14 equal; 2/14 TAS better.	6/14 EP had normal TAS.	4/14 EP had normal TVS.
Clinical and sonographic F/U, histological examination.	TVS more useful information in 31% of EP, 52% of IUP. Gestational sac seen in 90% of IUP with TVS and TAS, One false pos EP by each technique.	Ectopic embryo missed in 8 patients with EP. Ectopic sac missed in 10 patients with EP.	Adnexal mass missed in 4 patients with EP.
Surgical diagnosis of EP in 6 patients.	TVS: tubal ring 13/16; false pos 3.	Not evaluated.	Empty uterus and free fluid: 3/16 patients.
Surgical diagnosis of EP in 32 patients.	TVS: 29/70 correct diagnosis of EP.	Ten false results. Failure rates 13.1%.	Three EP missed; 7 suspected EP could not be confirmed or excluded.
Surgically proven EP in 22 patients.	Adnexal mass consistent with EP (TVS N = 20, TAS N = 11). Two false positive adnexal masses for TVS.	Adnexal mass not identified in 11 patients.	Two EP missed.
Surgical diagnosis in 41 patients. Clinical F/U in remainder.	TVS: better anatomical detail 76%; unique diagnostic information 15%.	6 simple cysts and 4 complex pelvic masses not seen.	None.

Combination of Ultrasound and Biochemical Tests

Pelvic sonography and maternal urine or serum pregnancy testing are commonly combined in clinical practice to evaluate early pregnancy and its complications. In this section we shall review the recent literature pertaining to this combination, to assess whether or not it provides additional information of clinical importance over the two techniques used in isolation.

Gestational sacs larger than 2–4 mm in diameter are visible by TVS in pregnancies of 4–5 weeks duration. The last 10 years has seen the threshold hCG level (Table 11.2) at which a gestational sac is always seen fall from 6500 to around 1000 IU/l (First IRP), although it should be emphasised that in terms of menstrual age this represents approximately a week, since hCG levels rise exponentially. Lowering of the discriminatory hCG zone is a function of the technical quality of the ultrasound equipment used, the reliablity and reproducibility of laboratory hCG testing and, of course, the skills of the ultrasound operator. It therefore follows that there will come a point beyond which, with the current state-of-the-art ultrasound equipment, it will not be possible to identify an intrauterine gestational sac. Presently, the lowest hCG level at which a gestational sac is consistently visible is 1000 IU/l (First IRP). This figure should be divided by 2.2 to convert to the second International Standard for hCG. However, there are reports such as that by Bernaschek et al. (1988) in which TVS correctly identified intrauterine pregnancies at the much lower hCG level of 300 IU/l (2nd IS) At this stage (the second day after the missed period), the mean sac diameter was 2 mm. These remarkable results will need to be repeated by those units choosing to rely on such low hCG levels as discriminatory values, since their introduction into clinical practice is clearly operator and equipment dependent. Indeed the authors recommended that the TVS be repeated after 2 days, when the gestational sac diameter would be expected to have increased by 2 mm (and hence become consistently visible) and the hCG level risen to 750 IU/l (2nd IS).

Even when low serum hCG levels can be accurately determined, their interpretation is limited unless the exact length of gestation is known. Moreover, many patients in clinical practice present with symptoms of pregnancy or its complications at a stage too early for TVS to identify an intrauterine gestational sac. A similar problem was encountered by those proponents of the algorithm for the diagnosis of ectopic pregnancy based on serial quantitative hCG assays (Romero et al. 1985). A substantial proportion of patients at risk for ectopic pregnancy presented with an initial hCG value below the then accepted discriminatory level of 6500 IU/l (First IRP). Clearly, as the discriminatory hCG level falls, so will the proportion of patients who fall into this category. The study of Stiller et al. (1989) identified 13% of patients at risk for ectopic gestation with an initial hCG value of less than 1300 IU/l (First IRP), while in the retrospective study of DiMarchi et al. (1989), approximately half the patients with ectopic pregnancy at 35 to 86 days gestation had hCG levels greater than 750 IU/l (2nd IS), sufficient to use a vaginal sonographic hCG discriminatory zone to assist diagnosis.

Does lowering the hCG threshold value improve the ability of ultrasound to diagnose ectopic pregnancy? Certainly it allows the exclusion of ectopic pregnancy more often by visualising an intrauterine gestational sac at an earlier stage than is possible with TAS. However if the initial hCG level exceeds 1000 IU/l (First IRP), the absence of an intrauterine sac is not specific for ectopic pregnancy. A recent spontaneous abortion or indeed a molar pregnancy remain possibilities. However if serial hCG values are available, falling levels are typically found in spontaneous abortion, while the reverse will be the case with a molar pregnancy. Nevertheless, ectopic pregnancy is far more likely as well as more dangerous, and a diagnostic laparoscopy is mandatory.

To give a practical example of this problem, Stiller et al. (1989) reported on a group of 139 women at risk for ectopic pregnancy managed with TVS and hCG estimations, using a discriminatory level of 1300 IU/l (First IRP). TVS alone correctly identified 64% of the women with ectopic pregnancy (14/22), based on the identification of an extrauterine sac in the absence of an intrauterine sac. In 4 patients with ectopic pregnancy the TVS findings were normal but an hCG greater than 1300 IU/l allowed them to be correctly identified laparoscopically. In the remaining 4 patients with ectopic pregnancy, the TVS findings were either normal or equivocal, but an hCG value less than 1300 IU/l did not allow a definitive diagnosis to be made. Of the total study group at risk for ectopic pregnancy, 18 (13%) could not be definitively diagnosed by TVS (sac not visualised at an hCG level less than 1300 IU/l). Serial hCG, repeat ultrasound or both were needed to correctly diagnose ectopic pregnancy (4), early intrauterine pregnancy (4) and complete abortion (10).

If these results hold true in other studies, it would appear that the use of TVS alone will correctly resolve the majority of cases of suspected ectopic pregnancy, although the remaining cases will require additional and often repeated investigation with both biochemical and sonographic modalities. The choice of which diagnostic test to use in clinically stable women should depend on the facilities available in the given institution, although the cost of repeated quantitative hCG estimations will militate against their routine use.

Management of Ectopic Pregnancy

In spite of the dramatic increase in the incidence of ectopic pregnancy in recent years, there has been a fall in the number of fatalities. This is, in part, due to the widespread introduction of diagnostic tests and an increasing appreciation by patients and their doctors of the serious nature of this disease. In one unit, for example, the rate of tubal rupture (and hence dramatic presentation with life-threatening symptoms and signs) was only 20% (Pansky et al. 1991). Whether or not this is similar in other parts of the world remains uncertain. What is clear is the increasing need for conservative and/or expectant forms of management to deal with that large group of women who present with subacute ectopic pregnancy i.e., our Group 3 patients.

The basis of expectant management is the fact that a substantial proportion of ectopic pregnancies diagnosed in the western world are at a very early stage, at which time some at least would be expected to resolve spontaneously. In their recent review, Pansky et al. (1991) reported on a total of 61 patients treated expectantly. They concluded that the role for this form of non-treatment is probably limited to that small subgroup of patients who are minimally symptomatic and in whom serum hCG levels are clearly falling.

Medical treatment of ectopic pregnancy with systemic drugs (e.g., methotrexate, actinomycin D, mifepristone) has recently been introduced into clinical practice. Ultrasound or laparoscopic directed aspiration and/or local injection with drugs such as potassium chloride, methotrexate and adrenaline, as well as prostaglandin E2 and F2 alpha into the gestational sac is also possible. Recently, the administration of these medications by trans-cervical tubal cannulation under sonographic control has been performed successfully (Risquez et al. 1990). The advantage of ultrasound is that it does not require general anaesthesia, but this may be countered by the risk of accidental puncture of blood vessels. Most of the literature has been in the form of case reports describing the indications, dosage and expected adverse reactions of these therapeutic regimes. The key to success using medical therapy as a whole is the selection of suitable patients based on features such as the size of the pregnancy (less than 3 cm), an unruptured tube without active bleeding, serum hCG levels less than 1500 IU/l and a sonographically non-viable pregnancy. It is anticipated that only a quarter of all ectopic pregnancies are suitable for non-surgical management. Analysis of the published results of medical treatment reveals that most have very similar success rates of 80%–90%, which is hardly surprising since the selection criteria for medical treatment are fairly uniform. It should be emphasised that only those departments with access to quantitative hCG and good ultrasound should be using one of these treatment modalities. Which one to use depends to a certain extent on personal choice and practical skills, until such time as controlled randomised prospective studies indicate which technique is superior in terms of adverse reactions and effects on future fertility.

At exploratory laparoscopy the surgeon must determine the exact location of the pregnancy, the condition of the involved tube, that of the opposite tube and ovary and the importance of any existing pelvic abnormalities. Since most tubal pregnancies occur in the ampulla, the surgical treatment of choice in the unruptured tube is a salpingotomy-type procedure performed either laparoscopically or via microsurgical laparotomy. Two surgical procedures are available to the surgeon confronted with a mid tubal ectopic pregnancy. The first, salpingotomy, is useful when the tube is intact and can be performed either laparoscopically or via microsurgical laparotomy. The second procedure, mid tubal resection with or without end-to-end anastomosis is necessary when the tube has ruptured or when bleeding control is felt to be inadequate.

Laparoscopic surgery can be used in the vast majority of cases, the only relative contraindications to its use being massive intra-abdominal bleeding and extensive intra-abdominal adhesions. There are a variety of methods available to open the tube e.g., electrocautery, laser or surgical instruments. The trophoblast is removed and suction/irrigation used for evacuation. The most difficult aspect of a laparoscopic approach is occasional inability to achieve complete haemostasis at the site of placental attachment on the interior tubal wall. All bleeding points must be secured by meticulous point electrocoagulation. If this cannot be achieved then laparotomy is essential. Surgery on the opposite tube noted to be damaged at the time of conservative surgery is probably best deferred in order to take advantage of surgical experience and the availability of microsurgical tools.

The histopathology of the developing tubal pregnancy suggests that extraluminal spread of trophoblast takes place in a large proportion of cases (Budowick et al. 1980). The fact that the vast majority of the conceptuses lie between the tube and the peritoneum mitigates against the deceptively simple process of "milking" out the tube. This may also account for the approximately 5%–10% risk of persistent trophoblast tissue remaining after conservative surgery (a figure which is remarkably similar for all forms of non-radical surgery). Typically there is a latency of 1–4 weeks before symptoms appear. Therefore serial hCG measurements are recommended until non-pregnant levels are reached (Lundorff et al. 1991).

The philosophy behind conservative treatment is that preserving the tube increases the chance of subsequent live births. In fact the results of conservative surgery suggest that irrespective of the surgical technique used, the condition of the contralateral tube is the most significant factor in terms of future fertility. Comparison between the numerous published series is hampered by the fact that some have grouped together patients in whom the contralateral tube was normal and abnormal. Recurrent ectopic pregnancy is the major risk of any technique, occurring in approximately 10%–15% of patients. It appears that this is as likely to occur in the opposite, presumably normal tube, as in the tube operated on conservatively.

Salpingectomy is indicated in patients with a large ectopic pregnancy (more than 2–3 cm in diameter), when the tube has ruptured, when haemoperitoneum is associated with shock or when bleeding is uncontrolled. The sole desire for sterilisation is not generally accepted as the primary indication for radical surgery, unless this has been documented in previous records. The reported subsequent intrauterine pregnancy rates vary from 23%–70% and the incidence of repeat ectopic pregnancy ranges from 10%–30%. These wide variations in pregnancy rates are largely due to differences in reporting characteristics. For example, by calculating the incidence of pregnancy as a percentage of all patients who were operated on, it is possible to underestimate the true incidence. This is probably best expressed as a proportion of the number of women who desire pregnancy after the procedure. Using this denominator approximately 35% of women desirous of pregnancy will have a subsequent intrauterine pregnancy and 15% will have a repeat ectopic pregnancy.

Conclusion

Ectopic pregnancy occurs in approximately 1% of all maternities and remains the major cause of maternal mortality in the first trimester. Early diagnosis relies on maintaining a high index of suspicion. TVS in combination with quantitative hCG estimations may allow a more conservative therapeutic approach.

Acknowledgements.   Figures 11.2 and 11.4b were supplied by Dr. K. Harrington and Mr T. Bourne, and Dr N. Amso, respectively.

References

Andolf E, Jorgensen C (1990) A prospective comparison of transabdominal and transvaginal ultrasound with surgical findings in gynecologic disease. J Ultrasound Med 9:71–75

Atrash HK, Friede A, Hogue CJR (1987) Ectopic pregnancy mortality in the United States, 1970–1983. Obstet Gynecol 70:817–822

Beral V (1975) An epidemiological study of recent trends in ectopic pregnancy. Br J Obstet Gynaecol 82:755–782

Bernaschek G, Rudelstorfer R, Csaicsich P (1988) Vaginal sonography versus serum hCG in early detection of pregnancy. Am J Obstet Gynecol 158:608–612

Braunstein GD, Asch RH (1983) Predictive value analysis of measurements of hCG, pregnancy specific beta-1-glycoprotein, placental lactogen and cystine amniopeptidase for the diagnosis of ectopic pregnancy. Fertil Steril 39:62–67

Bree LR, Edwards M, Bohm-Velez M, Beyler S, Roberts J, Mendelson AB (1989) Transvaginal sonography in the evaluation of normal early pregnancy: correlation with hCG level. AJR 153:75–79

Budowick M, Johnson TRB, Genadry R, Parmley TH, Woodruff JD (1980) The histopathology of the developing tubal ectopic pregnancy. Fertil Steril 34:169–171

Buhi WC, vanWert JW, Alvarez IM et al. (1989) Synthesis and secretion of proteins by postpartum human oviductal tissue in culture. Fertil Steril 51:75–80

Cacciatore B, Ylostalo P, Stenman UH, Widholm O (1988) Suspected ectopic pregnancy: ultrasonic findings and hCG levels assessed by an immunofluorometric assay. Br J Obstet Gynaecol 95:497–502

Cacciatore B, Stenman UH, Ylostalo P (1989) Comparison of abdominal and vaginal sonography in suspected ectopic pregnancy. Obstet Gynecol 73:770–774

Cacciatore B, Tiitinen A, Stenman UH, Ylostalo P (1990) Normal early pregnancy: serum hCG levels and vaginosonographic findings. Br J Obstet Gynaecol 97:899–903

Center for Disease Control (1986) Ectopic pregnancy in the USA: 1970–1983, CDC Surveillance summaries. MMWR 35:29

Coleman BG, Arger PH, Grumbach K et al. (1988) Transvaginal and transabdominal sonography: prospective comparison. Radiol 166:639–634

Dashefsky SM, Lyosn EA, Levi CS, Lindsay DJ (1988) Suspected ectopic pregnancy: endovaginal and transvesical ultrasound. Radiol 169:181–184

deCrespigny LC (1988) Demonstration of ectopic pregnancy by transvaginal ultrasound. Br J Obstet Gynaecol 95:1253–1256

Degenhardt F (1988) Endosonographie bei Extrauteringravidität. Geburtshilfe Frauenheilkd 48:352–354 (English Abstract)

Department of Health and Social Security (1990) Report on confidential enquiries into maternal deaths in the United Kingdom. 1985–1987. HMSO, London

Di Marchi JM, Kosas TS, Hale RW (1989) What is the significance of hCG value in ectopic pregnancy? Obstet Gynecol 74:851–855

Emmrich P, Kopping H (1981) A study of placental villi in extrauterine gestation: a guide to the frequency of blighted ova. Placenta 2:63–70

Fossum GT, Davajan V, Kletzky OA (1988) Early detection of pregnancy with transvaginal ultrasound. Fertil Steril 49:788–791

Funk A, Fendel H (1988) Verbesserte Diagnostik der Extrauteringravidität durch die Endosonographie. Z Geburtshilfe Perinatol 192:49–53 (English Abstract)

Gelder MS, Boots LR, Younger JB (1991) Use of a single random progesterone value as a diagnostic aid for ectopic pregnancy. Fertil Steril 55:497–500

Goldstein SR, Snyder JR, Watson C, Danon M (1988) Very early pregnancy detection with endovaginal ultrasound. Obstet Gynecol 72:200–204

Hahlin M, Wallin A, Sjoblom P, Lindblom B (1990) Single progesterone assay for early recognition of abnormal pregnancy. Human Reprod 5:622–626

Hahlin M, Sjoblom P, Lindblom B (1991) Combined use of progesterone and hCG for differential diagnosis of very early pregnancy. Fertil Steril 55:492–496

Hamori M, Stuckensen JA, Rumpf D et al. (1989) Early pregnancy wastage following late implantation of embryos after IVF-ET. Human Reprod 4:714–717

Hill LM, Kislak S, Martin JG (1990) Endovaginal sonographic evaluation of pseudogestational sac associated with ectopic pregnancy. Proceedings 34th Annual Convention AIUM, J Ultrasound Med 9:558

Hubinont CH, Thomas C, Schwers JF (1987) Luteal function in ectopic pregnancy. Am J Obstet Gynecol 156:669–673

Iffy L (1963) The role of premenstrual post mid cycle conception in the aetiology of ectopic gestation: An evaluation of the reflux theory. J Obstet Gynaecol Br Cmwlth 70:996–1000

Jain KA, Schiller VL, Perrella RR, Sutherland ML, Grant EG (1988) Transabdominal versus endovaginal pelvic sonography: prospective study. Radiol 170:553–556

Lande IM, Hill MC, Cosco EE et al (1988) Adnexal and cul-de-sac abnormalities: transvaginal sonography. Radiol 166:325–332

Leibman JA, Kruse B, McSweeney MB et al. (1988) Transvaginal sonography: comparison with transabdominal sonography in the diagosis of pelvic masses. AJR 151:89–92

Lindblom B, Hahlin M, Sjoblom P (1989) Serial hCG determinations by fluoroimmunoassay for differentiation between intrauterine and ectopic gestation. Am J Obstet Gynecol 161:397–400

Liu HC, Jones G, Kreiner D, Jones H, Muasher SH, Rosenwaks Z (1988) Beta hCG as a monitor of pregnancy outcome in IVF-ET patients. Fertil Steril 50:89–94

Lower AM, Tyack AJ (1989) Heterotopic pregnancy following IVF-ET. Two case reports and a review of the literature. Human Reprod 4:726–728

Lower AM, Yovich JL, Hancock C, Shenton P, Grudzinskas JG (1992) Is luteal function maintained by factors other than hCG in early pregnancy? Submitted.

Lundorff P, Hahlin M, Sjoblom P, Lindblom B (1991) Persistent trophoblast after conservative treatment of tubal pregnancy: prediction and detection. Obstet Gynecol 77:129–133

Maguiness SD, Djahanbakhch O, Grudzinskas JG (1992) Assessment of the Fallopian tube. Obstet Gynecol Survey. In Press.

Mendelson EB, Bohm-Velez M, Joseph N et al. (1988) Gynecologic imaging: comparison of transabdominal and transvaginal sonography. Radiol 166:321–324

Meunier K, Guichard A, Mignot TM, Zorn JR, Maria B, Cedard L (1991) Predictive value of active renin assay for the diagnosis of ectopic pregnancy. Fertil Steril 55:432–435

Nyberg DA, Filly RA, Mahoney BS, Monroe S, Laing FC, Jeffrey RB (1985) Early gestation: correlation of hCG levels and sonographic identification. AJR 144:951–954

Nyberg DA, Mack LA, Jeffrey RB, Laing FC (1987) Endovaginal sonographic evaluation of ectopic pregnancy: a prospective study. AJR 149:1181–1186

Nyberg DA, Mack LA, Laing FC, Jeffrey RB (1988) Early pregnancy complications: endovaginal sonographic findings correlated with human chorionic gonadotrophin levels. Radiol 167:619–622

Nyberg DA, Hughes MP, Mack L, Wang KW (1991) Extrauterine findings of ectopic pregnancy at transvaginal ultrasound: importance of echogenic fluid. Radiol 178:823–826

Pansky M, Golan A, Bukovsky I, Caspi E (1991) Non surgical management of tubal pregnancy. Necessity in view of the changing clinical appearance. Am J Obstet Gynecol 164:888–895

Pedersen JF, Sorensen S, Ruge S (1991) Serum level of secretory endometrial protein PP14 in intact ectopic pregnancy. Br J Obstet Gynaecol 98:414

Pennell RC, Baltarowich OH, Kurtz AB, Vilaro MM (1987) Complicated first trimester pregnancies: evaluation with endovaginal versus transabdominal technique. Radiol 165:79–83

Poulsen HK, Westergaard JG, Teisner B, Bolton AE, Grudzinskas JG (1987) Undetectable circulating placental proteins in some women with ectopic gestation. J Obstet Gynaecol 7:274–276

Pulkkinen MO, Jaakkola UM (1989) Low serum progesterone levels and tubal dysfunction – A possible cause of ectopic pregnancy. Am J Obstet Gynecol 161:934–937

Riddle AF, Sharma V, Masson B et al. (1987) Two years experience of ultrasound directed oocyte retrieval. Fertil Steril 48:454–460

Risquez F, Mathieson J, Zorn J-R (1990) Tubal cannulation via the cervix: a passing fancy or here to stay? J IVF-ET 7:301–303

Risk B, Tan SL, Morcos S, Riddle A, Brinsden P, Mason B, Edwards RG (1991) Heterotopic pregnancies after IVF and ET. Am J Obstet Gynecol 164:161–164

Romero R, Kadar N, Jeanty P et al. (1985) The diagnosis of ectopic pregnancy: the value of the hCG discriminatory zone. Obstet Gynecol 66:357–360

Sauer MV, Sinosich MJ, Yeko TR et al. (1989) Predictive value of a single PAPP-A or progesterone in the diagnosis of abnormal pregnancy. Hum Reprod 4:331–334

Shapiro BB, Cullen M, Taylor KJW, deCherney AH (1988) Transvaginal ultrasound for the diagnosis of ectopic pregnancy. Fertil Steril 5:425–429

Stabile I (1988) *Pregnancy Associated Plasma Protein A in complications of early pregnancy with particular reference to ectopic gestation.* PhD thesis, University of London

Stabile I, Grudzinskas JG (1990) Ectopic pregnancy: a review of incidence, etiology and diagnostic aspects. Obstet Gynecol Survey 45:335–347

Stabile I, Campbell S, Grudzinskas JG (1988) Can ultrasound reliably diagnose ectopic pregnancy? Br J Obstet Gynaecol 95:1247–1252

Stabile I, Olajide F, Chard T, Grudzinskas JG (1989a) Maternal serum alpha-fetoprotein levels in anembryonic pregnancy. Human Reprod 4:204–205

Stabile I, Olajide F, Chard T, Grudzinskas JG (1989b) Maternal serum alpha-fetoprotein levels in ectopic pregnancy. Human Reprod 4:835–836

Stabile I, Howell R, Teisner B, Chard T, Grudzinskas JG (1989c) Circulating levels of PP12 in complications of first trimester pregnancy. Arch Gynecol Obstet 246:201–206

Stabile I, Teisner B, Chard T, Grudzinskas JG (1990) Circulating levels of PP12 in ectopic pregnancy. Arch Gynecol Obstet 247:149–153

Stiller RJ, de Regt RH, Blair E (1989) Transvaginal sonography in patients at risk for ectopic pregnancy. Am J Obstet Gynecol 161:930–933

Tessler FN, Schiller VL, Perrella PR, Sutherland ML, Grant EG (1989) TAS versus endovaginal pelvic sonography: prospective study. Radiol 170:553–556

Timor-Tritsch IE, Rottem S, Thaler I (1988) Review of transvaginal sonography: a description with clinical application. Ultrasound Quarterly 8:1–34

Tornehave D, Chemnitz J, Westergaard JG et al. (1986) Placental proteins in peripheral blood and tissues of ectopic pregnancies. Gynecol Obstet Invest 23:97–102

Tuomivaara L, Kauppila A, Puolakka J (1986) Ectopic pregnancy–An analysis of the etiology, diagnosis and treatment in 552 cases. Arch Gynaecol 237:135–139

Verhage HG, Fazleabas AT, Donnelly K (1988) The in vitro synthesis and release of proteins by the human oviduct. Endocrinol 122:1639–1645

Vilaro MM, Rifkin MD, Pennell RG et al. (1987) Endovaginal ultrasound: a technique for evaluation of non follicular pelvic masses. J Ultrasound Med 6:697–701

Westergaard JG, Teisner B, Stabile I, Grudzinskas JG (1988) Diagnostic aspects of ectopic pregnancy. In: Tomoda S, Mizutani S, Narita O, Klopper A (eds) Endometrial and placental proteins: Basic concepts and clinical applications. VSP International Scientific Publishers, Netherlands, pp 615–622

Westrom L (1975) Effect of acute pelvic inflammatory disease on fertility. Am J Obstet Gynecol 121:707–713

Yeko TR, Gorrill MW, Hughes LH et al. (1987) Timely diagnosis of ectopic pregnancy using a single blood progesterone measurement. Fertil Steril 48:1048–1050

12. Surgical Treatment of Spontaneous Abortion

M. Macnaughton

The question of recurrent abortion is considered in Chapter 7. This chapter will deal with two aspects of surgery in association with abortion. The first is the place of cervical cerclage in the treatment of abortion and the second is the use of curettage in the management of the condition.

Cervical Cerclage in the Management of Cervical Incompetence

Cervical incompetence is usually associated with spontaneous abortion occurring after 12–14 weeks. It is seldom a cause of spontaneous abortion before this time. The basis for considering the operation of cervical cerclage is the possibility that a congenital or traumatically acquired weakness of the cervix or multiple pregnancy may cause premature dilatation of the cervix, which leads to spontaneous second trimester abortion or pre-term delivery. This incompetence may present as silent dilatation of the cervix without painful uterine contractions. The membranes bulge through the cervical canal and eventually rupture spontaneously. In practice, the clinical diagnosis of cervical incompetence relies heavily on the history of previous abortions. The classical picture is of sudden spontaneous rupture of the membranes with little or no bleeding, followed by a relatively painless expulsion of the pregnancy (Palmer and Lacomme 1949). There is no true diagnostic test of cervical incompetence and the decision to insert a cervical suture is usually based on past obstetric history or clinical examination of the cervix during pregnancy. Past obstetric history is not, however, a strong predictor of subsequent early delivery. About 85% of women who have had one previous delivery at 20–30 weeks gestation will carry a subsequent pregnancy to term and even after two such events the term delivery rate is still as high as 70% (Bakketeig et al. 1979; Carr-Hill and Hall 1985).

Several techniques have been recommended to diagnose cervical incompetence between pregnancies. These include inspection of the cervix to detect a widely gaping internal os, determining the largest dilator which will pass through the cervix without meeting resistance (Palmer 1950), radiological hysterography (Rubovitz et al. 1953) and studies with balloons to demonstrate dilatation of the internal os and uterine isthmus (Mann 1959). More recently, ultrasound has been used to measure the diameter of the internal os (Brook et al. 1981). In the technique devised by Anthony et al. (1982), the force required to dilate the cervix with serial, graduated dilators of diameters 3–8 mm inclusive is recorded on an instrument previously described by Fisher et al. (1981). This value is described as the "cervical resistance index" (CRI). In general, those patients whose history points to cervical incompetence have a low CRI while those whose history is of bleeding and pain before abortion have a normal CRI.

There are, therefore, great difficulties in making a diagnosis of cervical incompetence and as a result the use of cervical cerclage varies widely between different units. In a survey of British obstetricians in 1979, the incidence of cervical cerclage varied from 0%–8% of pregnancies (Interim Report of the MRC/RCOG Working Party 1988). The high degree of uncertainty amongst obstetricians about the place of cerclage in the prevention of abortion and pre-term delivery was the indication for randomised controlled trials to assess the results of this procedure.

Operative Procedures for Cervical Incompetence

There are 2 main procedures which are commonly used for cervical cerclage. The simplest and most widely used was described by MacDonald (1957). The other and more complicated operation was described by Shirodkar (1960). In a survey of British obstetricians, the ratio of the use of the MacDonald to the Shirodkar suture was 3:1 and the use of tape to monofilament nylon 12:1.

In the MacDonald procedure a suture of No. 2 prolene is used to encircle the cervix under the cervical skin. This is inserted using a curved needle. The suture is tightened sufficiently to reduce the diameter of the cervical canal to a few millimetres and is then securely tied. This is the simplest procedure available and is the one to be recommended in most cases. In the Shirodkar procedure the anterior skin of the cervix is incised and the bladder is pushed up prior to encirclement of the cervix with Dacron tape using a special needle. This is a more traumatic procedure than the MacDonald operation and is now seldom used. Furthermore, there is less blood loss, less scarring of the cervix and less likelihood of cervical dystocia with the MacDonald procedure.

Both procedures are best performed in the first trimester of pregnancy and certainly before dilatation of the cervix commences. Bleeding and cramping pains are contra-indications to surgery. Should the patient continue to abort following the insertion of the suture, the suture must be removed.

For the woman with a typical history of repeated abortions caused by an incompetent cervix, Lash and Lash (1950) devised an operation to be performed when the woman was not pregnant. In this procedure, the skin of the cervix is dissected from the anterior lip and an elliptical incision is made in the anterior lip between the internal and external os. A small amount of tissue is removed and the defect closed with interrupted sutures. The problem with this procedure has been that the patient may be rendered infertile, so it is seldom performed.

Transabdominal cervical cerclage is sometimes employed in unusual cases such as following cervical amputation, deep cervical or uterine lacerations or in cases of congenital shortening of the cervix. This is a much more major procedure than the first two but has a place in special cases (Anthony and Price 1986).

Choice of Patients

The selection of patients for cervical cerclage is usually based on past obstetric history. In addition the operation is performed when there is clinical or ultrasound evidence that the cervix is either being "taken up" or that actual dilatation is occurring, sometimes with bulging membranes. When this has occurred it is probably too late and certainly the results in this situation are poor. This is particularly the case when the membranes are bulging and have to be pushed back since rupture or subsequent infection are very likely to occur.

The indications for cerclage are shown in Table 12.1. These are the common considerations which determine whether or not cervical cerclage should be performed. They are wide ranging and probably account for the difficulties in assessing whether or not the operation achieves its intended effect. They also account for the wide variation in the number of sutures inserted by those who are uncertain of the advantages of the procedure but who wish to do everything possible to avert the possibility of a further miscarriage or pre-term labour. The wishes of the patient should also be considered. Many have read or heard that the operation could be of advantage in a woman who has suffered repeated miscarriages. Patients are not really interested in statistics or probabilities but want to feel that everything that might possibly help has been done. If the woman thinks that "stitching in the baby" might help she will want the procedure; this has been an important indication for the operation, particularly if it was also done in a previous pregnancy.

Table 12.1. Indications for cervical cerclage (Interim Report of the Medical Research Council/Royal College of Obstetricians and Gynaecologists Multicentre Randomised Controlled Trial)

Previous pre-term deliveries
Previous second trimester miscarriages
Previous early miscarriages
Previous induced abortions
Previous pre-term delivery or second trimester miscarriage
Past cervical history
   Cone biopsy
   Cervical amputation
   Previous cervical suture
Other indications
   "Abnormal" cervix
   Uterine abnormality
   Twins
   Other

Value of the Procedure

Cervical cerclage as a preventitive strategy has been poorly assessed. It has been recognised that in rare cases the operation may have serious adverse effects and that there is no good evidence of its efficacy. Various claims of the success of this procedure have been made and according to Beischer and Mackay (1986) if performed before 20 weeks and without rupturing the membranes there is a good chance of a successful outcome (between 40% and 90%). Stray-Pedersen and Stray-Pedersen (1984) found a similar success rate (70%). These, however, were not properly controlled trials so the results must be viewed with some degree of scepticism. Beta-mimetic drugs were often given intravenously for a day or two after the operation and then orally until the pregnancy was clearly seen to be progressing satisfactorily.

Table 12.2 shows the results of cervical cerclage as reported by MacDonald (1980). These results show more live births after prophylactic suture than ligation after membranes were bulging with the MacDonald, Shirodkar and abdominal approaches. However, this trial was not controlled.

Table 12.2. Results of cervical cerclage (MacDonald 1980)

Type of Suture	No. of cases	No. of live births	Percentage
MacDonald suture	} 148	128	86.5
Prophylactic suture at 14 weeks			
Ligation after membranes bulging	76	36	47.4
Shirodkar ligature	37	27	72.9
Abdominal ligature	8	6	75.6
Total	269	197	70.5

Randomised Controlled Trials

The encouraging results of the non-controlled trials and the uncertainty among obstetricians stimulated the Medical Research Council (MRC) of Great Britain and the Royal College of Obstetricians and Gynaecologists (RCOG) to mount a multicentre, randomised trial of cervical cerclage. The aim of the trial was to assess whether cervical cerclage in women deemed to be at risk of cervical incompetence does indeed prevent spontaneous abortion and prolong pregnancy and thereby improve fetal and neonatal outcome. The problem with other trials had been the small numbers, and the results of a randomised controlled trial from South Africa (Rush et al. 1984) and France (Lazar et al. 1984) illustrated the need for larger randomised trials of the operation if a precise assessment of its effects was to be made.

South African Trial

The South African trial included 194 subjects who were at high risk (30%) of pre-term delivery. The pre-term delivery rate was slightly higher in the cerclage group

(Table 12.3) but because of the relatively small number of subjects the confidence limits were large and the real effect might have been anything between a 62% increase and a 27% decrease in the relative risk of pre-term delivery. A decrease in the relative risk by as much as 27% would clearly be clinically important. However, the South African trial could only conclude that the effect was not greater than 27%.

Table 12.3. Pre-term deliveries in cerclage and control groups of two randomised controlled trials of cervical cerclage

	Cerclage	Control
South African Trial	33/96 (34.4%)	31/98 (31.6%)
French Trial	18/268 (6.7%)	13/238 (5.5%)

French Trial

The French Trial included 506 subjects recruited from four centres with a relatively low risk of pre-term delivery (6%). As Table 12.3 illustrates, the cerclage group again appeared to be at increased risk of early delivery.

The French investigators were surprised to find that more women in the cerclage group were admitted to hospital for reasons other than the operation and more received oral tocolytic therapy. The South African cerclage group similarly spent more time in hospital and received more tocolytic therapy. They were also more likely to experience puerperal pyrexia.

Both trials, then, suggest some adverse effects of the operation even if spontaneous abortion is prevented. The findings emphasised the need for more clear-cut evidence of benefit if the current use of cerclage is to continue. However, the South African and French trials were too small to demonstrate or exclude such an effect, with confidence. The lack of evidence for the effectiveness of cervical cerclage based on past obstetric history has raised questions about the place of the operation in those patients in whom a diagnosis of cervical incompetence is made on the basis of physical signs before and during pregnancy. There have been calls for randomised trials in these circumstances but such cases are rare; few centres could recruit sufficient numbers to make any meaningful comparison.

The MRC/RCOG Randomised Cervical Cerclage Trial

A randomised trial to assess the effects of the operation was established by the MRC and the RCOG. The trial involved 200 obstetricians in 9 countries. A total of 905 cases with complete records were available for analysis. A woman was eligible for entry to the trial if her obstetrician was uncertain whether to advise her to have cervical cerclage or not. Basic identifying and descriptive data were given over the telephone and a random allocation was made to one of two clinical policies: either a recommendation to insert a cervical suture (unless a clear contra-indication arose subsequently) or a recommendation to avoid suture (unless a clear indication arose). A request was made to keep ancillary treatment with beta-mimetics and bed-rest to a minimum for all women; otherwise subsequent care was left entirely to the clinician responsible. The prime measures of outcome were length of pregnancy, deliveries before 33 completed weeks and deliveries "pre-term" (i.e., before 37 completed weeks), and the status of the baby at the time of completion of the form. A successful continuation of the pregnancy meant that spontaneous abortion had been prevented. The reasons for inclusion in the trial are given in Table 12.1. The type of operation was not specified in advance.

Results of the MRC/RCOG Trial

As in previous trials there was increased intervention during the MRC/RCOG trial, judged by admission to hospital, use of oral beta-mimetics, induction of labour and caesarean section in cervical cerclage patients. By contrast with other trials the MRC/RCOG trial suggested a beneficial effect of cerclage on length of gestation and vital outcome. There were 5% fewer deliveries between 20 and 32 weeks gestation. If real, this would be equivalent to the prevention of 1 pre-term delivery for every 20 sutures inserted. But the results were only marginally significant and were within a wide range of possible outcomes.

In spite of the large numbers, this trial still leaves much uncertainty as to whether there is any real benefit and whether the operation prevents spontaneous abortion.

Dor et al. (1982), in a small randomised controlled trial of cervical cerclage in twin pregnancy with ultrasound evidence of cervical incompetence, showed no difference between the suture and the control groups. Lazar et al. (1984) recruited women with singleton pregnancies with an overall pre-term delivery rate of only 6%. In conclusion, the value of cervical cerclage in the prevention of spontaneous abortion is minimal; probably only one case of pre-term delivery would be prevented for every 20 sutures inserted.

Management of Spontaneous Abortion

Curettage is indicated in spontaneous abortion after the diagnosis of incomplete abortion has been made or if a dead or absent fetus is diagnosed in the case of threatened abortion.

The management of abortion in the first trimester has been revolutionised by the development of ultrasound (Robinson 1972a). Threatened abortion can be differentiated from an incomplete or complete abortion, thereby avoiding unnecessary treatment by bed-rest or evacuation of the uterus. Robinson (1972b, 1978) also showed that the fetal heart beat could normally be demonstrated by 7 weeks gestation.

About half of all pregnancies complicated by threatened abortion have a successful outcome (Stabile et al. 1987) but if the fetal heart beat is identified after

9 weeks outcome is successful in 90% of cases (Bennett and Kerr-Wilson 1980; Jouppila et al. 1980). Increased bleeding, rhythmical uterine contractions and a loss of clear fluid suggest that abortion is inevitable. At this stage ultrasound assessment can identify whether the fetus is alive or dead. If the fetus is dead and unless complete expulsion of the uterine contents follows rapidly, the uterus should be emptied surgically under general anaesthesia.

Ultrasound can be used to ascertain if the uterus is empty following abortion. The author has found this to be unsatisfactory because blood clot and retained products appear very similar. Curettage is essential to ensure that the uterus is indeed empty, otherwise haemorrhage, infection and later complications such as Ascherman's syndrome may occur. In the case of incomplete abortion the cervix is dilated and placental debris may lie free in the lower uterine segment. The products of conception may protrude through the external cervical os. In this case the uterine size is smaller than would be expected from the calculated period of gestation. There is frequently heavy bleeding and the vagina may be full of blood clot. When the cervix is dilated with placental debris protruding from the os it may be possible to remove these products without general anaesthesia. The uterine cavity may also be evacuated, without anaesthesia, with a suction curette. In most cases, however, evacuation of an incomplete abortion requires general anaesthesia to ensure that the uterine cavity is completely cleared.

Abortion in the second trimester is managed in the same way as in the first trimester. If the fetus is alive and normal as demonstrated by ultrasound, treatment is aimed at maintaining the pregnancy (see below). All cases of bleeding after a period of amenorrhoea should now be subjected to ultrasound examination so that threatened abortion, incomplete abortion and ectopic pregnancy may be identified.

Dilatation and Curettage

Dilatation of the cervix is usually an essential preliminary to uterine curettage. Equipment for the procedure includes a vaginal speculum, a uterine sound, a toothed vulsellum forceps, a pair of narrow ovum forceps and small, medium and large uterine curettes as well as a suction curette. A series of dilators should also be available.

The speculum is inserted into the vagina and the size and position of the uterus is assessed by bi-manual examination. The anterior lip of the cervix is grasped with a vulsellum forceps, thus drawing it down to the introitus. This has the effect of straightening the cervical canal and easing the passage of the instruments. The toothed variety of vulsellum forceps may cause bleeding due to vascularity of the cervix in pregnancy, but this is usually minimal and easily controlled. Alternatively, an ovum forceps may be applied to the cervix. This causes less trauma but does not allow strong traction.

A uterine sound is inserted to measure the length of the uterine cavity. Great care must be taken here to avoid perforating the soft uterine fundus. In many cases of abortion the cervix is already open and no further dilatation is required. If the cervix has closed, dilatation may be necessary, but this should be kept to the minimum needed to evacuate the uterus completely. The uterine fundus is very soft in these cases and perforation is not uncommon. The surgeon should be able to feel the dilator gently touch the fundus of the uterus as each dilator is inserted.

The dilator should never be passed for a greater distance than the sounded length. Judgement of pressure required can only be acquired by practice. A dilatation of 9–11 mm should be adequate in most cases; the greater the degree of dilatation, the greater is the likelihood of damage to the cervix.

Complications of Dilatation and Curettage

Tearing and Laceration of the Cervix

The soft pregnant cervix is easily damaged. An ovum forceps is less likely to tear the cervix than a vulsellum. If dilatation leads to bleeding from a cervical tear a suture or a pressure pack may be required. If bleeding continues it may occasionally be necessary to split the cervix to identify the bleeding point. Very rarely, continued bleeding may necessitate hysterectomy.

Perforation of the Uterus

The usual site of perforation is at the fundus. Perforation of the uterus is especially likely if the uterus is retroverted. The sound or dilator then penetrates the anterior wall of the uterus into the peritoneal cavity or the bladder. If perforation is suspected, laparoscopy is essential to ascertain the extent of the injury; if there is bleeding into the peritoneal cavity laparotomy will be required.

Most perforations produce no major or long-term sequelae provided they are recognised at the time. However, infection may progress to peritonitis. Symptoms of abdominal pain and discomfort may be delayed for one or two days. Antibiotic therapy should be instituted and laparotomy may be essential to assess the full extent of the complication.

Bowel Damage

Damage to the bowel may accompany perforation of the uterus. The ovum forceps may deliver unrecognised pieces of bowel and omentum. Recognition of this damage should lead to immediate laparotomy and repair of the bowel.

Perforation into the Broad Ligament

Perforation into the broad ligament is usually secondary to laceration of the cervix at or close to the internal os. Lateral rupture of the uterus into the broad ligament occurs, often involving the uterine artery with formation of a broad ligament haematoma. Pain is the commonest initial symptom followed by signs of acute blood loss. Bi-manual examination reveals a mass on the affected side. Conservative treatment is the best option as the pressure from the broad ligament will usually cause the bleeding to stop. The haematoma will usually resolve over a period of weeks. Only occasionally is it necessary to resort to laparotomy to stop the bleeding.

Perforation of the Bladder

Perforation of the bladder may occur when the sound or dilator is pushed through the anterior wall of a retroverted uterus, particularly if the bladder has not been emptied prior to operation. If there is a flow of urine into the vagina, laparotomy and repair of the fistula is indicated.

Infection

Peritonitis may follow perforation or occasionally simple dilatation. The peritonitis is usually localised to the pelvis. Rarely the infection becomes severe and signs of bacteraemia and septic or endotoxic shock appear. In the Report on Confidential Enquiries into Maternal Deaths in England and Wales in 1979–1981 (Report on Confidential Enquiries into Maternal Deaths 1986) one death occurred from sepsis following spontaneous abortion.

Infection after spontaneous abortion may result in tubal occlusion.

Asherman's Syndrome – Intrauterine Adhesion

Adhesions can cause partial or complete obliteration of the uterine cavity. This can lead to menstrual abnormalities, amenorrhoea and abortion. The commonest cause is curettage for incomplete abortion (March and Israel 1981). Schenker and Margalioth (1982) showed that 66.7% of cases of adhesions followed curettage after abortion.

To minimise this complication, curettage should be gentle and superficial, not extending deeply into the uterine lining. It is best to use the suction curette initially, followed by gentle sharp curettage.

Haemorrhage

Haemorrhage from the uterine cavity is a common complication of abortion. The uterus should be evacuated under general anaesthesia as rapidly as possible. Administration of an oxytocic drug in the interval before evacuation is helpful; blood transfusion may be necessary.

References

Anthony GS, Calder AA, Macnaughton MC (1982) Cervical resistance in patients with previous spontaneous mid-trimester abortion. Br J Obstet Gynaecol 89:1046–1049

Anthony GS, Price JL (1986) Successful use of transabdominal isthmic cerclage in the management of cervical incompetence. Eur J Obstet Gynaecol Reprod Biol 22:379–382

Bakketeig LS, Hoffman HJ, Harley EE (1979) The tendency to repeat gestational age and birth weight in successive births. Am J Obstet Gynecol 135:1086–1103

Beischer NA, Mackay EV (1986) Bleeding in early pregnancy. In: Beischer NA, Mackay EV (eds.) Obstetrics in the Newborn. Baillière Tindall; London, pp 140–166

Bennett MJ, Kerr-Wilson RHJ (1980) Evaluation of threatened abortion by ultrasound. Internat J Gynaecol Obstet 17:382–384

Brook I, Femgold M, Schwartz A, Zakut H (1981) Ultrasonography in the diagnosis of cervical incompetence in pregnancy. A new diagnostic approach. Br J Obstet Gynaecol 88:640–643

Carr-Hill RA, Hall MH (1985) The repetition of spontaneous pre-term labour. Br J Obstet Gynaecol 92:921–928

Dor J, Shalev J, Mashiach G, Blankstein J, Serr D (1982) Elective cervical suture of twin pregnancies diagnosed ultrasonically in the first trimester following induced ovulation. Gynaecol Obstet Invest 13:55–60

Fisher J, Anthony GS, McManus TJ, Coutts JRT, Calder AA (1981) Use of a force measuring instrument during cervical dilatation. J Med Eng Tech 5:194–195

Interim Report of the Medical Research Council/Royal College of Obstetricians and Gynaecologists Working Party Multicentre Trial of Cervical Cerclage (1988) Br J Obstet Gynaecol. 95:437–445

Jouppila P, Huhtaniemi I, Tapaneinen J (1980) Early pregnancy failure: a study by ultrasonic and hormonal methods. Obstet Gynecol 55:42–47

Lash AF, Lash SR (1950) Habitual abortion: the incompetent internal os of the cervix. Am J Obstet Gynecol 59:68–76

Lazar P, Guegan S, Dreyfus J, Renaud R, Pontonnier G, Papiernik E (1984) Multicentre controlled trial of cervical cerclage in women at moderate risk of pre-term delivery. Br J Obstet Gynaecol 91:731–735

MacDonald IA (1957) Suture of the cervix for inevitable miscarriage. J Obstet Gynaecol Br Emp 64:346–350

MacDonald IA (1980) Cervical cerclage. Clin Obstet Gynaecol 3:461–479

Mann EC (1959) Habitual abortion. Am J Obstet Gynecol 77:706–718

March CM, Israel R (1981) Gestational outcome following hysteroscopic lysis of adhesions. Fertil Steril 36:455–459

Palmer R (1950) Physiology of the uterine isthmus and its part in sterility and habitual abortion. Rev Fr Gynecol Obstet 45:218–220

Palmer R, Lacomme M (1940) La beance de l'orifice interne. Gynecol Obstet (Paris), 47: 905–906

Report on Confidential Equiries into Maternal Deaths in England and Wales 1979–1981 (1986) Her Majesty's Stationery Office, London

Robinson HP (1972a) Sonar in the management of abortion. J Obstet Gynaecol Br Commonwth 79:90–94

Robinson HP (1972b) Detection of fetal heart movements in the first trimester of pregnancy using pulsed ultrasound. Br Med J 4:466–468

Robinson HP (1978) Normal development in early pregnancy. In: de Vlieger M, Kazner E, Kossot G et al. (eds), Handbook of Clinical Ultrasound. Wiley, New York, pp 121–134

Rubovitz FE, Cooperman NR, Lash AF (1953) Habitual abortion. A radiographic technique to demonstrate the incompetent internal os of the cervix. Am J Obstet Gynecol 66:269–280

Rush RW, Isaacs S, McPherson K, Jones L, Chalmers I, Grant A (1984) A randomised controlled trial of cervical cerclage in women at high risk of spontaneous preterm delivery. Br J Obstet Gynaecol 91:724–730

Schenker JG, Margalioth EJ (1982) Intrauterine adhesions: An updated appraisal. Fertil Steril 37:593–610

Shirodkar VM (1960) Contributions to obstetrics and gynaecology. Churchill Livingstone, Edinburgh, pp 1–16

Stabile I, Campbell S, Grudzinskas JG (1987) Ultrasonic assessment in complications of first trimester pregnancy. Lancet ii:1237–1240

Stray-Pedersen B, Stray-Pedersen S (1984) Etiologic factors and subsequent reproductive performance in 195 couples with a prior history of habitual abortion. Am J Obstet Gynecol 148:140–146

13. Endocrine Treatment in the Prevention and Management of Spontaneous Abortion

A. M. Lower and J. G. Grudzinskas

Introduction

It is generally held that at least one pregnancy in four will fail during the first trimester. Although the majority of women will subsequently achieve a successful pregnancy, the prospect of recurrent miscarriages and the despair of reproductive failure is a reality for some. Preventive measures have failed to achieve a significant impact on the prevalence of spontaneous miscarriage, reflecting partly the heterogeneous nature of the condition. Fetal chromosomal abnormalities are thought to be responsible for most miscarriages (Lauritsen 1976; Boué et al. 1975; Simpson 1980; Hassold et al. 1980), the majority being due to early embryonic arrest, previously termed "blighted ovum". At least 50% of all abortuses from clinically recognised pregnancies following IVT-ET also have abnormal karyotypes. An abnormal chromosome complement may result from abnormal sperm (approximately 10% of human sperm successfully karyotyped by Martin (1988) after hamster ovum penetration test showed chromosomal anomalies); from abnormal oocytes (up to 50% of human oocytes examined after ovarian stimulation contain chromosomal anomalies, the incidence increasing dramatically with advancing maternal age (Wramsby et al. 1987; Plachot et al. 1986)); and also from errors created during fertilisation, the most common being trisomy. This anomaly has been reported in association with spontaneous abortion for every human autosome except chromosome 1 (Simpson and Bombard 1987), although trisomy for that chromosome has been reported in an 8-cell embryo (Watt et al. 1987). Pregnancies affected by chromosomal abnormalities are not likely to respond to treatment aimed at preventing spontaneous abortion once conception has occurred. As the majority of early pregnancy losses are unavoidable, the efficacy of the therapeutic measures discussed below should be judged in this context.

This chapter will address the use of endocrine treatment in the prevention of spontaneous abortion and assess whether there is a place for such therapy in the management of incomplete or missed abortion.

Prevention

Spontaneous abortion represents the end point of a range of heterogeneous processes affecting early pregnancy, only some of which may be amenable to treatment. Some generalised metabolic and endocrine disorders have been associated with pregnancy failure. The associations are not especially firm, since the diverse causes of spontaneous abortion hamper the conduct of conclusive studies. However reproductive outcome will generally be improved with control of the underlying disorder. Conditions characterised by the relative deficiency or excess of reproductive hormones have been of particular interest and it is in this area that the majority of research has been concentrated.

A further confounding variable in studies of early pregnancy failure has been the high rate of response to placebo. Stray-Pedersen and Stray-Pedersen (1984) carried out a trial in which women with recurrent abortion were randomised to receive either full and sensitive counselling and encouragement or a rather shorter, more detached treatment. The subsequent obstetric outcome was improved in those women who received the greater input in terms of counselling and emotional support.

Systemic Disorders

Diabetes Mellitus

There has been some controversy over whether women with diabetes mellitus are at increased risk of spontaneous abortion (Coustan 1988; Sutherland and Pritchard 1987), since some of the early trials were flawed by retrospective design, unsystematic recruitment of patients and variable periods of follow-up. The recent multicentre "Diabetes in Early Pregnancy Study" coordinated by the National Institute of Child Health and Human Development concluded that diabetic women with good metabolic control were no more likely than non-diabetic women to miscarry, whereas those with elevated blood glucose and glycosylated haemoglobin levels in the first trimester (suggesting poor control) had a significantly increased risk of spontaneous abortion (Mills et al. 1988). This prospective study was well designed, most (75%) of the 818 subjects being recruited prior to conception and the remainder within 21 days of conception. Those who had spontaneous abortions had higher fasting ($p<0.01$) and post-prandial ($p<0.005$) glucose levels in the first trimester than those whose pregnancies continued. Moreover where glycaemic control was poor, the rate of pregnancy loss increased by 3.1% for each increase in the serum level of glycosylated haemoglobin of 1 S.D. above the normal range throughout the first trimester.

Pre-pregnancy counselling has made important contributions to decreasing the rate of spontaneous abortion among diabetic women: firstly by ensuring that diabetic control is optimal at the time of conception and maintained as such throughout the pregnancy; secondly, by ensuring that appropriate contraception measures are used, so that pregnancies can be planned with optimal diabetic control during organogenesis. Furthermore the decrease in incidence of spontaneous abortion in this group may also have a significant impact on the incidence of fetal congenital abnormality (Green et al. 1989).

Thyroid Disease

It is customary to perform tests of thyroid function as part of the range of investigations for recurrent miscarriage, although the rationale for this is poorly documented and hence questionable. The first connection between thyroid dysfunction and miscarriage was revealed in studies using basal metabolic rate and butanol-extractable iodine, in which an increased rate of miscarriage was seen in those women with chemical hypothyroidism (Litaenberg and Carey 1929). Subsequently Montoro and colleagues (1981) reported the successful delivery of 9 infants from 11 women with untreated hypothyroidism. Stagnaro-Green and his colleagues (1990) reported a higher miscarriage rate among women with thyroid auto-antibodies compared with those who were antibody-negative. There were no significant differences in gestational age, maternal age or past obstetric history between the two groups. Moreover none of the antibody-postitive women were clinically hypothyroid and fewer than half had elevated levels of thyroid stimulating hormones (TSH). The authors concluded that thyroid antibodies are an independent marker of at-risk pregnancy, although the sensitivity (34%) and positive predictive value (17%) were very low, reflecting once again the heterogenous nature of spontaneous abortion.

These results do not exclude the possibility that the presence of thyroid auto-antibodies is part of a more generalised maternal auto-immune condition. It is also possible that the auto-antibodies reflected a response to the impending pregnancy loss rather than the cause. Moreover antithyroid antibodies are commonly detected in the maternal circulation after normal term deliveries (Ramsey 1986).

Coagulation Disorders

Lupus Anticoagulant.   The inappropriately named Lupus anticoagulant is an uncommon cause of recurrent abortion which may be amenable to various therapies (Scott et al. 1987). This is discussed in detail in Chapter 10. At present no endocrine treatment has been demonstrated to be of specific benefit to this group of patients.

Factor XIII Deficiency. Factor XIII deficiency is an even more uncommon condition and is amenable to anticoagulation therapy but not to endocrine treatment (Schubring et al. 1990; Rodeghiero et al. 1987).

Reproductive System Disorders

Abnormalities of Secretion of Luteinising Hormone

Various groups have suggested an association between elevated serum levels of luteinising hormone (LH) and poor reproductive performance (Homburg et al. 1988; Stanger and Yovich 1985; Polson et al. 1988). Recently, Regan and her colleagues (1990) have convincingly demonstrated this relationship in a prospective study of women attending a pre-pregnancy counselling clinic. In their study, miscarriage rates of 65% were recorded in women with serum LH levels greater and 12% in those with LH levels less than 10 IU/l in blood taken in the mid-follicular phase. The exact mechanism by which elevated levels of serum LH affect pregnancy outcome is not clear. It has been suggested that LH may act by stimulating premature reactivation of meiosis in the preovulatory oocyte. The extended interval between completion of the first meiotic division and fertilisation may lead to karyotypic abnormalities and death of the fetus or embryo (Tsafriri 1988; Baker 1982).

Polycystic ovary syndrome (PCO) is an important cause of elevated serum LH levels. Strong associations between PCO and recurrent abortion have been reported (Johnson and Pearce 1990; Homburg et al. 1988; Sagle et al. 1988). The diagnosis has been made using ultrasound criteria in 80% of women with recurrent abortion (Sagle et al. 1988) but only in 23% of healthy women of reproductive age (Polson et al. 1988). PCO is a condition with a spectrum of severity ranging from minor ultrasonic changes and endocrine disturbances to the full clinical presentation of obesity, oligomenorrhoea and hirsutism originally described by Stein and Leventhal (1985). It has been suggested that amongst women with PCO syndrome, those with elevated levels of serum LH are more likely to be infertile and to have recurrent miscarriage than those without (Homburg et al. 1989; Conway et al. 1989).

The use of gonadotrophin-releasing-hormone (GnRH) antagonists such as Buserelin to decrease levels of LH in the serum during the follicular phase is theoretically attractive. Johnson and Pearce (1990) have shown a miscarriage rate of 9% after pituitary down-regulation and stimulation with pure follicle stimulating hormone (FSH) compared with 48% for pregnancies conceived on clomiphene citrate. Unfortunately they did not state the absolute levels of serum LH in their study although all subjects had an LH/FSH ratio >3 and ultrasound evidence of PCO. Clomiphene citrate leads to an increase in serum LH (in addition to the beneficial rise in FSH) which may account for the high rate of miscarriage in this study. Nonetheless, there may be an advantage in terms of conception rate and miscarriage rate to pregnancies conceived with Buserelin and FSH. The major disadvantages are the cost of exogenous gonadotrophin therapy, especially when combined with GnRH analogues such as Buserelin, as well as the stringent monitoring required. In women who fail to conceive or have recurrent miscarriages after clomiphene this may be the treatment of choice. Further studies are urgently needed to clarify this issue.

The beneficial effects of surgical treatment (wedge resection and laparoscopic ovarian diathermy) for polycystic ovarian syndrome may be mediated via a reduction in serum LH levels. These are discussed further in Chapter 10.

Corpus Luteum Deficiency

The corpus luteum is essential for the establishment and maintenance of a successful pregnancy. The importance of the ovarian contribution to progesterone synthesis in the earliest weeks of pregnancy was first established by Csapo and colleagues (1972). They also demonstrated that exogenous progesterone ensures continuation of the pregnancy following luteectomy at this time (Csapo et al. 1983). The corpus luteum appears to respond to the luteotrophic effects of circulating human chorionic gonadotrophin (hCG) synthesised by the gestational trophoblast. We and others have speculated that the corpus luteum may be influenced by additional factors from either the embryo or the endometrium (Norman et al. 1988; Lower et al. 1992).

Various groups have proposed that deficiency in progesterone synthesis by the corpus luteum may be an important cause of early pregnancy failure and have suggested the use of progestational agents to prevent abortion (Daya 1989). The theory is attractive although no clear benefit has been demonstrated in randomised trials of progestogens or hCG, including a meta-analysis of the combined data (Goldstein et al. 1989). However, the design of the trials was often unsatisfactory in that therapy was started late in some cases and ultrasonic confirmation of a viable pregnancy prior to the commencement of treatment was often lacking. Furthermore, recent ultrasound studies suggest that "anembryonic pregnancies" may account for up to 60% of all first trimester losses (Stabile et al. 1987). These pregnancies cannot be expected to respond to progestational support. The inclusion of such pregnancies in studies of the efficacy of progestogen or other endocrine therapy would significantly diminish the observed benefits of any treatment regimen.

Implantation failure and subclinical pregnancy losses may be regarded as very early spontaneous abortions and their treatment largely follows that outlined here for similar reasons. Many groups have attempted to demonstrate that deficient corpus luteum function following ovarian hyperstimulation may be responsible for failure to conceive due to early embryonic arrest or implantation failure. Again it is noteworthy that of the many studies which have been established to test this hypothesis, most have failed to demonstrate any advantage. The Southampton study is exceptional in that a statistically significant increase in the pregnancy rate was shown in the group which received hCG for luteal phase support (Smith et al. 1989). In this study all patients received similar ovarian stimulation including the use of gonadotrophin-releasing-hormone (GnRH) agonists. It has been suggested that the down-regulation effect of GnRH agonists on the pituitary-ovarian axis may be prolonged during the early luteal phase, thus causing an abnormal luteal response which is responsible for the poor pregnancy rates following such therapy. Most fertility clinics now advocate the routine use of luteal support following assisted conception especially if GnRH agonists are employed.

Empirical Treatment

The routine use of progestogens and/or hCG has been recommended as empirical therapy in women with recurrent abortion, those over the age of 35 years and in cases of threatened miscarriage. Taking into consideration the above arguments concerning the difficulty in establishing objective proof of the benefit of these treatments, if there is a place for empirical treatment, it should be limited to women in these categories. The cost of such treatment is small and the known side effects are minimal. In particular, progestational agents such as medroxyproges-terone acetate have been shown to have no long-term consequences in infants born to women treated during early pregnancy (Yovich et al. 1988). Neither has endocrine therapy been found to prolong pregnancies with abnormal chromosomes inappropriately, nor is there an associated increase in the incidence of chromosomal abnormalities at term compared with the incidence in untreated pregnancies (Yovich et al. 1988). Moreoever a strong placebo effect has been demonstrated in many women (Stray-Pedersen and Stray-Pedersen 1984), and it may be that this is responsible for much of the claimed effectiveness of empirical therapy.

Timing of Treatment

The major criticism of the trials previously described is that therapy was commenced relatively late in the pregnancy. In order to be of proven benefit endocrine therapy should be commenced at or before the time of implantation. However this strategy will present difficulty in interpretation of the results since a large proportion of preimplantation pregnancies are destined to fail due to chromosomal abnormality. Recent studies have shown that in excess of 95% of pregnancies will survive to the stage of viability once embryonic heart activity has been demonstrated at ultrasound (Stabile et al. 1987). Therefore, if therapy is delayed until fetal heart activity has been demonstrated, beneficial effects could only be seen in less than 5% of cases even if the treatment was 100% successful.

In order to be able to offer early treatment, patients would need to be assessed and counselled prior to conception. Women attending fertility and recurrent abortion clinics would be in an ideal position to benefit from such therapy, being at high risk of miscarriage and selected prior to conception. Those women conceiving following assisted conception or in monitored cycles would be especially suitable since the timing of ovulation and fertilisation is precisely known. Randomised controlled trails are required to determine whether preconception clinics can successfully identify women at risk of spontaneous abortion and whether endocrine therapy early in the luteal phase is of benefit to this group.

Endocrine Treatment of Incomplete or Missed Abortion

The definitive treatment of spontaneous abortion is surgical evacuation if the loss is identified prior to 13 weeks of gestation, the aims being to achieve prompt and complete removal of the retained tissues, to prevent infection and to arrest haemorrhage. Alternatives to curettage may avoid some of the associated risks, and offer financial savings if hospital admission can be avoided (Whittaker et al. 1989).

Pregnancy failure at a more advanced gestation is managed medically. Avoiding delay in removing the dead fetus reduces the risk of coagulopathy. Prostaglandins and oxytocic agents are used to produce cervical dilatation and uterine contractions. The adminstration of prostaglandins via a number of routes (oral, intravenous, intra- and extra-amniotic infusions and vaginal pessaries, creams and gels) has been described with variable success. Oxytocin is used to induce uterine contractions in the third trimester, but cannot be relied upon to achieve the complete expulsion of the abortus during the first or second trimesters when used alone.

The principal action of prostaglandins is direct stimulation of uterine muscle. In addition they may have a luteolytic effect. The effects mediated at a cellular level have recently been reviewed by Smith (1989). Karim and Filshie (1970) pioneered much of the early work in inducing abortion in otherwise healthy pregnancies. Initially natural prostaglandins were given by intravenous infusion. This was associated with a high incidence of side effects and incomplete abortion and the time from administration to expulsion of the conceptus was unreliable. More recently, intra-amniotic and extra-amniotic administration have been used with some success in the second trimester for inducing labour for both therapeutic termination and after spontaneous fetal demise. The use of prostaglandins for first trimester terminations has not been popular as success rates have not been clinically acceptable in comparison with those obtained with surgical treatment.

Recently the progesterone antagonist RU 486 (Mifepristone, Roussell, UK) has been used in conjunction with prostaglandin pessaries for the induction of early therapeutic termination (Rodger and Baird 1987). RU 486 is usually administered as a single oral dose of between 400 and 800 mg. When this is followed 48 h later by a synthetic prostaglandin analogue (0.5–1 mg by vaginal pessary; Gemeprost, May & Baker, UK) an abortion rate of 95% has been reported in women with gestation of less than 56 days. The primary action of RU 486 seems to be a competitive blockade of progesterone receptor sites leading to decidual necrosis. RU486 has also been reported to stimulate prostaglandin synthesis by endometrial stromal cells in vitro (Kelly et al. 1986), and it may be through this mechanism that it mediates myometrial contractions and softening of the uterine cervix.

The possibility of extending the use of progesterone antagonists to out-patient medical management of missed abortions or early embryonic demise is attractive. There would be financial savings, with fewer hospital admissions and for many women surgery with the attendant risks of anaesthesia and surgical complications could be avoided. However this treatment requires early access to ultrasound facilities and would only be appropriate for those cases in which pain and bleeding were not significant factors. In addition careful follow-up would be essential in order to ensure complete expulsion of the products of conception. Asch and colleagues (1990) have recently reported three spontaneous abortions in which curettage was avoided by the complete expulsion of gestational products following treatment with RU 486.

Conclusion

We have discussed the possible endocrine treatments available for spontaneous abortion. There are a number of possible preventive measures but these would benefit only a small proportion of cases. Furthermore, in most cases the cause is unknown or unpreventable (caused by chromosomal anomalies). There is a significant placebo effect.

Both patients and their medical attendants should be aware that a large proportion of spontaneous abortions represent the efficient operation of natural selection and for these no treatment can be offered other than a sympathetic ear and reassurance that future conceptions are unlikely to end in a similar fashion.

References

Asch RH, Weckstein LN, Balmaceda JP, Rojas F, Spitz IM, Tadir Y (1990) Non-surgical expulsion of non-viable early pregnancy: a new application of RU 486. Hum Reprod 5:481–483

Baker TG (1982) Oogenesis and ovulation. In: Austin CR, Short RV (eds). Reproduction in mammals, part 1: germ cells and fertilisation, 2nd Edn. Cambridge University Press, Cambridge, pp 17–45

Boué J, Boué A, Lazar P (1975) Retrospective and prospective epidemiological studies of 1500 karyotyped spontaneous human abortions. Teratology 12:11–26

Conway GS, Honour JW, Jacobs HS (1989) Heterogeneity of the polycystic ovary syndrome: clinical, endocrine and ultrasound features in 556 patients. Clin Endocrinol 30:459–470

Coustan DR (1988) Pregnancy in diabetic women (editorial). N Engl J Med 319:1663–1665

Csapo AI, Ruttner B, Sauvage JP, Wiest WG (1972) The significance of the human corpus luteum in pregnancy maintenance. Am J Obstet Gynecol 112:1061–1067

Csapo AI, Pulkkinen MO, Wiest WG (1973) Effects of luteectomy and progesterone replacement therapy in early pregnant patients. Am J Obstet Gynecol 115:759–765

Daya S (1989) Efficacy of progesterone support for pregnancy in women with recurrent miscarriage. A meta-analysis of controlled trials. Br J Obstet Gynaecol 96:275–280

Goldstein P, Berrier J, Rosen S, Sacks HS, Chalmers TC (1989) A meta-analysis of randomized control trials of progestational agents in pregnancy. Br J Obstet Gynaecol 96:265–274

Greene MF, Hare JW, Cloherty JP, Benacerraf BR, Soeldner JS (1989) First-trimester haemoglobin A1 and risk for major malformation and spontaneous abortion in diabetic pregnancy. Teratology 39:225–231

Hassold T, Chen N, Funkhouser J et al. (1980) A cytogenetics study of 1000 spontaneous abortions. Ann Hum Genet 44:151–178

Hollingsworth DR, Jones OW, Resnik R (1984) Expanded care in obstetrics for the 1980s: Preconception and early postconception counselling. Am J Obstet Gynecol 149:811–814

Homburg R, Armar NA, Eshel A, Adams J, Jacobs HS (1988) Influence of luteinising hormone concentrations on ovulation, conception, and early pregnancy loss in polycystic ovary syndrome. Br Med J 297:1024–1026

Homburg R, Eshel A, Armar NA (1989) One hundred pregnancies after treatment with pulsatile luteinising hormone releasing hormone to induce ovulation. Br Med J 298:809–812

Johnson P, Pearce JM (1990) Recurrent abortion and polycystic ovarian disease: comparison of two regimens to induce ovulation. Br Med J 300:154–156

Karim SM, Filshie GM (1970) Therapeutic abortion using prostaglandin F2alpha. Lancet i:157–159

Kelly RW, Healy DL, Cameron MJ, Cameron IT, Baird DT (1986) The stimulation of prostaglandin production by two antiprogesterone steroids in human endometrial cells. J Clin Endocrinol Metab 62:1116–1123

Lauritsen JG (1976) Aetiology of spontaneous abortion. A cytogenetic and epidemiological study of 288 abortuses and their parents. Acta Obstet Gynecol Scand Suppl 52:1–28

Litaenberg JC, Carey JB (1929) The relation of basal metabolism to gestation. Am J Obstet Gynecol 17:550–552

Lower AM, Yovich JL, Hancock C, Shenton P, Grudzinskas JG (1992). Is luteal function maintained by factors other than human chorionic gonadotrophin in early pregnancy. Submitted.

Martin RH (1988) Human sperm karyotyping: A tool for the study of aneuploidy. In: Vig BK, Sandberg AA (eds) Aneuploidy, Part B: induction and test systems, Alan R Liss Inc, New York, pp 297–316

Mills JL, Simpson JL, Driscoll SG et al. (1988) Incidence of spontaneous abortion among normal women and insulin-dependent diabetic women whose pregnancies were identified within 21 days of conception. N Engl J Med 319:1617–1623

Montoro M, Collea JV, Frasier SD, Mestman JH (1981) Successful pregnancy outcome in women with hypothyroidism. Ann Int Med 94:31–34

Norman RJ, Buck RH, Kemp MA, Joubert SM (1988) Impaired corpus luteum function in ectopic pregnancy cannot be explained by altered human chorionic gonadotropin. J Clin Endocrinol Metab 66:1166–1170

Plachot M, Junca A-M, Mandelbaum J, de Grouchy J, Salat-Baroux J, Cohen J (1986) Chromosome investigations in early life. I. Human oocytes recovered in an IVF programme. Hum Reprod 1:547–551

Polson DW, Wadsworth J, Adams J, Franks S (1988) Polycystic ovaries: a common finding in normal women. Lancet ii:870–872

Ramsay I (1986) Postpartum thyroiditis – an underdiagnosed disease. Br J Obstet Gynaecol 93:1121–1123

Regan L, Owen EJ, Jacobs HS (1990) Hypersecretion of luteinising hormone, infertility, and miscarriage. Lancet 336:1141–1144

Rodeghiero F, Castaman GC, Di Bona E, Ruggeri M, Dini E (1987) Successful pregnancy in a woman with congenital factor XIII deficiency treated with substitutive therapy. Report of a second case. Blut 55:45–48

Rodger MW, Baird DT (1987) Induction of therapeutic abortion in early pregnancy with mifepristone in combination with prostaglandin pessary. Lancet ii:1415–1418

Sagle M, Bishop K, Ridley N et al. (1988) Recurrent early miscarriage and polycystic ovaries. Br Med J 297:1027–1028

Schubring C, Grulich Henn J, Burkhard P, Kloss HR, Selmayr E, Muller Berghaus G (1990) Firbrinolysis and factor XIII in women with spontaneous abortion. Eur J Obstet Gynecol Reprod Biol 35:215–221

Scott JR, Rote NS, Branch DW (1987) Immunologic aspects of recurrent abortion and fetal death. Obstet Gynecol 70:645–656

Simpson JL (1980) Genes, chromosomes, and reproductive failure. Fertil Steril 33:107–116

Simpson JL, Bombard AT (1987) Chormosomal abnormalities in spontaneous abortions: Frequency, pathology and genetic counselling. In: Edmonds DK, Bennett MJ (eds) Spontaneous abortion. Blackwell, London

Smith EM, Anthony FW, Gadd SC, Masson GM (1989) Trial of support treatment with human chorionic gonadotrophin in the luteal phase after treatment with buserelin and human menopausal gonadotrophin in women taking part in an in vitro fertilisation programme. Br Med J 298:1483–1486

Smith SK (1989) Prostaglandins and growth factors in the endometrium. Baillieres Clin Obstet Gynaecol 3:249–270

Stabile I, Campbell S, Grudzinskas JG (1987) Ultrasonic assessment of complications during first trimester of pregnancy. Lancet 2:1237–1240

Stagnaro Green A, Roman SH, Cobin RH, el Harazy E, Davies TF (1990) Detection of at-risk pregnancy by means of highly sensitive assays for thyroid autoantibodies (see comments). JAMA 264:1422–1425

Stanger JD, Yovich JL (1985) Reduced in-vitro fertilization of human oocytes from patients with raised basal luteinizing hormone levels during the follicular phase. Br J Obstet Gynaecol 92:385–393

Stein IF, Leventhal ML (1935) Amenorrhoea associated with bilateral polycystic ovaries. Am J Obstet Gynecol 29:181–191

Stray-Pedersen, B, Stray-Pedersen S (1984) Etiologic factors and subsequent reproductive performance in 195 couples with a prior history of habitual abortion. Am J Obstet Gynecol 148:140–146

Sutherland HW, Pritchard CW (1987) Increased incidence of spontaneous abortion in pregnancies complicated by maternal diabetes mellitus. Am J Obstet Gynecol 156:135–138

Tsafriri A (1988) Local nonsteroidal regulators of ovarian function. In: Knobil E, Neill J (eds) The physiology of reproduction. Raven Press, New York, pp 527–565

Watt JL, Templeton A, Messinis I (1987) Trisomy 1 in an eight cell human pre-embryo. J Med Genet 24:60

Whittaker PG, Stewart MO, Taylor A, Lind T (1989) Some endocrinological events associated with early pregnancy failure. Br J Obstet Gynaecol 96:1207–1214

Wramsby H, Fredga K, Liedholm P (1987) Chromosome analysis of human oocytes recovered from preovulatory follicles in stimulated cycles. N Engl J Med 316:121–124

Yovich JL, Turner SR, Draper R (1988) Medroxyprogesterone acetate therapy in early pregnancy has no apparent fetal effects. Teratol 38:135–144

14. Immunotherapy of Recurrent Spontaneous Miscarriage

W. D. Billington

Introduction: Maternal Immunity in Normal Pregnancy

Pregnancy is associated with a number of changes in the immunological status of the female. The nature, extent and significance of there changes are, however, controversial. Much of the difficulty has resulted from the need to rely upon in vitro assays on samples obtained from only limited stages of gestation. In addition, ethical constraints have restricted most studies to assays on peripheral blood samples. It is now clear that systemic levels are rarely an adequate reflection of local immune responses (Westermann and Pabst 1990). The allogeneic (genetically alien) conceptus in its intrauterine environment needs to be evaluated with respect to its own specialised milieu. Parameters of systemic immunity could be misleading downstream indicators of local immune reactions.

It is not the purpose here to review the scattered, and often conflicting, literature on maternal immune responses in pregnancy. This has been attempted elsewhere (Billington 1988, 1992b). Despite substantial endeavour, the central question as to whether the successful establishment and maintenance of pregnancy is dependent upon maternal immunoregulatory mechanisms is unanswered. The introduction into the female organism of male foreign antigens, expressed on the components of seminal fluid and any embryo, would be expected to initiate antagonistic maternal immune responses. There is, however, a widely held view that such responses are not only normally avoided but that a beneficial, indeed essential, protective immunity is generated. This concept has its origins in the demonstration of a host–antibody response that can block the anticipated attack by lymphocytes on certain types of tumour cells (Hellström and Hellström 1974). A number of factors, of both specific (antibody) and non-specific nature, have been identified in pregnancy sera that have blocking activity in assays of cellular immune function in vitro (see Davies 1986). Whether such activity is expressed in vivo is unknown. An important point, not often appreciated, is that there is no evidence for the existence of maternal cytotoxic T lymphocytes showing sensitisation to the allogenic conceptus (Bell and Billington 1983; Sargent et al. 1987, 1988). If blocking factors have any functional role it must be in the inhibition of the *generation* of potentially deleterious immunity rather than in the suppression of its effector activities. Antibody is, hence, less likely to be a blocking agent than some of the more recently described, but not yet fully characterised, factors of placental trophoblast (Chaouat 1987) and/or uterine decidual origin (Clark et al. 1987).

There is the further possibility that the alterations of maternal immune reactivity in pregnancy are merely epiphenomena, arising as a trivial consequence of genetic incompatibilities between mother and fetus. The fetal trophoblast forms a continuous and unbroken barrier between the conceptus and the maternal tissues from the time of blastocyst implantation onwards. If this barrier expresses no antigens capable of acting as targets for any maternal immune effector agents, this alone would explain the survival of the allogeneic conceptus and render irrelevant any consideration of the need for a protective maternal response. Unfortunately, the antigenic status of the trophoblast has not been easy to define. It exists in a variety of sub-populations and in close juxtaposition to maternal cells in the uterus. None of these sub-populations express the classical Class I or II major histocompatibility complex (MHC) antigens (HLA-A, B, C, DR) that are involved in rejection reactions in tissue transplantation (Bulmer and Johnson 1985). Thus, although trophoblast may be an immunologically inert barrier, it also contains other antigens, of both non-classical Class I MHC (HLA-G) (Ellis et al. 1990; Kovats et al. 1990) and tissue-associated (trophoblastic) nature (Johnson et al. 1981; Faulk and McIntyre 1983; Davies and Browne 1985a). It is possible, that these could render trophoblast a target for maternal immunity. Current immunological dogma would imply that MHC antigens are required for T-lymphocyte recognition of other target cell antigens but tropho-blast could represent a special case. It cannot be susceptible to natural killer (NK) cells, which exhibit non-MHC-restricted killing, as it does not possess the appropriate NK targets (King et al. 1990).

Rationale for Immunotherapy in Pregnancy Loss

It is far from certain that maternal recognition leading to a protective immune response is a necessary condition for successful pregnancy. However, this has prompted the assumption that unexplained recurrent spontaneous miscarriage (RSM) is due to a failure of maternal immune control. Upon this assumption is founded the rationale for the immunotherapy of RSM. Elicitation of the supposedly missing immune responses has been attempted by immunisation procedures with fetal and adult antigenic material. As the specificity of the immune response(s) has not been defined, the antigen(s) required to initiate this is not known. It is, however, generally assumed to be one or more of the trophoblast-associated antigens. Any manipulation of the immune response must obviously be directed towards the relevant antigen(s). Maternal immunity to antigens of the fetus other than those expressed on trophoblast must be irrelevant, as there is no convincing evidence for the passage of maternal immune effector cells or anti-paternal cytotoxic alloantibody (fetal HLA-specific for the extant pregnancy) across the trophoblast and into the fetal circulation in normal pregnancy (Billington 1992a). The logic of immunotherapy is therefore only tenable with respect to the manipulation of immune responses targeted against the trophoblast.

Definition of Recurrent Pregnancy Loss

An important issue concerns the criteria for selection of patients who might benefit from immunotherapy. As many as 80% of women suffering RSM (McIntyre et al. 1989), have been considered to have an underlying immunological defect.

The clinical definition of recurrent miscarriage is generally agreed to be three or more consecutive pregnancy losses, with a primary group in whom all previous pregnancies have failed and a secondary group consisting of women who have had one successful pregnancy (commonly the first) followed by consecutive losses (Stirrat 1990a; see also Chapter 10). Partner-specific miscarriage in both groups is considered as potentially treatable by immunotherapy although it should be borne in mind that the miscarriages could have different causes. It is advisable, therefore, to identify, and treat the two groups independently. It must also be borne in mind that even without intervention the chance of achieving a successful pregnancy after three or more consecutive losses is relatively high (60%, possibly even up to 75%) (Stirrat 1990b). This introduces further difficulty in the interpretation of results of any form of therapy (see below).

Methods of Treatment

The different forms of treatment have reflected the bias of the investigative group as to the precise nature of the immunological defect. By far the most common procedure is immunisation with leucocytes of either paternal (partner-specific) or third party origin, but treatments with trophoblast, seminal plasma and immunoglobulin preparations have been reported (Table 14.1).

Table 14.1. Immunotherapeutic approaches to the treatment of recurrent pregnancy loss

A *Active immunisation*
Paternal (partner-specific) leucocyte injection
Donor (third-party) leucocyte injection
Trophoblast microvillous membrane infusion
Donor seminal plasma: vaginal suppositories

B *Passive immunisation*
Intravenous injection of pooled immunoglobulin

Leucocyte Immunisation

This was the first form of immunotherapy described for repeated pregnancy loss. Taylor and Faulk (1981) reported that three women, each with a history of repeated miscarriage, produced normal healthy babies following multiple transfusions throughout pregnancy with pooled leucocyte-enriched plasma from erythrocyte-compatible donors. The treatment was based upon the premise that the observed HLA antigen sharing between husband and wife in these cases mirrored compatibility of their postulated trophoblast-leucocyte cross-reacting (TLX) antigen(s) (Faulk et al. 1978). There antigens were, therefore, not able to stimulate a maternal protective immune response unless provided by injection with unrelated donor leucocytes. Evidence had also been presented that recurrent aborters lacked the inhibitors of cell-mediated immunity demonstrable in the blood of women during normal pregnancy (Rocklin et al. 1976; Stimson et al. 1979; McIntyre and Faulk 1979), thus initiating the concept of "blocking factors" in pregnancy.

In a study similar to that of Taylor and Faulk, Beer and his colleagues (1981) also achieved successful pregnancies in women given leucocyte immunotherapy, but in this case using cells obtained from the male partner and injected intradermally. The HLA antigen sharing in these couples was shown to be commonly associated with hyporeactivity in one-way mixed lymphocyte culture reactions using female responder and male stimulator cells. Although these studies were taken to indicate that MHC homozygosity may predispose to reproductive wastage, it was also recognised by these authors that it could merely reflect homozygosity at some other relevant, non-MHC, locus (or loci).

The immunogenetic basis of RSM has since been addressed by numerous studies. It is now claimed that there are no significant data to support the view that there is any relevant specific HLA allele sharing in couples experiencing recurrent pregnancy loss (Adinolfi 1986; Johnson and Ramsden 1988; Christiansen et al. 1989). Similarly, there appears to be no convincing evidence for any significant HLA locus homozygosity in women suffering RSM. It has been concluded that there is little justification for continuing with HLA tissue typing in either the identification or management of RSM patients (Cowchock et al. 1990). However, it is difficult to draw conclusions from conflicting data generated in different centres. The discrepant results could be due to differences in patient and selection criteria and numbers, and to different tissue typing methodologies.

Following the early encouraging reports on the success of leucocyte immunotherapy and a small preliminary study of their own, Mowbray and his colleagues embarked upon a controlled trial of treatment using paternal cells. They reported a success rate of 78% in women immunised with their husband's lymphocytes compared to 37% in the group given their own cells (Mowbray et al. 1985). In all cases the women were not pregnant at the time of treatment, which consisted of multiple injections of 3 ml of lymphocyte cell suspension given intravenously and 0.5 ml into each of two intradermal and two subcutaneous sites on the forearm. Primary and secondary RSM groups were included in the trial, but women who were rhesus-negative or who had detectable cytotoxic antibody against paternal T or B lymphocytes were excluded, the latter on the assumption that these would not be expected to benefit from further sensitisation.

Not all treatment centres use pre-existing cytotoxic antibody as an exclusion criterion. The presence of such antibody is not essential for the initiation or maintenance of normal pregnancy, indeed it is detectable in only a minority of pregnancies and even then only in the second trimester or beyond (Regan and Braude 1987; Billington 1988). Cytotoxic anti-paternal antibody is clearly not a consistent feature of normal pregnancy; its absence cannot be a valid indicator of maternal immunological deficiency or causally related to recurrent pregnancy loss. Nor can it be used with confidence for monitoring immunotherapy and predicting pregnancy outcome; in the controlled trial described above, seroconversion did not occur in all immunised women. Pregnancy success or failure following immunisation does not correlate with the presence or absence of cytotoxic antibody (Regan 1988).

The occurrence and relevance of anti-paternal cytotoxic antibody in pregnancy is part of a much wider issue. Standard tests for cytotoxic antibodies will not detect the many other antibodies that do not fix complement. Although anti-fetal alloantibody responses are not a consistent feature of pregnancy, either in man or in other species (Bell and Billington 1983; Billington 1988), the nature and kinetics of maternal antibody production elicited against the full spectrum of fetal antigens has not been fully investigated. A recent report has also shown that although anti-HLA antibodies can be detected as early as the 8th week of pregnancy these may be masked by complexing with soluble HLA antigens or by the development of anti-idiotypic (anti-anti-HLA) antibodies (Reed et al. 1991).

Interest in leucocyte immunotherapy developed from the mid-1980s with a rapidly expanding literature. Most centres employed a protocol similar to that described by Mowbray but without a randomised double-blind placebo-controlled design. Success rates have commonly been within the range 70%–80%, but have been as low as 50%, depending upon the nature of the treated group (e.g. Beer et al. 1985; Unander and Lindholm 1986; McIntyre et al. 1986; Smith and Cowchock 1988; Gatenby et al. 1989; Carp et al. 1990). A rather consistent feature has been the high rate of pregnancies in control groups, where these were included. It is notable that the Mowbray trial would not have reached a statistically significant conclusion if the control group had had a pregnancy rate typical of that observed in almost all other centres.

The need for a further fully controlled trial became evident with the increasing lack of confidence in the validity of the differences between treated and control patient groups, and of both selection criteria and therapeutic regimes.

Two recent studies attempted to overcome some of the difficulties in interpretation of results from treatment lacking appropriate control groups. Cauchi and his colleagues (1991) conducted a paired sequential double-blind trial in order to determine whether 10^7–10^8 paternal mononuclear cells were more effective in preventing miscarriage than normal physiological saline injected in the same volume and in an identical manner. Both primary and secondary RSM groups were taken into the trial but patients with anti-paternal cytotoxic antibodies, auto-antibodies (including anti-cardiolipin), immunised group and abnormal coagulation test results, were excluded. No significant difference was observed in the rate of pregnancy success between those immunised with paternal cells (62%) and those receiving saline (76%), although the numbers were relatively small (21 patients in the experimental group and 25 in the control group). In a second study, Ho and collaborators (1991) investigated the effects of immunising primary and secondary RSM groups with husband's or third party lymphocytes and compared these to patients immunised with their own lymphocytes. The study group came from an ethnically homogeneous Chinese population in

Taiwan; they were screened for normal auto-antibody levels and then randomly assigned to the three treatment groups, each receiving $100–200 \times 10^6$ cells intradermally into several sites. The results of this controlled study showed no differences between the two immunised groups (50 women) and the control group (44 women) injected with their own cells, with respect to numbers of live births, ongoing pregnancies or further abortions, whether analysed individually for primary and secondary RSM groups or collectively for both groups combined. The presence of an MLR blocking effect and anti-paternal cytotoxic antibody did not relate to the success or failure of post-immunisation pregnancies.

Both of these recent studies have therefore failed to demonstrate any beneficial effect of immunisation on the outcome of pregnancy. They highlight again the fact that successful pregnancies can be achieved in a high percentage of control groups of women. However, neither study replicated precisely the conditions of the Mowbray trial; it could therefore be argued that the minor differences were the reason for the discrepant findings. Important factors might include the number of cells injected and the route of immunisation, with some protocols providing less (or more) than the optimal immunogenic challenge; Smith and his colleagues (1990) showed that the number of cells in the inoculum influences pregnancy outcome.

Trophoblast Membrane Infusion

The rationale for this form of treatment is that trophoblast directly and continuously confronts the maternal immune system and must, therefore, be a major contributor to any immunoregulatory system. As this fetal tissue lacks classical Class I and II MHC antigens it also provides a means of establishing whether these antigens are essential in determining the success of pregnancy. Additionally, it avoids the potential hazards associated with maternal immunisation using allogeneic nucleated cells, and possibly bearing pathogenic viruses (see below).

The trophoblastic preparation consists of syncytiotrophoblast microvillous plasma membranes obtained from term placentae by the method described originally by Smith and colleagues (1974). Immunotherapy of women with unexplained recurrent miscarriage by infusion of trophoblast membranes was first reported by Johnson and his group in 1988. A single intravenous infusion consisting of 100 mg of total protein obtained from two separate membrane preparations from donors who were blood-group matched with the recipient was given in an open trial on 50 women. Of the 21 women in whom pregnancy was subsequently established, 16 (76%) had a live birth or were more than 28 weeks of gestation at the time of the report. However, in a follow-up randomised double-blind placebo-controlled trial on clinically defined subgroups of unexplained RSM there was no significant difference in outcome between the treated and control groups (Johnson et al. 1991). When data from their open study were included with those from the trial, pregnancy success was 58% following trophoblast infusion and 68% in those women receiving placebo (1:600 dilution of intra-lipid emulsion) or no treatment. This is consistent with the epidemiological evidence on the likelihood of successful pregnancy with no treatment following three consecutive failures.

It would appear that trophoblast infusion is not effective in the immunotherapy of RMS. However, the data obtained were from one particular protocol. Also, there was no evidence of any immune response to the infusion: antibodies to trophoblast were not detected by ELISA in the serum of the treated women (Johnson et al. 1988). The existence of anti-trophoblast antibodies in normal pregnancy is debatable because of difficulties with the techniques employed for their detection (Johnson et al. 1985; Hole et al. 1987), and the fact that they may exist as free antibodies (Davies and Browne 1985b; Kajino etal. 1988a), immune complexes (Davies 1985), or anti-idiotypic antibodies (Torry et al. 1989). Thus it would be expected that any effective form of immunotherapy should induce a detectable change in some parameter of maternal immunity. It would be premature to dismiss the potential of trophoblast membrane infusion therapy until other protocols are examined, perhaps involving higher dose levels, repeated infusions and/or continued treatment of patients with early established pregnancies.

Seminal Plasma

Seminal plasma, rendered cell- and spermatozoa-free by centrifugation, has been reported to contain trophoblast-lymphocyte cross-reactive (TLX) antigens. These were detected by ELISA and immunochemical assays using rabbit antisera to human syncytiotrophoblast microvillous membranes (Kajino et al. 1988b). The TLX antigens in seminal plasma are insoluble and probably membrane-associated. They could also be associated with platelets in the semen as these are capable of absorbing anti-TLX antibody activity and have been shown to express the TLX antigen(s) (Kajino et al. 1987). Seminal plasma TLX antigens may contribute, with the placental trophoblast, to the stimulus to the production of maternal anti-TLX antibodies. Such antibodies could be important in the maintenance of pregnancy, acting as blocking agents, but are difficult to detect because they induce the formation of auto-anti-idiotypic (anti-TLX) antibodies (Faulk and McIntyre 1986; Torry et al. 1989).

The identification of TLX antigen in seminal plasma and the belief that the allotypic TLX system plays an important role in reproductive success led to the novel immunotherapeutic use of seminal plasma vaginal suppositories. Seminal plasma is screened for infections, pooled and aliquoted into 1-ml gelatin capsules; placebo capsules contain lubrication jelly instead of seminal plasma. Preliminary data from a double-blind trial indicate that pregnancies can be achieved and maintained in patients receiving supposititories on three separate occasions in the menstrual cycle and continued twice weekly up to 30 weeks of gestation. However, the numbers reported are too small to allow attribution of pregnancy success to the treatment (McIntyre et al. 1989; Coulam et al. 1991).

The existence of TLX antigens, their proposed role in immunoregulation in pregnancy, and their potential for immunotherapy has been promoted by only a single group of workers. Moreover, TLX antigen has not been biochemically defined, other than by an anti-trophoblast monoclonal antibody (H316) that identified a possible determinant of TLX carried on two sialylated glycoproteins of M_r 65000 and 55000 (Stern et al. 1986). Independent confirmation of the nature and function of the TLX system is urgently required.

Recent studies have thrown a rather different light on this area. It has been reported that the TLX antigen is actually a complement regulatory protein known as MCP (membrane cofactor protein); both are identified by a monoclonal antibody that defines the CD46 molecule (Purcell et al. 1990). The presence of MCP on the surface of some forms of trophoblast implies a functional role, either in preventing complement-dependent antibody-mediated cytolysis (although the evidence for a potentially damaging maternal cytotoxic antibody directed against known specific antigens expressed on trophoblast is unconvincing) or, more likely, in an anti-coagulatory role. Whether the allotypy reported with TLX is also exhibited by MCP remains to be determined, as does the presence of MCP in seminal plasma.

Intravenous Immunoglobulin (IVIG)

This therapy for RSM is based on the premise that maternal blocking antibodies are essential in normal pregnancy, and that antibody formation is an indicator of effective immunisation and successful pregnancy outcome following leucocyte immunotherapy. The immunoglobulin is prepared form a large pool of donors and is assumed to contain preformed antibodies of similar specificities to those seen in leucocyte-immunised patients. The first report on the use of IVIG in RSM showed a success rate of 82% in a group of 20 women infused with 30 g at 5 weeks of gestation, treatment was repeated (20 g) every three weeks up to 22–24 weeks of gestation (Mueller-Eckhardt et al. 1989). In the only other reported study, four RSM patients were given IVIG 0.5 mg/kg/month beginning prior to conception (Coulam et al. 1990). All four women achieved successful pregnancies.

This form of passive immunotherapy requires further evaluation. There are several potential advantages, including avoidance of the HLA sensitisation inherent in leucocyte therapy and elimination of risk of viral transmission by use of appropriately prepared samples. Application is needed only after establishment of pregnancy and in all patients irrespective of their immune response status, i.e., their individual level of ability to respond to injected antigens.

The mechanism of this treatment is obscure. Almost all IVIG preparations contain antibodies capable of inhibiting immune phagocytosis and probably MHC specificity (Neppert et al. 1986). This does not readily equate with the lack of classical Class I and II MHC antigens on trophoblast. More likely is that IVIG contains Fc receptor-blocking antibodies, which may play an important role in normal pregnancy (Stewart et al. 1984) and be valuable indicators of successful outcome following leucocyte immunization (Kuhn et al. 1991).

Assessment of Outcome of Treatment: Difficulties of Interpretation

It is impossible to compare the results from different centres, owing to the variety of selection criteria, study designs, the nature of the control groups (if any), and the specific therapeutic regimens. A prominent factor, however, is the high success rate in control groups in the small populations of women studied.

A number of non-immunological procedures have been used to treat RSM.

These include injection of human chorionic gonadotropin from the earliest diagnosis of pregnancy until 16 weeks gestation (Harrison 1988), cervical cerclage at 7 weeks gestation following detection of fetal heart activity (Edmonds 1988) and psychotherapy (Stray-Pedersen and Stray-Pedersen 1988). Remarkably high levels of success have been achieved in all cases (100%–10/10; 94%–34/37 and 85%–99/116, respectively). The findings with psychotherapy are particularly intriguing. This consisted of "tender loving care" (TLC) treatment: psychological support with weekly medical and ultrasound examinations and the recommendation to avoid heavy work, travelling and sexual intercouse until 3–4 weeks beyond the stage at which the previous miscarriage occurred. 42 women in the same unknown aetiology group received no special care and produced only 15 pregnancies (36%). However, caution must be exercised in interpreting these results. This was not a double-blind controlled trial involving random assignment of comparable patients to the two study groups, but a selective process based upon the offer of TLC treatment only to those women living within reasonable distance of the hospitals involved. Although there was no explanation of the underlying mechanisms, the success of alternative forms of treatment indicates that the chances of a normal pregnancy are increased by providing some form of medical attention rather than none. This is supported by the finding of a significant placebo effect in the immunotherapy studies.

On present evidence it appears likely that patients with RSM, however they are partitioned by clinical assessment and by laboratory test, still represent a heterogeneous group with respect to underlying cause. The apparent efficacy of treatment might reflect an ability to influence outcome in particular subgroups, presently undefined.

Potential Hazards of Immunotherapy

A number of theoretical hazards have been suggested, mainly associated with the use of leucocytes as the immunogenic agent (Table 14.2). However, in the 10 years since the introduction of immunotherapy, there has been no clear evidence that any are sufficiently serious to justify withholding this treatment. One of the earliest fears, that of induction of graft-versus-host disease (GVHD), has not materialised. To affect the fetus the injected leucocytes would have to cross the

Table 14.2. Potential hazards of immunotherapy

Graft-versus-host reactions in immunised women
Graft-versus-host disease in fetus
Intrauterine fetal growth retardation
Virus transmission
HLA sensitisation
ABO and other blood group antigen sensitisation
Platelet sensitisation
Autoimmunity induction by cross-reacting epitopes
Anaphylaxis
Serum sickness

placenta, which does not occur in normal pregnancy (Billington 1992a) and only rarely under pathological circumstances (Pollack et al. 1982). Furthermore, the frequency of intrauterine growth retardation (IUGR), which is higher in RSM patients in the group having had one live birth, may actually be reduced following successful immunotherapy (Mowbray 1987; Ho et al. 1991). Careful screening should reduce (but not entirely prevent) the likelihood of virus transmission by infected leucocytes or serum. Blood group matching when using third party leucocytes would similarly limit the possibility of sensitisation by any contaminating erythrocytes. The induction of auto-immune reactions by recognition of antigens (or rather, epitopes) on the injected leucocyte cell surface shared by host somatic cells is theoretically possible but has no supporting evidence.

An awareness of potential hazards is a sensible precaution for any intended immunotherapeutic approach but should not preclude consideration of treatment.

Future Requirements

Above all else, it is necessary to establish clearly the extent to which maternal immune recognition of the allogenic embryo is an important determina of pregnancy success. Only then will it be possible to state that some forms of unexplained recurrent pregnancy loss may have an immunological basis that can be expected to be manipulated by immunotherapy. An intact maternal immune system is not *essential* for normal pregnancy. Certain forms of immunodeficiency in humans, and severe experimentally-induced immune defects in laboratory animals, do not preclude normal reproductive function (Good and Zak 1956; Rodger 1985; Sulila et al. 1988).

Although it is tempting to accept the rather fragile evidence of an immunological basis for the apparent success of immunotherapy (Beer and Kwak 1991; Clark and Daya 1991), this cannot be taken for certain. We do not know whether any of the alterations in immune responsiveness in normal gestation are the determinants or merely the result of pregnancy success. Nor do we know whether those changes seen in aborters are immunological causes or effects.

If the blocking antibodies purported to be critical for the maintenance of pregnancy (Takeuchi 1990) are involved in preventing a cytotoxic T-cell-mediated attack on the normal conceptus, then these cells should be evident in patients undergoing pregnancy failure. This has not been demonstrated. It would require a prospective study of a cohort of patients, comparing those who maintained their pregnancies with those who lost them. Peripheral blood samples would give only limited information) more relevant would be analysis of cell populations from placental bed biopsies, but ethical constraints would render this difficult. However, as in vitro expanded mouse cytotoxic T-cells are unable either to kill trophoblast cultures or adversely to affect normal gestation following injection into pregnant mice (Kamel and Wood 1991), it appears unlikely that this form of immune response is actually relevant. There are undoubtedly alterations in the relative proportions of circulating T-lymphocyte subsets following leucocyte immunotherapy (Sugi et al. 1991; Takakuwa et al. 1991) but the significance of these remains to be determined.

The fetal targets for any maternal immune attack must be identified and characterised. Although several studies have indicated that the induction of MLR blocking antibodies is predictive of pregnancy success (e.g., Takakuwa et al. 1990; Unander et al. 1991) the specificity of these antibodies has not been determined. The continuing preoccupation with the role of the HLA system must be justified by the demonstration of specificity related to this system.

The evidence from experimental animals has implicated non-antigen-specific mediators (NK cells and cytokines) in pregnancy loss (Clark 1989). Although human trophoblast does not express NK target molecules (King et al. 1990), it would appear important to obtain further information on cytokines (both lymphokines derived from activated lymphocytes and monokines from activated macrophages) in normal and aborting pregnancies (Hill 1990). Cytokines play a central role in the regulation of the immune system. Their presence in the uterus and placenta (Hunt 1989) indicates that they have a function in the immunological interrelationships between mother and fetus. Disturbances at this level could underly pregnancy failure, although the events that might initiate such disturbances are undefined. They could be antigen-specific, induced by cell-mediated responses to fetal antigens, or non-antigen-specific, triggered by leukocyte/macrophage/monocyte activation in reponse to stimuli such as infection.

The diversity of the immunotherapeutic approaches, and of the various protocols of leucocyte immunisation, has made it impossible to compare studies. Numerous variables could have an influence on pregnancy outcome, these variables include especially patient selection, dose of immunising cells and interval to pregnancy (Smith and Cowchock 1988; Smith et al. 1990; Cowchock et al. 1990) (see Table 14.3). Following an initiative from the American Society for the Immunology of Reproduction, workshops have been held to review the data and to suggest ways to determine unequivocally whether immunotherapy can be an efficacious treatment. The consensus of opinion from a workshop on unification of immunotherapy protocols was that a new controlled study was required: proposals were made both for inclusion and exclusion criteria and for an immunisation protocol (Coulam 1991). It has since been argued that procedures for a new trial can be identified with information from a statistical analysis of all existing data (a meta-analysis) (Clark and Daya 1991). This considerable undertaking has been agreed in principle but will depend upon the efforts of a co-ordinating group and the co-operation of all centres. The time scale of the meta-analysis, its translation into agreed procedures, the initiation of a trial and the collation and analysis of data will, if put into effect, be of the order of five years.

Table 14.3. Variables in leucocyte immunotherapy that could affect pregnancy outcome

Previous obstetric history
Unknown heterogeneity (especially immunological and genetic) of patients
Patient selection procedure: inclusion and exclusion criteria
Degree of HLA antigen sharing (Class I and Class II) between partners
Pre-existing allo-antibodies and auto-antibodies
Number of cells injected
Route of immunisation
Frequency of immunisation – booster doses
Interval between immunisation and conception
Degree of induction of anti-paternal antibodies and/or MLR blocking factors

Conclusions

The immunoregulatory processes associated with normal pregnancy are not fully defined. It is not known for certain that they are essential for the successful implantation and development of the allogenic embryo. Deficiency in immuno-regulation as a causal basis for pregnancy failure is therefore still in the realms of hypothesis and not fact. There is also a need to establish the specific nature of any immunological changes associated with recurrent miscarriage and to determine whether these are the cause or the effect of pregnancy loss.

Reproducible laboratory assays are required to examine the immunological parameters in order to identify the nature of any defect, to determine the appropriate treatment, to monitor the effects of treatment, and to predict the outcome. Some progress is being made, for example, by the use of two colour flow cytometry cross-match for identification of antibodies to T-lymphocytes in leucocyte immunised women (Gilman-Sachs et al. 1990). For the present, immunotherapy should be considered as an experimental procedure of no proven benefit. If offered, it should be only on that basis, following exhaustion of all other possibilities, and conducted only in centres with protocols designed to provide data that can usefully contribute to an understanding of the problem.

A meta-analysis of available data on patients who have undergone leucocyte immunotherapy should identify an agreed procedure for the selection and treatment of a large group of women who will be willing to enter a new randomised controlled double-blind trial. Other immunotherapeutic approaches also require to be validated by much larger controlled studies. Efficacy is defined by the difference in pregnancy outcome between experimental and control groups; it is therefore essential to reduce patient heterogeneity to a minimum, and to reduce the effect of unknown variables by use of large numbers. In the case of RSM, this latter could well be of the order of 400–800 couples.

Finally, it remains possible that unexplained recurrent pregnancy failure is partly a genetic problem. MHC-linked genes affecting fetal growth and develop-ment have been identified in laboratory animals and postulated, albeit on the controversial basis of a significantly increased level of HLA-sharing in aborters, to exist in humans (Ho et al. 1990). It has been suggested that most RSMs have a genetic basis, involving either chromosomal abnormalities or homozygosity for recessive, lethal genes (Gill 1992). This further underlines the importance of seeking the nature of the subgroups of the heterogeneous population of patients currently labelled as unexplained recurrent spontaneous primary and secondary aborters. Treatment appropriate to the identified defect(s) might then be provided. This is unlikely to be a realistic prospect before the end of this century.

References

Adinolfi M (1986) Recurrent habitual abortion, HLA sharing and deliberate immunization with partner's cells: a controversial topic. Human Reprod 1:45–48
Beer AE, Kwak JYH (1991) What is the evidence for immunologic pregnancy loss? Lymphocyte immunization: the supportive view. Colloque INSERM 212:285–293

Beer AE, Quebbeman JF, Ayers JWT, Haines RF (1981) Major histocompatibility complex antigens, maternal and paternal immune responses, and chronic habitual abortions in humans. Am J Obstet Gynecol 141:987–999

Beer AE, Semprini AE, Xiaoyu Z, Quebbeman JF (1985) Pregnancy outcome in human couples with recurrent spontaneous abortion: HLA antigen profiles, HLA antigen sharing, female serum MLR blocking factors and paternal leukocyte immunization. Exp Clin Immunogenet 2:137–153

Bell SC, Billington WD (1983) Anti-fetal allo-antibody in the pregnant female. Immunol Rev 75:5–30

Billington WD (1988) Maternal-fetal interactions in normal human pregnancy. Baillière's Clinical Immunology and Allergy, Vol 2/3:527–549

Billington WD (1992) Transfer of antigens and antibodies between mother and fetus. In: Coulam CB, Faulk WP, McIntyre JA (eds). Immunological obstetrics. WW Norton & Co, New York (in press)

Billington WD (1992) The normal feto-maternal immunological relationship. In: The Immune System in Disease, (eds Stirrat GM, Scott JR), Baillière's Clinical Obstetrics and Gynaecology, WB Saunders Co. London (in press)

Bulmer JN, Johnson PM (1985) Antigen expression by trophoblast populations in the human placenta and their possible immunobiological relevance. Placenta 6:127–140

Carp HJA, Toder V, Gazit E, Orgad S, Mashiach S, Nebel L, Serr DM (1990) Immunization by paternal leucocytes for prevention of primary habitual abortion: results of a matched controlled trial. Gynecol Obstet Invest 29:16–21

Cauchi MN, Lim D, Young DE, Kloss M, Pepperell RJ (1991) Treatment of recurrent aborters by immunization with paternal cells – controlled trial. Am J Reprod Immunol 25:16–17

Chaouat G (1987) Placental immunoregulatory factors. J Reprod Immunol 10:179–188

Christiansen OB, Riisom K, Lauritsen JG, Grunnet N (1989) No increased histocompatibility antigen-sharing in couples with idiopathic habitual abortions. Hum Reprod 4:160–162

Clark DA (1989) What do we know about spontaneous abortion mechanisms? Am J Reprod Immunol 19:29–37

Clark DA, Daya S (1991) Trials and tribulations of recurrent spontaneous abortion. Am J Reprod Immunol 25:18–24

Clark DA, Croy BA, Wegmann TG, Chaouat G (1987) Immunological and paraimmunological mechanisms in spontaneous abortion: recent insights and future directions. J Reprod Immunol 12:1–12

Coulam CB (1991) Unification of immunotherapy protocols: workshop report. Am J Reprod Immunol 25:1–9

Coulam CB, Peters AJ, McIntyre JA, Faulk WP (1990) The use of intravenous immunoglobulin for the treatment of recurrent spontaneous abortion. Am J Reprod Immunol 22:78

Coulam CB, Faulk WP, McIntyre JA (1991) Immunotherapy for recurrent spontaneous abortion and its analogies to treatment for cancer. Am J Reprod Immunol 25:114–119

Cowchock FS, Smith JB, David S, Scher J, Batzer F, Corson S (1990) Paternal mononuclear cell immunization therapy for repeated miscarriage: predictive variables for pregnancy success. Am J Reprod Immunol 22:12–17

Davies M (1985) The formation of immune complexes in primiparous and multiparous pregnancies. Immunol Lett. 10:199–205

Davies M (1986) Blocking factors and human preganancy: an alternative explanation for the success of lymphocyte transfusion therapy in abortion-prone women. Am J Reprod Immunol Microbiol 10:58–63

Davies M, Browne CM (1985a) Identification of selectively solubilized syncytiotrophoblast plasma membrane proteins as potential antigenic targets during normal human pregnancy. J Reprod Immunol 8:33–44

Davies M, Browne CA (1985b) Anti-trophoblast antibody responses during normal human pregnancy. J Reprod Immunol 7:285–297

Edmonds DK (1988) Use of cervical cerclage in patients with recurrent first trimester abortion. In: Beard RW, Sharp F (eds) Early pregnancy failure: mechanisms and treatment. The Peacock Press Ltd, UK, pp 411–419

Ellis SA, Palmer MS, McMichael AJ (1990) Human trophoblast and the choriocarcinoma cell line BeWo express a truncated HLA Class I molecule. J Immunol 144:731–735

Faulk WP, McIntyre JA (1983) Immunological studies of human trophoblast: markers, subsets and functions. Immunol Rev 75:139–175

Faulk WP, McIntyre JA (1986) Role of anti-TLX antibody in human pregnancy. In: Clark DA, Croy BA (eds) Reproductive immunology. Elsevier, Amsterdam, pp 106–114

Faulk WP, Temple A, Lovins R, Smith NC (1978) Antigens of human trophoblast: a working hypothesis for their role in normal and abnormal pregnancies. Proc Nat Acad Sci USA 75:1947–1951

Gatenby PA, Moore H, Cameron K, Doran TJ, Adelstein S (1989) Treatment of recurrent spontaneous abortion by immunization with paternal lymphocytes: correlates with outcome. Am J Reprod Immunol 19:21–27

Gill TJ (1992) MHC-linked genes affecting reproduction, development and susceptibility to cancer. In: Coulam CB, Faulk WP, McIntyre JA (eds) Immunological obstetrics. WW Norton & Co, New York (in press)

Gilman-Sachs A, Harris D, Beer A, Beaman KD (1990) Inhibition of binding of anti-CD3 antibodies to paternal lymphocytes correlates with failure of immunotherapy for treatment of recurrent spontaneous abortions. J Reprod Immunol 17:41–51

Good RA, Zak SJ (1956) Disturbances in gamma globulin synthesis as "experiments of nature". Paediatrics 18:109–149

Harrison RF (1988) Early recurrent pregnacy failure: treatment with human chorionic gonadotrophin. In: Beard RW, Sharp F (eds) Early pregnancy loss: mechanisms and treatment. The Peacock Press Ltd, UK, pp 421–431

Hellström KE, Hellström I (1974) Lymphocyte-mediated cytotoxicity and blocking serum activity to tumor antigens. Adv Immunol 18:209–277

Hill JA (1990) Immunological mechanisms of pregnancy maintenance and failure: a critique of theories and therapy. Am J Reprod Immunol 22:33–42

Hill JA (1991) The rationale for leukocyte immunization in women with recurrent spontaneous abortion: fact or fiction? Colloque INSERM 212:263–269

Ho H-N, Gill TJ, Nsieh R-P, Hsieh H-J, Lee T-Y (1990) Sharing of human leukocyte antigens (HLA) in primary and secondary recurrent spontaneous abortions. Am J Obstet Gynecol 163:178–188

Ho H-N, Gill TJ, Hsieh H-J, Jiang J-J, Lee T-Y, Hsieh C-Y (1991) Immunotherapy for recurrent spontaneous abortions in a Chinese population. Am J Reprod Immunol 25:10–15

Hole N, Cheng HM, Johnson PM (1987) Antibody activity against human trophoblast antigens in the context of normal pregnancy and unexplained recurrent miscarriage? Colloque INSERM 154:213–224

Hunt JS (1989) Cytokine networks in the uteroplacental unit: macrophages as pivotal regulatory cells. J Reprod Immunol 16:1–17

Johnson PM, Ramsden GH (1988) Recurrent miscarriage. Baillière's clinical immunology and allergy. Vol 2/3:607–624

Johnson PM, Cheng HM, Molloy CM, Stern CMM, Slade MB (1981) Human trophoblast-specific surface antigens identified using monoclonal antibodies. Am J Reprod Immunol 1:246–254

Johnson PM, Cheng HM, Stevens VC, Matangkasombut P (1985) Antibody reactivity against trophoblast and trophoblast products. J Reprod Immunol 8:347–352

Johnson PM, Chia KV, Hart CA, Griffith HB, Francis WJA (1988) Trophoblast membrane infusion for unexplained recurrent miscarriage. Br J Obstet Gynaecol 95:342–347

Johnson PM, Ramsden GH, Chia KV, Hart CA, Farquharson RG, Francis WJA (1991) A combined randomised double-blind and open study of trophoblast membrane infusion (TMI) in unexplained recurrent miscarriage. In: Cellular and molecular biology of the materno-fetal relationship. Colloque INSERM 212:277–284

Kajino T, Faulk WP, McIntyre JA (1987) Antigens of human trophoblast: trophoblast-lymphocyte cross-reactive (TLX) anigens in platelets. Am J Reprod Immunol Microbiol 14:70–78

Kajino T, McIntyre JA, Faulk WP, Dent SC, Billington WD (1988a) Antibodies to trophoblast in normal pregnant and secondary aborting women. J Reprod Immunol 14:267–282

Kajino T, Torry DS, McIntyre JA, Faulk WP (1988b) Trophoblast antigens in human seminal plasma. Am J Reprod Immunol Microbiol 17:91–95

Kamel S, Wood GW (1991) Failure of in vitro-expanded hyperimmune cytotoxic T lymphocytes to affect survival of mouse embryos in vivo. J Reprod Immunol 19:69–84

King A, Kalra P, Loke YW (1990) Human trophoblast cell resistance to decidual NK lysis is due to lack of NK target structure. Cell Immunol 127:230–237

Kovats S, Main EK, Librach C, Stubblebine M, Fisher SJ, DeMars R (1990) A Class I antigen, HLA-G, expressed in human trophoblasts. Science 248:220–223

Kuhn U, Blasczyk R, Hojnacki B et al. (1991) Fc receptor blocking antibodies after active immunization for the treatment of recurrent spontaneous abortion. J Reprod Immunol 20:141–151

McIntyre JA, Faulk WP (1979) Maternal blocking factors in human pregnancy are found in plasma not serum. Lancet ii:821–823

McIntyre JA, Coulam CB, Faulk WP (1989) Recurrent spontaneous abortion. Am J Reprod Immunol 21:100–104

McIntyre JA, Faulk WP, Nicholas-Johnson VR, Taylor CG (1986) Immunologic testing and immunotherapy in recurrent spontaneous abortion. Obstet Gynecol 67:169–175

Mowbray JF (1987) Genetic and immunological factors in human recurrent abortion. Am J Reprod Immunol Microbiol 15:138–140

Mowbray JF, Gibbings C, Liddell H, Reginald PW Underwood JL, Beard RW (1985) Controlled trial of treatment of recurrent spontaneous abortion by immunization with paternal cells. Lancet i:941–943

Mueller-Eckhardt G, Heine O, Neppert J, Kunzel W, Mueller-Eckhardt C (1989) Prevention of recurrent spontaneous abortion by intravenous immunoglobulin. Vox Sang 56:151–154

Neppert J, Clemens M, Mueller Eckhardt C (1986) Immune phagocytosis inhibition by commercial immunoglobins. Blut 52:67–72

Pollack MS, Kirkpatrick D, Kapoor N, Dupont B, O'Reilly RJ (1982) Identification by HLA typing of intra-uterine derived maternal T cells in four patients with severe combined immunodeficiency. N Engl J Med 307:662–666

Purcell DFJ, McKenzie IFC, Lublin DM, et al. (1990) The human cell-surface glycoproteins Hul Y-m5, membrane co-factor protein (MCP) of the complement systems, and trophoblast leucocyte-common (TLX) antigen, are CD46. Immunology 70:155–161

Reed E, Beer AE, Hutcherson H, King DW, Suciu-Foca N (1991) The alloantibody response of pregnant women and its suppression by soluble HLA antigens and anti-idiotypic antibodies. J Reprod Immunol 20:115–128

Regan L (1988) A prospective study of spontaneous abortion. In: Beard RW, Sharp F (eds) Early pregnancy loss: mechanisms and treatment. The Peacock Press Ltd, UK, pp 23–42

Regan L, Braude PR (1987) Is antipaternal cytotoxic antibody a valid marker in the management of recurrent abortion? Lancet ii:1280

Reznikoff-Etievant MF, Durieux I, Huchet J, Salmon C, Netter A (1988) Human MHC antigens and paternal leucocyte injections in recurrent spontaneous abortions. In: Beard RW, Sharp F (eds) Early pregnancy loss: mechanisms and treatment. The Peacock Press Ltd, UK, pp 375–387

Rocklin RE, Kitzmiller J, Carpenter B, Garovoy M, David JR (1976) Maternal-fetal relation: absence of an immunologic blocking factor from the serum of women with chronic abortions. N Engl J Med 295:1209–1213

Rodger JC (1985) Lack of a requirement for a maternal humoral immune response to establish or maintain successful allogeneic pregnancy. Transplantation 40:372–375

Sargent IL, Arenas J, Redman CWG (1987) Maternal CMI to paternal HLA may occur but is not a regular event in normal human pregnancy. J Reprod Immunol 10:111–120

Sargent IL, Wilkins T, Redman CWG (1988) Maternal immune responses to the fetus in early pregnancy and recurrent miscarriage. Lancet ii:1099–1104

Smith JB, Cowchock FS (1988) Immunological studies in recurrent spontaneous abortion: effects of immunization of women with paternal mononuclear cells on lymphocytotoxic and mixed lympho-cyte reaction blocking antibodies and correlation with sharing of HLA and pregnancy outcome. J Reprod Immunol 14:99–113

Smith JB, Cowchock FS, Lata JA, Hankinson BT, Eftekhar A, Rote NS (1990) Pregnancy outcome after immunotherapy is influenced by the number of cells in the inoculum. Am J Reprod Immunol 22:88

Smith NC, Brush MG, Luckett S (1974) Preparation of human placental surface membranes. Nature 252:302–303

Stern PL, Beresford N, Thompson S, Johnson PM, Webb PD, Hole N (1986) Characterization of the human trophoblast-leukocyte antigenic molecules defined by a monoclonal antibody. J Immunol 137:1604–1609

Stewart GM, Mason RJ, Thomson MAR, MacLeod AM, Catto GRD (1984) Non-cytotoxic antibodies to paternal antigens in maternal sera and placental eluates. Transplantation 38:111–115

Stimson WH, Strachan AF, Shepherd A (1979) Studies on the maternal immune response to placental antigens: absence of a blocking factor for the blood of abortion-prone women. Br J Obstet Gynaecol 86:41–45

Stirrat GM (1990a) Recurrent miscarriage I: definition and epidemiology. Lancet 336:673–675

Stirrat GM (1990b) Recurrent miscarriage II: clinical associations, causes and management. Lancet 336:728–733

Stray-Pedersen B, Stray-Pedersen S (1988) Recurrent abortions: the role of psychotherapy. In: Beard RW, Sharp F (eds). Early pregnancy loss: mechanisms and treatment. The Peacock Press Ltd, UK, pp 433–442

Sugi T, Makino T, Maruyama T, Kim WK, Iizuka R (1991) A possible mechanism of immunotherapy for patients with recurrent spontaneous abortions. Am J Reprod Immunol 25:185–189

Sulila P, Holmdahl R, Hansson I, Bernadotte F, Mattsson A, Mattsson R (1988) An investigation of allogeneic pregnancy in multiparous mice subjected to in vivo depletion of CD8 (Ly2) – positive lymphocytes by monoclonal antibody treatment. J Reprod Immunol 14:235–245

Takakuwa K, Goto S, Hasegawa I et al. (1990) Result of immunotherapy on patients with unexplained recurrent abortion: a beneficial treatment for patients with negative blocking antibodies. Am J Reprod Immunol 23:37–41

Takakuwa K, Ueda H, Goto S et al. (1991) Influence of immunotherapy on the cellular immunity of unexplained recurrent aborters. J Reprod Immunol 20:153–163

Takeuchi S (1990) Is production of blocking antibodies in successful human pregnancy an epiphenomenon? Am J Reprod Immunol 24:108–119

Taylor C, Faulk WP (1981) Prevention of recurrent abortion with leucocyte transfusions. Lancet ii:68–70

Torry DS, Faulk WP, McIntyre JA (1989) Regulation of immunity to extra-embryonic antigens in human pregnancy. Am J Reprod Immunol 21:76–81

Unander AM, Lindholm A (1986) Transfusions of leucocyte-rich erythrocyte concentrates: a successful treatment in selected cases of habitual abortion. Am J Obstet Gynecol 154:516–520

Unander AM, Norberg R, Årfors L et al. (1991) Opinion on treatment for women with habitual abortion based on investigations for blocking antibody and autoantibodies. Am J Reprod Immunol 26:32–37

Westermann J, Pabst R (1990) Lymphocyte subsets in the blood: a diagnostic window on the lymphoid system? Immunol Today 11:406–410

Subject Index